Presentation of Clinical Data

Other Books by Bert Spilker

Guide to Clinical Studies and Developing Protocols
(Raven Press, 1984)

Guide to Clinical Interpretation of Data (Raven Press, 1986)

Guide to Planning and Managing Multiple Clinical Studies
(Raven Press, 1987)

*Multinational Drug Companies: Issues in Drug Discovery
and Development* (Raven Press, 1989)

Quality of Life Assessments in Clinical Trials (Editor)
(Raven Press, 1990)

Inside the Drug Industry (with Pedro Cuatrecasas,
Prous Science Publishers, 1990)

Presentation
of
Clinical Data

Bert Spilker, Ph.D., M.D.

Director, Project Coordination, Burroughs Wellcome Co.
Research Triangle Park, North Carolina
Adjunct Professor of Pharmacology and Clinical Associate Professor of Medicine
University of North Carolina
Clinical Professor of Pharmacy
University of North Carolina School of Pharmacy
Chapel Hill, North Carolina

and

John Schoenfelder, Ph.D.

Associate Director of Biostatistics, Glaxo Inc.
Research Triangle Park, North Carolina
Adjunct Assistant Professor of Biostatistics
University of North Carolina School of Public Health
Chapel Hill, North Carolina

Raven Press 🖎 **New York**

Raven Press, Ltd., 1185 Avenue of the Americas, New York, New York 10036

Made in the United States of America

Library of Congress Cataloging-in-Publication Data

Spilker, Bert.
    Presentation of clinical data / Bert Spilker, John Schoenfelder.
       p.   cm.
    Includes bibliography.
    ISBN 0-88167-566-0
    1. Communication in medicine—Charts, diagrams, etc. 2. Clinical medicine—Charts, Diagrams, etc. I. Schoenfelder, John.
II. Title.
    [DNLM: 1. Data Display. W 26.5 S756p]
    R118.S75 1989
    616′.0021—dc20
    DNLM/DLC
    for Library of Congress   89-10801
                                           CIP

9 8 7 6 5 4 3 2 1

For my mother, Sara, and the memory of my father,
Victor Spilker

* * *

For my parents and family,
Bob and Margaret,
and Carol, Brian, Jason, and Laura Schoenfelder

Preface

The way that data are displayed has a great influence on how they are interpreted. Questions often arise before, during, and especially after clinical studies about how the data obtained will be presented. Answers vary from "I don't know" to "There's only one way," but many factors influence the final decision. One or more relevant factors are often overlooked. In addition, many accepted methods for generating figures and tables are unknown to those responsible for presenting data.

Current methods of choosing formats to present data often appear haphazard in the medical literature. Nonetheless, some general rules and systematic approaches can be used. By providing examples of prototype tables and figures and indicating appropriate uses, this book helps authors either to develop a systematic approach or to evaluate formats they might not have considered. Most examples have either real or mocked-up data to illustrate how clinical information may be presented and are accompanied by brief comments indicating why the table or figure is included in this catalogue.

The purpose of this book is to illustrate formats that may be used for the presentation, rather than the analysis, of data. Data analyses and statistical presentations are not described. The choice of the most appropriate statistical test is usually determined by the type of data collected, the specific null hypothesis of interest, and the professional biases (e.g., parametric or nonparametric, classical or Bayesian) of the analyst. The proposed presentations are intended to display data so that the basis for its interpretation is clear. The book is *not* a treatise on the logic underlying graphic illustrations or how graphs are visually perceived. Graphs and figures reprinted from the literature contain the original legends, except in a few cases where minor modifications were made to suit this book.

These tables, graphs, and figures are intended as a catalogue of major choices for academic, industrial, and government investigators and students who present data. No distinction is made between displays intended for use by any of these audiences. Nonetheless, academicians tend to use summary presentations of single studies rather than presentations of data from individual patients or across-study summaries. These latter approaches, however, are important for regulatory submissions prepared by pharmaceutical companies.

Numerous variations of all tables and figures may be created. Most variations and complex presentations are not included in this book to conserve both space and the reader's patience. Readers who desire to review types of visual presentations other than those presented in this book should consult books by Lockwood (1969), Spear (1969), Simmonds (1980), Tufte (1983), and/or Reynolds and Simmonds (1984).

* * * * *

Note to Readers

Readers are encouraged to send us any novel approaches or interesting variations on materials presented in this book. Please address all correspondence to Dr. Spilker (Burroughs Wellcome Co., 3030 Cornwallis Road, Research Triangle Park, North Carolina 27709) for inclusion. Contributors of materials included in future editions will be acknowledged.

Acknowledgments

The authors are pleased to acknowledge the help of Dr. Imogene McCanless and Dr. Allen Lai for reviewing portions of the manuscript and making several valuable suggestions.

Several graphs and tables are based on unpublished works by scientists and clinicians who kindly allowed us to modify their presentations. These people are Dr. Martha M. Abou-Donia, Mr. Richard DeAngelis, Dr. Michael F. Frosolono, Dr. Dannie King, Dr. Sandra Nusinoff Lehrman, Dr. Charles G. Lineberry, Mr. Alfred Guaspari, Mr. G. David Rudd, Dr. Richard L. Tuttle, Dr. J. Neal Weakly, and Dr. John Whisnant.

This work could not have been completed without the able assistance and help of Mrs. Joyce Carpunky and Mrs. Brenda Price with administrative details and Ms. Judy Appleton and others who typed the manuscript's several drafts. Many thanks are due to Ms. Thomasine Cozart for technical assistance.

The bibliography was prepared by Mr. Allen Jones who also helped us obtain details for permission to publish. We appreciate the help of Ms. Linda Byrd, whose Research Graphics Department at Burroughs Wellcome Co. cheerfully prepared all of the illustrations in this book. The illustrators are Ms. Linda Byrd, Ms. Linda DeLeon, Mr. Scott Hosa, Ms. Edie Johnson, Ms. Elizabeth Majors, Ms. Beverly Nobles, and Ms. Susan Sadler-Redmond, who also handled the coordination.

Contents

How to Use This Book

The book is organized into 13 chapters that depict different types of data that are often encountered in clinical presentations. We have presented formats within the chapters in the following order: tables, then graphs, and finally figures. A further division is sometimes made into formats illustrating individual patient data followed by formats illustrating group data. In addition to allowing readers readily to focus their attention on the most relevant formats, this consistent ordering allows readers to readily identify a selected format in a chapter and to compare it with similar formats in the same or other chapters.

Printed above most tables, graphs, and figures is a brief statement in bold type that identifies our reason for incorporating it in the book. At the end of many of these statements we have identified (in parentheses) whether the format may be used to illustrate data from individual patients or groups of patients, and whether data are from a single site/study or from multiple sites/studies. It must be stressed that most formats may be used in multiple ways, i.e., formats illustrating multiple sites/studies may generally also be used for a single site or study (and vice versa). Underneath most tables, graphs, and figures are footnotes and/or bullets that indicate common variations, modifications, or points about that figure.

Only selected examples of all possible presentations may be included in a book. Many alternatives are indicated, however, by brief comments underneath tables, graphs, or figures. In addition, it would make little sense to repeat most examples in each chapter since the presentations used in one chapter can be generally readily adapted to different types of data. For example, readers should refer to several chapters on safety data to identify examples that may be pertinent to their data. Tables created by readers may have less (or more) data than shown in the examples. Most tables in this book are models and have a large amount of data because it is usually easier to remove than to add table columns and rows.

The first chapter reviews each of the types of formats included in this book, and also mentions a number of types of formats that are not included in other chapters. Chapter 2 presents the parameters used when selecting particular formats. Chapters 3 to 12 show prototype formats, and the final chapter, 13, provides examples of overly complex or confusing presentations, which authors are encouraged to avoid.

Presentation of Clinical Data

1

Tools of the Trade

Data displays (i.e., presentations of clinical data) are the interface between the statistician and the clinical interpreter of data. The former analyzes data and the latter interprets and extrapolates results of those analyses. Together they display data in such a way that the rationale underlying the interpretation is readily apparent to the reader. Most data displays are presented through one or more of three basic types of formats: tables, graphs, and figures.

All three of these vehicles may be used correctly or incorrectly. A correct use occurs when the resulting display accurately reflects the data and provides a basis for an appropriate interpretation. An incorrect use occurs when the display inadvertently or purposefully misleads the reader. A number of books [*How to Lie with Statistics* (Huff, 1954); *Aha! Gotcha: Paradoxes to Puzzle and Delight* (Gardner, 1982); *Flaws and Fallacies in Statistical Thinking* (Campbell, 1974); and *How to Tell the Liars from the Statisticians* (Hooke, 1983)] provide a multitude of examples of incorrect uses of tables, graphs, and figures. These books help readers learn how to critique and accurately evaluate displays. This book includes only a few examples of incorrect formats or distorted presentations (Chapter 13), but concentrates on techniques for accurately and objectively presenting clinical data. Purely statistical presentations of data (e.g., biplot, probit analysis, quantile-quantile plots, multivariate analyses, jittering) are not included in this book. A summary of the types of statistical analyses is found in Bailar and Mosteller (1986).

Most data displays presented in this book are intended to be generic and may be used with any study design. Since well-controlled clinical studies generally are randomized, double-blind, and parallel, that assumption is made in presenting the framework for most sample displays. Although the formats shown are suitable for other study designs, some modifications may be necessary.

COMMON FORMATS FOR PRESENTING CLINICAL DATA

Tables, graphs, and figures are the three overall categories used to display clinical data. Although graphs and figures overlap to some degree, the distinctions made in the following list are used in this book. Examples are given in this chapter for the types of tables and graphs described. Examples of figures are given either in this chapter or elsewhere in this book.

Tables

1. Row and column
2. Lists
3. Categorizations
4. Descriptions

Graphs (Two-Dimensional)

1. Histograms
2. Line graphs
3. Curvilinear graphs
4. Scattergrams (i.e., graphs consisting solely of multiple points, although a linear regression or other type of line may be superimposed)
5. Circular graphs (i.e., line graph variant that is useful to show a cyclical change)
6. Cumulative step-wise functions (e.g., cumulative survival from a life table)

Graphs (Three-Dimensional)

1. Histograms
2. Surfaces or volumes

Figures

1. Drawings
2. Algorithms
3. Flow diagrams or flow charts
4. Venn diagrams
5. Maps of various types
6. Photographs
7. Equipment outputs (e.g., electrocardiogram, echocardiogram, sonogram)
8. Schematic diagrams (e.g., metabolic pathways)
9. Filled-in squares
10. Pie charts
11. Decision trees
12. PERT charts (Program Evaluation and Review Technique)
13. Four-quadrant distribution charts
14. Gantt charts
15. Visual analogue charts
16. Timelines
17. Computer graphics
18. Vector analyses
19. Nomograms
20. X-rays
21. Genealogy trees
22. Pictographs
23. Calendars

TABLES

Types of information that may be put in a table include:

1. Numbers
2. Text
3. Codes for data or information
4. Symbols used to designate data, information, or change (e.g., arrows ↑   ↓ where the number, size, and direction of the arrows may be indicative of different meanings).
5. Abbreviations
6. Combinations of the above

Data may represent (1) directly measured numbers or observations, (2) indirectly measured or obtained numbers or observations, (3) derived numbers or observations using a preset formula, or (4) transformed numbers. Tables 1.1 to 1.8 are examples of basic methods, organizations, and types of tables.

Illustrates types and levels of data presented in tables.

TABLE 1.1. Methods to Present Data on One Variable Evaluated in a Study[a]

	Type of data[b]			
Level of data presented	Raw data	Combined data[c]	Derived data[d]	Transformed data
Single patient				
Single group of patients				
Single study site				
Multicenter study				
Multiple groups of patients				
Multiple studies				

[a]Examples of the variable could be age of patient, sex of patient, dose of drug, patients with severe disease, patients treated for at least X months.

[b]These categories do not necessarily include measures of variability such as standard deviations, standard errors, 95% confidence intervals, or ranges.

[c]Combined data refers to means, medians, and ranges.

[d]Derived data refers to parameters obtained from variables measured directly (e.g., total systemic resistance equals mean arterial pressure times 80 and divided by cardiac output; cardiac index equals cardiac output divided by body surface area.)

Illustrates basic organization of many tables containing numbers.

TABLE 1.2. Basic Organization of Most Tables Presenting Clinical Data

Types, categories, or groups whose data are shown[a]	Data[b] shown in columns from 1 to N[c]	Statistical analyses: either separated or next to data[e]
Individual patients[d]		
Groups of patients		
Categories of abnormalities		
Treatment rendered		

[a]Explanatory material is often placed in a footnote beneath the table.

[b]Data may be numbers or comments, raw figures, derived numbers, or transformed values.

[c]There is no theoretical limit to the number of columns shown.

[d]Horizontal lines are not absolutely necessary, but they help set headings apart from data and make tables more readily understood. Most journals have their own requirements as to specific details for table format.

[e]Statistical analyses varying from means and error measurements to sophisticated analyses are optional in tables presenting data. Tables may consist entirely of statistical analyses. Some statistical analyses (e.g., mean, median) may appear in both rows and columns.

• Repeated numbers (i.e., two independent observations) may be illustrated by putting a slash between the two values obtained.

• Rows and columns may be switched in any table. Practical considerations of the size of computer paper, a publication, or other report usually determines which parameter(s) is placed in columns and which in rows.

• Complex or large tables are often divided into two or more separate tables to make the material more clear to the reader (e.g., two separate categories of data may be placed in two separate tables).

Illustrates a simple list in table format.

TABLE 1.3. Drugs Known to Precipitate Attacks of Acute Intermittent Porphyria

Barbiturates
Aminopyrine
Chlordiazepoxide
Meprobamate
Sulfonamides
Phenytoin
Androgens
Estrogens
Oral contraceptives

   • Drugs may be listed in alphabetical order.
   • If a large number of drugs are listed they should be categorized either by type or by a different classification.
   • Specific drugs should all be listed by generic and/or trade names. Trade and generic names should not be mixed unless unavoidable, and then a clear differentiation should be used (e.g., trade names capitalized).

Illustrates a commonly used hybrid form of a table and figure.

TABLE 1.4. Diagnostic Categories of Anemias

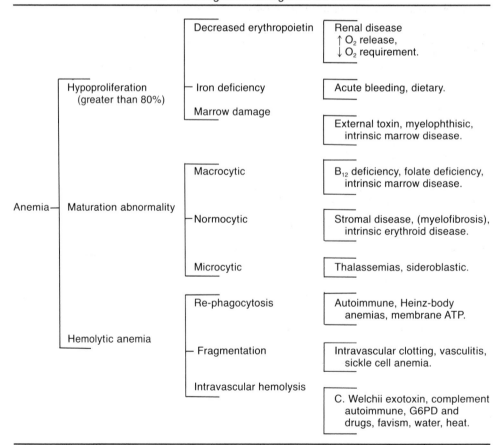

   • Presentation may also be ordered from top to bottom, as well as side to side (shown).

Illustrates a table of text elements instead of numbers.

TABLE 1.5. Approach to Differentiation of Anemias

		Reticulocyte Index	
Index > 3		Index < 2	
Test: smear indices	Hemolytic	Hypoproliferative	Maturation abnormalities
Cell size	macro-normo	normal	microcytic or macrocytic
Fragmentation	present or absent	absent	present
LDH	increased	normal	increased
Bilirubin	normal-elevated	low-normal	normal-elevated
Marrow	high (1 : 1 to 2 : 1)	normal (1 : 3 to 2 : 3)	high (1 : 1 to 2 : 1)
Morphology	hyperplastic- macro, normoblastic	normal	megaloblastic defect in hemoglobinization

Illustrates a table of text with five columns.

TABLE 1.6. Aspects of Immunity and Immunologic Disease

Type	Action and mechanism	Toxicity	Use	Examples
Active immunity	induce antibody formation	local inflammation, systemic malaise and fever	prevent infection	smallpox vaccine
Passive immunity	provide antibodies	hypersensitivity phenomena	treat infection	tetanus antitoxin
Histamine	stimulates (bronchial) or releases (vascular) smooth muscle	flushing, hypotension	diagnostic, gastric juice	histamine phosphate
Antihistamines	competitive interference with histamine at receptors	drowsiness, dizziness, dry mouth, nausea	hay fever, urticaria	tripelennamine
Anti-motion sickness	vestibular depression	same	motion sickness	dimenhydrinate

Illustrates a table of symbols rather than numbers or text.

TABLE 1.7. Changes in Blood Pressure Observed at Different Stages of Treatment

Age of treatment group	N	Relative change in blood pressure[a]				
		Day 1	Day 8	Day 15	Day 22	Day 29
14 to 18	75	0	↑	↑ ↑	↑	0
19 to 64	326	↓	↓ ↓	↓ ↓	↓ ↓	↓ ↓ ↓
Over 64	89	0	↓	↓	↓ ↓	↓ ↓

[a]0, change of 0 to 4; ↑, increase of 5 to 9; ↑ ↑, increase of 10 to 14; ↓, decrease of 5 to 9; ↓ ↓, decrease of 10 to 14; ↓ ↓ ↓, decrease of 15 to 19 mm Hg.

• Virtually any type of symbol may be used in a table as long as its meaning is identified.

Illustrates use of symbols in tables.

TABLE 1.8. Past, Present, and Future Uses of Hospital Services and Staff

	3 years ago	Present	2 years in future	5 years in future
Laboratory facilities	○	○	○	⊕
Pharmacy services	○	●	⊕	⊕
Consulting services	⊕	○	○	○
Emergency rooms	●	⊙	⊕	○
Operating rooms	⊕	⊕	⊕	○
Outpatient clinics	⊕	○	○	⊕
No. of nursing staff	⊙	⊙	⊙	●
Patient load factor	○	○	⊕	●

○, Adequate; ⊙, Area of concern; ⊕, Severe problem, and ●, Crisis.

Guidelines and Tips in Preparing Tables

1. Determine what information readers already have when they approach a table and what information they seek or the author wants to convey.
2. Row and column headings should relate to information the reader already possesses and the body of the table should contain information the reader seeks.
3. Present information in a sequence that will make sense to the reader. Thus, information is usually presented in order from left to right and from top to bottom.
4. When a reader is asked to compare items within a table, this is usually best done by scanning vertically, i.e., items to be compared should be listed above each other.
5. When there is a choice of placing a table's rows as columns or vice versa, list on the left the items about which the reader is most likely to want information. In some cases a large number of columns or rows will dictate the order that is used (a large number of one group is usually listed vertically).
6. Data that are related should be grouped together. A large table may be made easier to comprehend if categories of items are clustered together and separated by different heads (e.g., using body systems to categorize all adverse reactions into five or so groups). Lines may be used to divide a table into smaller parts that are easier to understand.
7. Scanning along a row is facilitated by sufficient space above and below the row. Likewise, scanning along a column is facilitated by space to its right and left. If sufficient space is impossible, then consider thin lines, bold type for alternate columns or rows, or adding background highlights or shading for certain columns or rows. Some computer paper is shaded in this manner.
8. Whenever possible present all data in a table that allows readers to find information they seek. Tables that present only part of the data and require the reader to interpolate may not be well received.
9. Eliminate columns of identical or nearly identical numbers in a table. For example, a column listing the number of patients assessed for a series of evalua-

tions may be identical and misdirect the reader's attention. The "N" and exceptions may be footnoted.
10. If a large amount of data is presented, group the results into ranges of responses or scores (e.g., instead of listing the number of times values from 1 to 100 obtained, list the number of times 0 to 9, 10 to 19, 20 to 29, etc., were obtained). Alternatively, list the degree of clinical change (e.g., mild, marked) and the range of scores each category represents, plus the number of responses in each category. Percent of total and cumulative percent columns may be added.
11. It is best to avoid vertical lines in the body of a table. They interfere with horizontal scanning along the rows.

GRAPHS

Graphs are initially discussed in terms of variables and axes.

Variables and Titles

Graphs illustrate the relationship between two or more variables. Variables are either independent or dependent. Independent variables usually change regularly (e.g., a series of equal time divisions) but are always unaffected by changes in the other. Dependent variables change irregularly and usually represent quantitative or percentage values such as activity or response. Dependent variables also may represent qualitative responses (e.g., change from severe to mild intensity).

The independent variable is usually calibrated or placed on the abscissa (x-axis) and the dependent variable on the ordinate (y-axis). Grid lines that illustrate units of measure along x and y axes are sometimes shown in the body of the curve. Grid lines should usually be light in weight.

Titles of tables, graphs, and figures should be brief and complete. They are usually placed above the material. They may be centered, or justified at either the right or left margins. Most styles are acceptable, but decorative lettering is usually inappropriate. Titles may be omitted or incorporated in a legend or in the text. Table titles must be distinct from column headings, either by spacing, use of bold lines, or with different style or size of lettering.

Orientation of Axes

Although values along an abscissa may be plotted in ascending order from right to left, it is the usual custom for ascending order to go from left to right (Fig. 1.1, top). For the ordinate it is also the custom to go from bottom to top with ascending values (Fig. 1.1, bottom). When values with a lower magnitude represent a more desirable clinical state, a decision must be made about whether to reverse the order of the values to show clinical improvement toward the upper part of the ordinate, or the right side of the abscissa. The authors' preference is to show clinical improvement in this way (Fig. 1.2), rather than showing clinical improvement as approaching the origin. This is based primarily on the traditional approach of presenting data and is consistent with the majority of graphs.

When labeling axes use equal increments throughout an arithmetic scale, unless a hatch mark is used to indicate a break in the scale. Log or semilog scales should be used when a wide distribution of values is to be plotted. If scale markings are close together, do not label each. Only label those that enhance clarity and comprehension. Unless there is a good reason to do otherwise, scales chosen and spacing used on axes should be planned so that the graph fills most of the available space.

Graphs with one to four axes are shown in Figs. 1.3 to 1.6. Appropriate data may be marked either on or above the axis. All axes could be identified with a scale (−) to (+), or (0) to (+). Scales may also be used to represent data obtained in the past on through to the future.

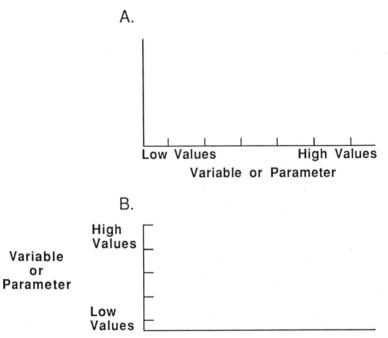

FIG. 1.1. Usual manner of assigning values to the abscissa or x-axis (panel A) and ordinate or y-axis (panel B).

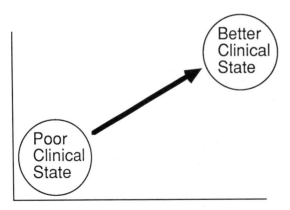

FIG. 1.2. Usual direction of graphing an improvement in clinical function.

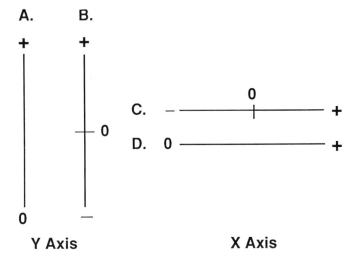

Y Axis   X Axis

FIG. 1.3. Examples of single-axis graphs.

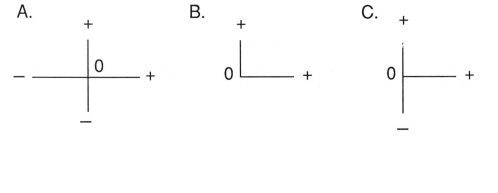

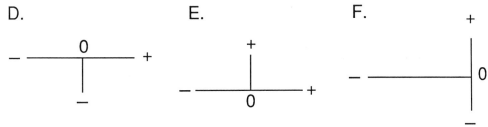

FIG. 1.4. Common examples of graphs with two axes.

A.

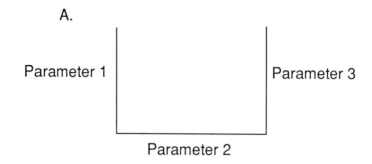

Parameter 1 | | Parameter 3

Parameter 2

B.

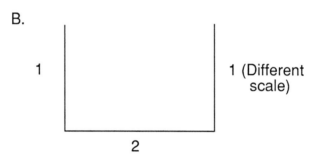

1 | | 1 (Different scale)

2

FIG. 1.5. Examples of graphs with three axes, showing three separate parameters (panel A), or two parameters where one is plotted using two scales (panel B).

A.

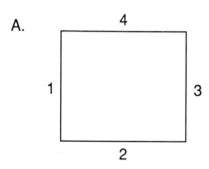

4

1 | | 3

2

B.

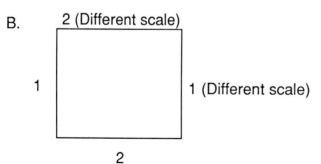

2 (Different scale)

1 | | 1 (Different scale)

2

FIG. 1.6. Examples of graphs with four axes. Numbers refer to different parameters.

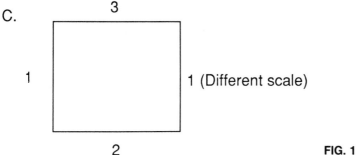

C.

3

1

1 (Different scale)

2

FIG. 1.6. *Continued.*

Potential Modifications of Axes

Modifications of single-axis graphs are shown in Fig. 1.7. Panels A and C start above zero and values become more positive. Panels B and D start below zero and values become more negative. Panel E shows changes from before to after (i.e., state 1 to 2), often for individual patients. Numerous variations of E exist (e.g., with mean or median values illustrated, with different groups of patients represented with different symbols).

Modifications of two-axis graphs are shown in Fig. 1.8. Panels A and B show axes where the origin is not illustrated. Panel C shows an axis with an additional line (*) to indicate the scale. Panel D shows an axis with broken scales. Panel E shows axes of unequal length. Panel F shows a line of equivalence (45° to each axis), assuming their scales are equal. In panels G and H the asterisk refers to a reference line that indicates a defined point. A different scale of the same data could be a log scale, one using different types of units (°F or °C), or may also represent a transformed scale of the data.

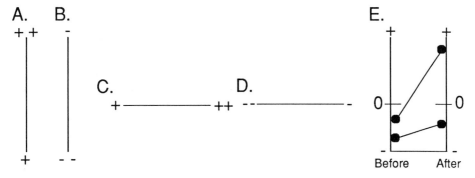

FIG. 1.7. Variations of single-axis graphs. Panels A to D illustrate variations where no "0" values are included. Panel E illustrates a common before and after treatment, where each line represents an individual patient. Scales may be placed along the axis and a scatterplot of values shown alongside the axis in panels A to D. Multiple points at a single value are often shown by stacking.

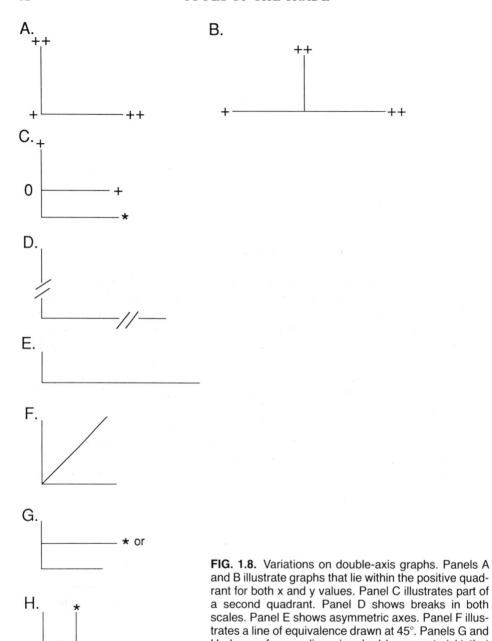

FIG. 1.8. Variations on double-axis graphs. Panels A and B illustrate graphs that lie within the positive quadrant for both x and y values. Panel C illustrates part of a second quadrant. Panel D shows breaks in both scales. Panel E shows asymmetric axes. Panel F illustrates a line of equivalence drawn at 45°. Panels G and H show reference lines (marked by an asterisk) that would be identified in the text.

How Does One Choose an Axis for a Parameter?

Conventions often exist as to which parameters should be on the abscissa (horizontal or x-axis) and which should be along the ordinate (vertical or y-axis) in a line graph. If no convention exists, then visual impact or other factors may be considered in assigning a parameter to a specific axis. A few examples are shown below.

A few types of graphs will be presented in greater detail to illustrate representative examples. Major types of graphs are histograms, line graphs, curvilinear graphs, scattergrams, cumulative step-wise functions, and three-dimensional graphs.

TABLE 1.9. Assigning an Axis to a Parameter (Selected Examples of Common Conventions)

Parameters that are usually plotted along the x-axis[a]		Parameters that are usually plotted along the y-axis
Dose of drug	versus	Response to drug (i.e., activity)
Time	versus	Concentration measured
Time	versus	Response to drug

[a]This is usually the independent variable.

Illustrates common parameters used to describe data.

TABLE 1.10. Selected Common Headings for Table Columns or Graph Axes

Number treated or number evaluatable
X effect at time y
Percent of patients with x effect at time y
Range of responses observed
Confidence intervals (e.g., 95%)
Number of patients or observations
Number of patients with clinically important results
Incidence rate
Time to onset of effect
Time to peak effect
Duration of effect
Peak response
Doses given
Parameters measured
Times (after drug) at which parameters were measured
Baseline values
Study number
Study site number
ED_{50}, ED_{95}, IC_{50}, EC_{50} (Effective dose to yield 50% of the total effect observed, same for 95%, inhibitory concentration that causes a 50% antagonism of a given response, effective concentration that causes 50% of the total effect observed.)
Relative risk
Comments
Total number of responses in terms of patients or events plus rates
Patients grouped by one or more demographic characteristics
Treatment group
Patient number
Ranking (i.e., rank order of data according to magnitude, frequency, or another characteristic)
Change in parameter for time 1 versus time 2
Weighted value
Transformed value (e.g., logarithmic transformation)

Guidelines and Tips in Preparing Graphs

1. Any graph (or figure) must have an overall structure. It is preferable when both the structure and illustrated data are simple rather than complex.
2. Avoid and eliminate all extraneous data and information. These details may be placed in a legend or text. Eliminate unnecessary lines or frames around a figure.
3. When particularly complex data must be presented, it is often desirable to build up to it using a series of separate graphs or figures. This issue is discussed in more detail in the discussion on preparing slides in Chapter 2.
4. The number of separate curves that may be included in any one graph depends on how close the curves are to each other and how many times the lines cross each other. If the number of curves to be placed on a graph must be determined, compare one or two curves per graphs with three or more. If the curves are to be compared, then it is generally preferable to place them on a single graph.
5. Figures with lines of different thickness are usually more attractive than those where all the lines are the same.
6. More emphasis should be placed on the data illustrated than on the axes. Curves or other lines illustrated on a graph should be thicker than lines used for axes.
7. Consider alternative details for drawing *error bars* (e.g., show one side only of the (+) and (−) part); *lines* (e.g., use different patterns such as hashes that clearly code the lines, especially those that cross each other), *lines crossing each other* (e.g., make one curve appear to go behind the other by having a small break on both sides of the line it crosses); and *calibrations* (e.g., insure they are outside the axis so that they do not interfere with the data presented, consider using calibration lines that go "behind" the data).
8. Do not superimpose different types of data if it adds confusion to the graph. Dividing the data into separate presentations is usually an appropriate solution.
9. Label the vertical axis (i.e., ordinate) so that the page does not have to be rotated to read it.
10. Use direct labeling of curves or data points whenever possible and try to avoid a key. If a key is necessary, then attempt to place it within the graph, or as close to the data as possible.

Maps

Maps may be used as a tool to illustrate many points.

1. Arrows of different sizes may be superimposed to show relative movements of different numbers of patients from region to region (e.g., in the spread of a disease).
2. Pie charts may be superimposed on individual states, countries, or other regions to illustrate clinical facets of an issue.
3. Symbols (e.g., dots, bars, circles, shading, colors) that relate to quantitative or qualitative parameters may be superimposed on a map.
4. Areas on maps may be distorted proportionally to a clinical attribute that relates to that area.

Histograms

Some authors differentiate between histograms, column charts, and bar graphs. Histograms are frequency distributions with vertical bars on an X axis with a continuous scale. Column charts and bar graphs (i.e., bar charts) are individual bars with space between bars that are aligned vertically (column chart) or horizontally (bar graph). Bar charts usually compare different quantities at one time point, whereas column charts compare one quantity at different times. The order of the columns may be chronological, ranked, or determined by another system. An arbitrary or random order also may be used. No distinction is made in this book between these three presentations. All bar presentations are described with the term histogram.

The following six figures illustrate numerous approaches to presenting data using histograms. In Fig. 1.9, panels A and B show single bars with and without standard deviation (SD) or standard error (SE) variation indicators. Panels C and D show

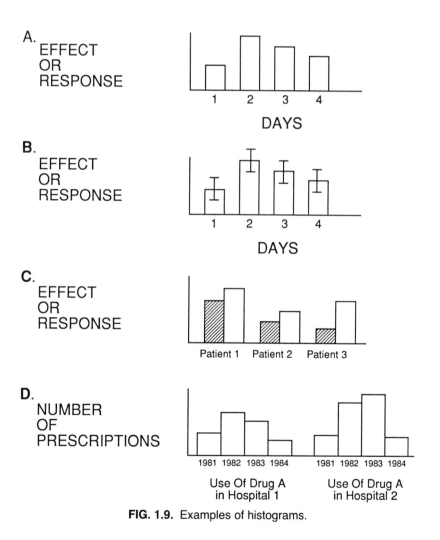

FIG. 1.9. Examples of histograms.

double or multiple bars used alongside each other to illustrate several aspects of each category (e.g., patient, hospital). Shading may represent "before" values. In Fig. 1.10, panel A illustrates components of the overall response on each single bar. Panel B shows a combination approach of histogram plus line graph. Panel C shows a continuous histogram. In Fig. 1.11, panels A and B are cumulative types of histograms, and panel C is a combination of histograms. Figure 1.12 shows two three-dimensional histograms (examples in Figs. 1.9 to 1.11 could each be illustrated in three dimensions). Figure 1.13 shows a percent change for two drugs and Fig. 1.14 shows SD bars in two axes.

Variations that May Be Incorporated in Histograms

1. Put a horizontal line across the graph either at a meaningful level or at a defined standard. This procedure illustrates those values that meet or exceed the level or standard of interest (Fig. 1.14).

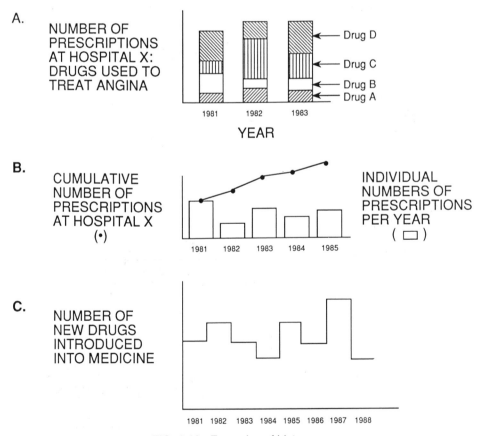

FIG. 1.10. Examples of histograms.

• A photograph, drawing, or shading could be put under the curve in panel C.

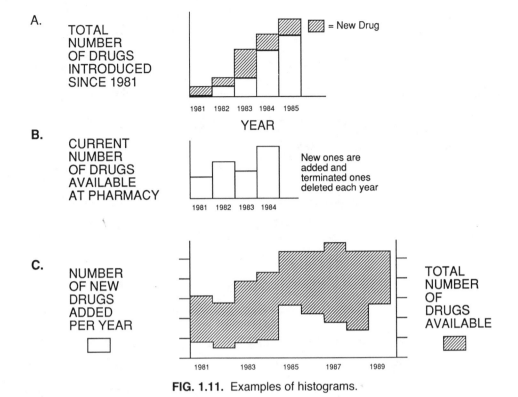

A. TOTAL NUMBER OF DRUGS INTRODUCED SINCE 1981

☑ = New Drug

1981 1982 1983 1984 1985

YEAR

B. CURRENT NUMBER OF DRUGS AVAILABLE AT PHARMACY

New ones are added and terminated ones deleted each year

1981 1982 1983 1984

C. NUMBER OF NEW DRUGS ADDED PER YEAR

TOTAL NUMBER OF DRUGS AVAILABLE

1981 1983 1985 1987 1989

FIG. 1.11. Examples of histograms.

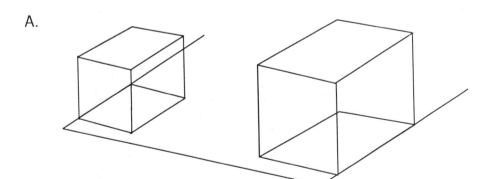

A.

FIG. 1.12. Examples of three-dimensional histograms.

B.

NUMBER
OF
STUDIES

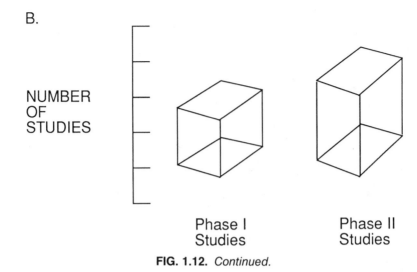

Phase I
Studies

Phase II
Studies

FIG. 1.12. *Continued.*

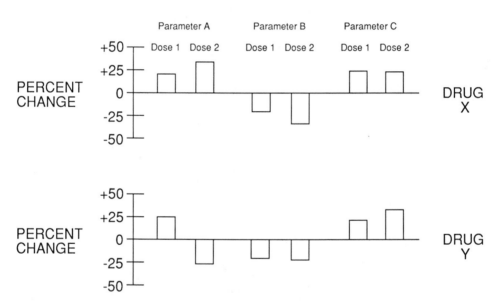

FIG. 1.13. Example of a histogram showing both positive and negative changes. Error bars of SD or SE could be added to provide additional data.

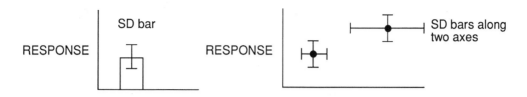

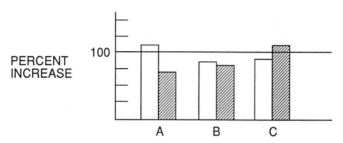

FIG. 1.14. Examples of error bars: upper graphs, and reference line (drawn at 100% response) in lower graph of grouped columns.

• Shading patterns or contrasting colors are used to differentiate each group's columns and to illustrate differences.

2. When two or more bars of a histogram are associated with a single question, patient, year, or other category, use contrasting colors or patterns in a consistent manner (Fig. 1.14).
3. Histogram bars may be rotated 90°, especially if this change enhances clarity.
4. Add numbers or symbols to a histogram to convey additional information. For example, where individual patients are shown, an asterisk could indicate those who dropped out or had characteristics not shared by all patients in the group.
5. Make each bar wider or narrower, closer or further from its neighbor, or adjust the axes dimensions to alter the appearance of the format. The space between bars should be less than their width. Care must be taken to present an appropriate and accurate graph.

Additional examples of histograms are shown below.

• Comparison histograms (Figs. 1.15 and 1.16C).
• Two-sided histograms (Figs. 1.15 to 1.18).
• Subdivided histograms (Figs. 1.16A, 1.19, and 1.20).
• Individual cases identified (Figs. 1.21 and 1.22).
• Combination (Figs. 1.10B, 1.21 bottom, and 1.23).
• Frequency distribution (Fig. 1.24).
• Scale placed behind histogram versus scale placed to one side (Fig. 1.25).
• Statistical comparisons shown diagrammatically (Fig. 1.26).
• Lines connecting similar parts of different columns to facilitate comparisons (Fig. 1.27).
• Three-dimensional with breakdown of each column (Fig. 1.28).

• Three-dimensional with two rows and vertical scale (Fig. 1.29) or three rows without vertical scale (Fig. 1.30).

• Three-dimensional histograms with one row of bars (Figs. 1.31 to 1.34).

• A photograph or drawing of the subject being discussed for the bars of the histogram (Figs. 1.35 and 1.36). This approach adds to the visual impact.

• Words as the bars of the histogram. This may add emphasis to the trend of data illustrated (Fig. 1.37).

• Use of a single bar demarcated into sections that are identified (Fig. 1.38).

Illustrates using a histogram to display individual patient data.

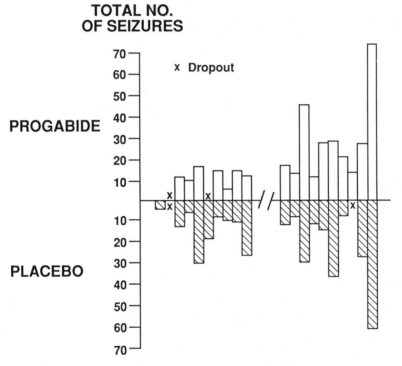

FIG. 1.15. The total number of seizures in each patient. The patients starting on placebo showed on average a lower number of seizures in both treatment periods. Reprinted from Dam et al. (1983) with permission.

• Cross-hatching each patient's placebo experience allows for easy interpretation.

• The "x" to indicate dropouts is an additional aid.

• It is unclear why the horizontal axis is broken; possibly it indicates a different treatment sequence.

• The ordinate could illustrate increases and decreases in a parameter. The abscissa could illustrate individual patients who would have either increases or decreases.

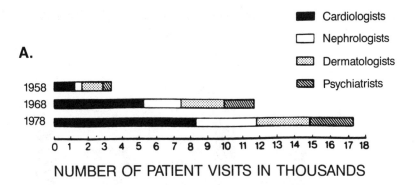

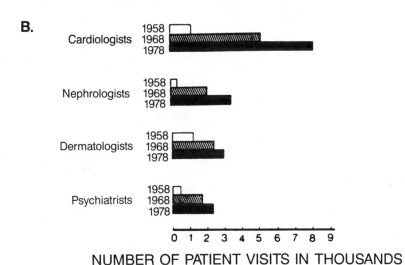

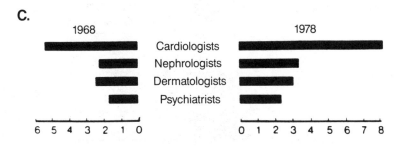

FIG. 1.16. Histograms where the same data are shown in three different formats.

• Panel A is the most difficult to read and interpret.
• Panel B shows grouped columns and enables one to readily read and interpret the data.
• Panel C's format only allows two periods to be compared.

Illustrates including error bars to indicate variability and the results of statistical comparisons in histogram.

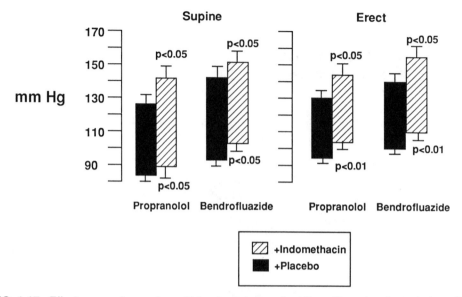

FIG. 1.17. Effects on supine and erect blood pressures of adding either placebo or indomethacin to treatment with propranolol or bendrofluazide. Reprinted from Watkins et al. (1980) with permission.

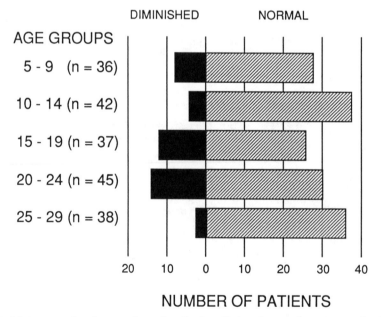

FIG. 1.18. Histogram showing number of patients with two types of responses for five separate groups of patients.

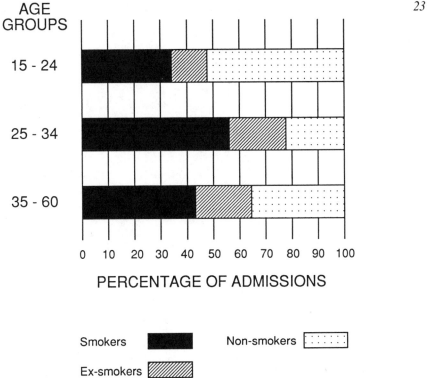

FIG. 1.19. Histogram with equal size bars divided by percents for different groups of patients.

• Vertical reference lines marking the scale are helpful.

Illustrates that many indicators may be incorporated into single patient displays.

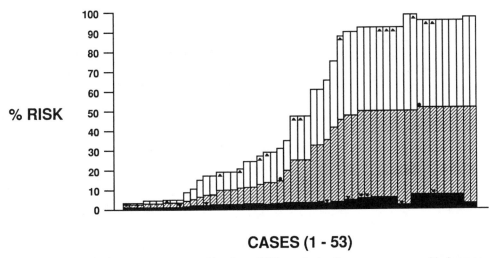

CASES (1 - 53)

FIG. 1.20. Alterations in fetal risk resulting from DNA analysis. Cases are arranged in increasing order of maternal carrier risk. Midline refers to risk to a male fetus based on sexing alone; upper and lower lines refer to risks to a male fetus carrying high and low risk, respectively. Reprinted from Cole et al. (1988) with permission.

Illustrates a histogram with individual cases.

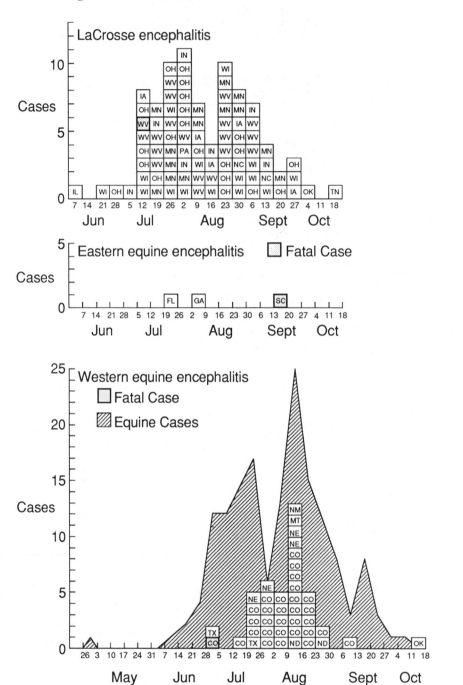

FIG. 1.21. Arboviral infections of the central nervous system—United States, 1987. Reprinted from Leads from the MMWR (1988a) with permission.

Illustrates a histogram with individual cases.

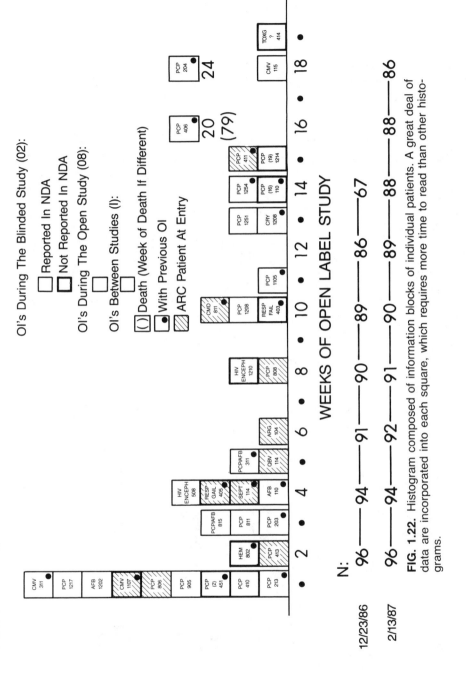

FIG. 1.22. Histogram composed of information blocks of individual patients. A great deal of data are incorporated into each square, which requires more time to read than other histograms.

25

Illustrates a means of superimposing data on a histogram.

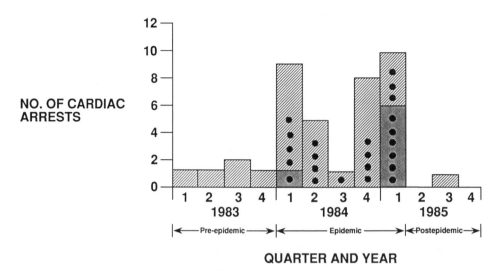

FIG. 1.23. Cardiac arrests that were unexpected in timing in patients with multiple arrests, by consistency with clinical course and by nurse, in intensive care unit, Maryland 1983–1985. Slashed bars indicate unexpected and consistent; cross-hatched bars, unexpected and inconsistent; and black bullet, nurse 14. Reprinted from Sacks et al. (1988) with permission.

Illustrates frequency type histogram with many separate bars providing overall patterns.

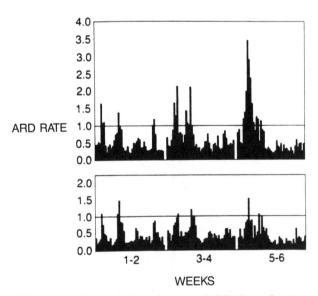

FIG. 1.24. Rates of febrile acute respiratory diseases (ARD) from October 1, 1982 through September 1, 1986, in modern (top panel) and old (bottom panel) barracks, by weeks of basic training cycle. Rates of ARD are shown for entire study period for each week-of-training–specific period. Reprinted from Brundage et al. (1988) with permission.

• Each thin bar could be replaced by a line. The resulting histogram is sometimes called a needle histogram.

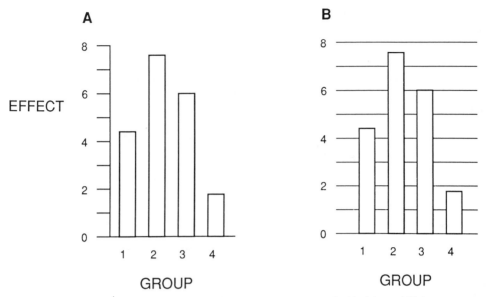

FIG. 1.25. Scales indicated to side of axis (panel A) or behind (panel B) bars.

• The width of bars may also be varied to represent another parameter.

Illustrates a statistical comparison of different groups shown with histograms.

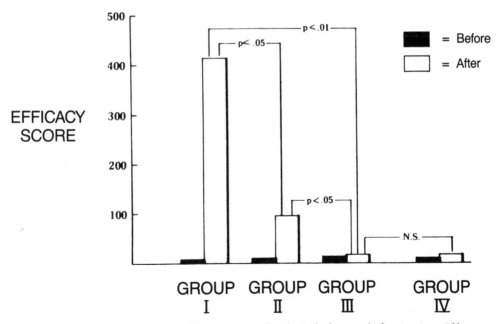

FIG. 1.26. Efficacy scores of four groups of patients before and after treatment X.

Illustrates use of dotted or solid lines connecting comparable parts of histogram bars to indicate changes of magnitude.

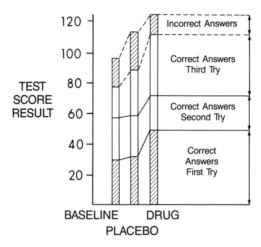

FIG. 1.27. Comparison of correct answers on three attempts, at baseline and on placebo or drug.

Illustrates using various shading schemes to demarcate distinct factors composing the bars of a histogram.

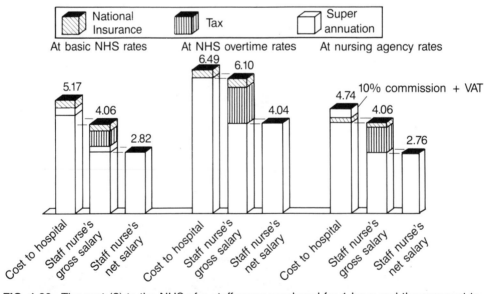

FIG. 1.28. The cost (£) to the NHS of a staff nurse employed for 1 hour and the payment to the nurse, assuming that the nurse is working 10 hours overtime a week and that the overtime rates are for Monday to Friday, exclusive of London week. Reprinted from Delamothe (1988a) with permission.

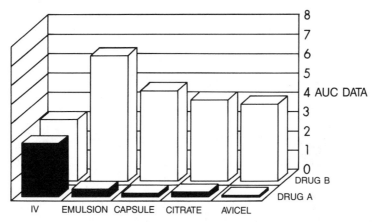

FIG. 1.29. Comparison of various formulations after oral administration.

• Horizontal lines are used to indicate reference values along the vertical axis.

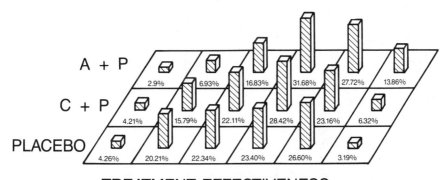

FIG. 1.30. Responses of three treatments given to six individual patients or groups of patients for two efficacy parameters (upper and lower graphs).

Illustrates two methods to overlap histograms.

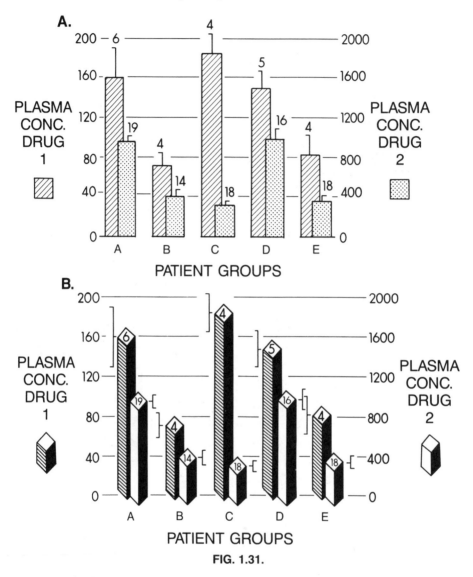

FIG. 1.31.

• Bar pairs in panel A are set in front and behind each other in two dimensions, whereas in panel B a third dimension is used.

• The degree of overlap of each pair of columns in panel A may be greater than shown here and is sometimes 50%.

Illustrates three-dimensional histograms in poster style.

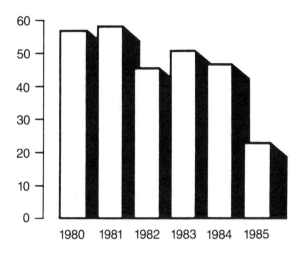

FIG. 1.32. A three-dimensional effect is provided. This approach is particularly useful for posters or dramatic presentations, but reading numbers off the y-axis is difficult. This effect is unsuitable for most presentations. Modified from Simmonds (1980) with permission.

Illustrates three-dimensional histograms in poster style.

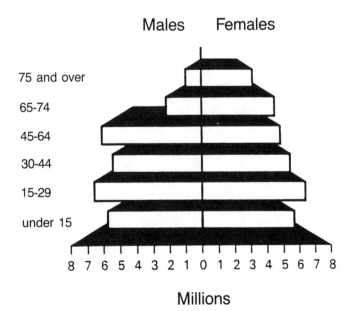

FIG. 1.33. This type of histogram with bars to the right and left of a center line is also referred to as a pyramid. In three dimensions (as shown) the same comments apply as for Fig. 1.32. Reprinted from Simmonds (1980) with permission.

Illustrates an inverted histogram in three dimensions.

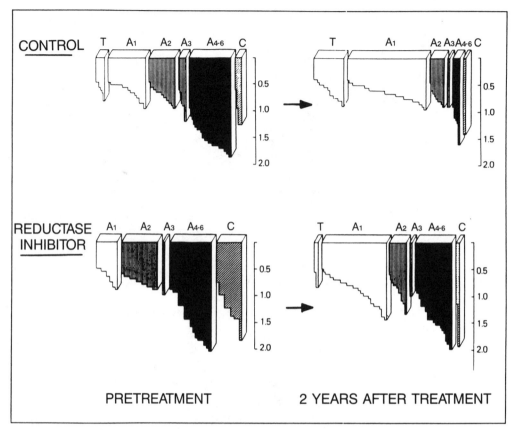

FIG. 1.34. 5α-Reductase inhibitor topical application in the frontal scalp of periadolescent macaques. Folliculograms of control animals changed to the pattern of bald scalp after 2 years, whereas those of treated animals show no change. T, telogen; A₁, early anagen. Reprinted from Uno (1987) with permission.

- The frame around the figure could be deleted.

Illustrates a histogram using symbolic elements.

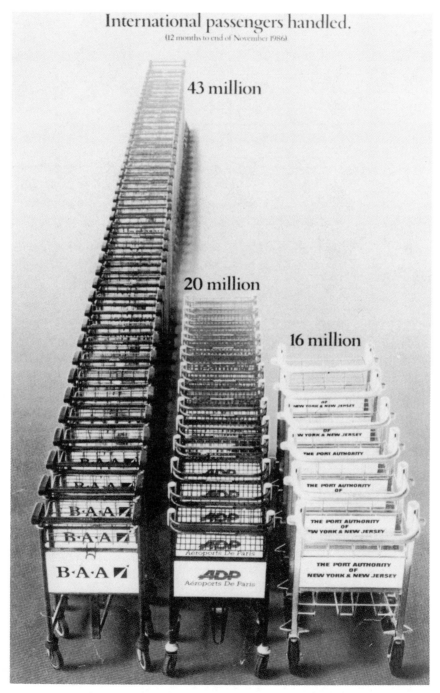

FIG. 1.35. Histogram with photograph related to items being compared.

Illustrates a histogram using symbolic elements.

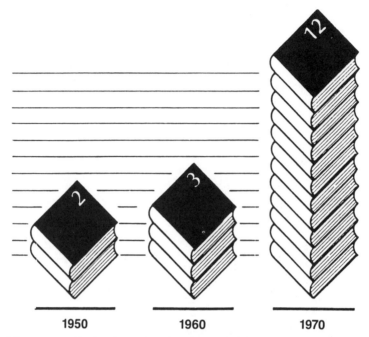

FIG. 1.36. Histogram with drawing related to items being compared. Reprinted from Simmonds (1980) with permission.

Advertisement

Since 1960, hormone levels

Pumping iron has replaced flower power. Pinstripes have replaced paisley. And Wall Street has replaced Woodstock.

But of all the major changes that have taken place since the 60's, one is hardly visible at all: the change that has taken place in the Pill.

In 1960, the Pill contained as much as 150 mcgs. of the hormone estrogen. Today, it's down to 35 mcgs. or less. That's a *fraction* of the original dosage.

Yet, today's Pill is as effective as yesterday's. In fact, it's still the most effective birth control available other than sterilization.

But is the Pill right for you? You should see your doctor to help you answer that. If the answer is yes, then the ultimate decision is yours. And it's important that you learn all you can about oral contraceptives.

First and foremost, what are the risks? Does the Pill cause cancer? Will it make you less fertile? Do you need to take a rest from it? These are just a few questions that have surrounded the Pill since 1960. Questions which must be addressed by you and your physician.

What about the Pill and breast cancer? Although there are conflicting reports concerning this issue, the Centers for Disease Control reported that women who took the Pill, even for 15 years, ran no higher risk of breast cancer than women who didn't. The CDC also reported that ovarian and uterine cancer are substantially *less* common among women who use oral contraceptives.

The Pill has been shown to have other health benefits as well. Pill users are less likely to develop pelvic inflammatory disease (tubal infections), benign breast disease, and iron deficiency anemia, not to mention menstrual cramps.

But if the Pill is so effective at preventing pregnancy, can it later prevent you from having a baby when you're ready to have one? Studies

in the Pill have

indicate that if you were fertile before you took the Pill, taking it will not affect your ability to have children later. Some women may experience a short period of readjustment after discontinuing the Pill. Even so, most women usually become pregnant soon.

One piece of advice you may have heard if you're on the Pill is that you should take an occasional rest from it. Yet there's no medical basis for this advice. Furthermore, a rest could turn out to be anything but restful, since switching to a less effective form of birth control increases your chances for unplanned pregnancy.

Now that you know what the risks aren't, you should know what the risks *are*. For example, if you are taking the Pill, you should not smoke. Especially if you are over 35. Cigarette smoking is known to increase the risk of serious and possibly life-threatening adverse effects on the heart and blood vessels from Pill use. What's more, women with certain conditions or medical histories should not use the Pill.

Even if you're already on the Pill, you should see your doctor at least once a year. And read the patient information regularly.

Taking the Pill is easy. Deciding whether or not to take it isn't. That's why it's so important for you to make an informed decision. Continue reading everything you can about birth control methods. Seek out reliable sources. Talk to your doctor.

You've already taken a step in the

dropped considerably.

right direction. Just think, since you began reading this, there's a good chance your knowledge level about the Pill has increased. Considerably.

A message from the Association of Reproductive Health Professionals through an educational grant from Ortho Pharmaceutical Corporation.

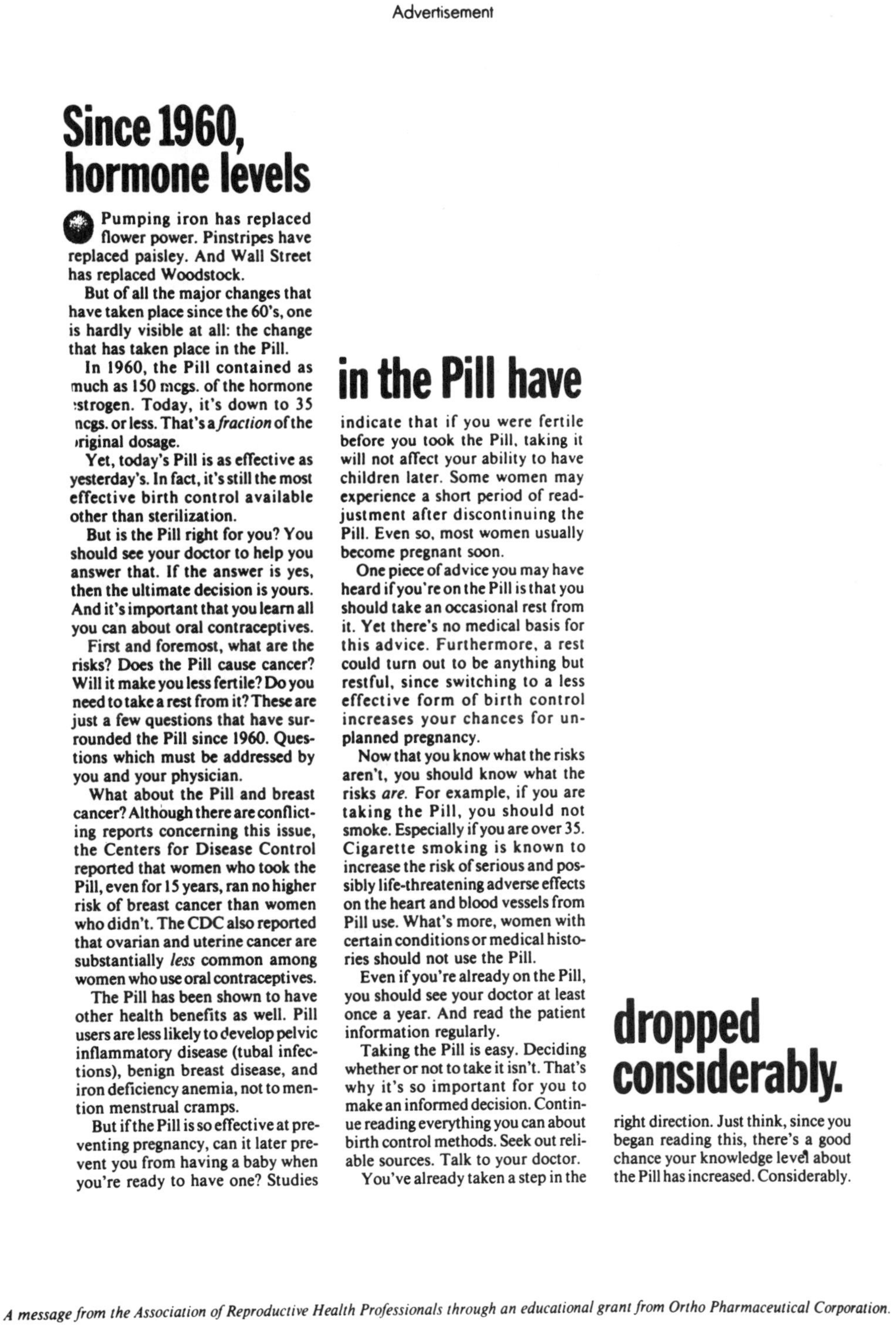

FIG. 1.37. Histogram with bars composed of words. In this example, the words relate to the decreasing size of the histogram bars. Reprinted from *Newsweek* with permission of Ortho Pharmaceuticals.

Illustrates a divided bar graph.

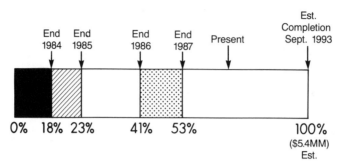

FIG. 1.38. Use of a single bar subdivided into sections. Modified from Spilker (1988b) with permission.

• This type of chart, as well as a pie chart, is often used to portray components of a 100% total.

Scattergrams (Point Graphs)

Each datum point is illustrated in this type of graph. Data are shown on a plot, usually with one or more points per patient, per time, or per other parameter. The calculated or estimated line of best fit is sometimes measured to calculate a correlation of the data and the significance of that correlation. This line may be superimposed on the graph (Fig. 1.39, panel A). Other lines may be illustrated on the graph to show other statistical evaluations, such as lines encompassing the observed ranges (Fig. 1.39, panel B) or lines delineating 95% confidence bands (Fig. 1.39, panel C).

Illustrates scattergrams with superimposed lines.

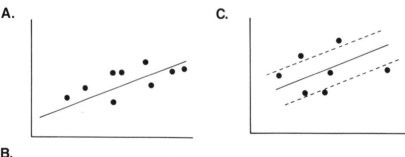

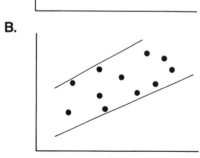

FIG. 1.39. Three examples of a scattergram (discussed in text).

• Each point or group of points on the graph may be represented by a different symbol, letter, or word.

• Each point may be proportional to a third variable.

Illustrates a scattergram with related points connected.

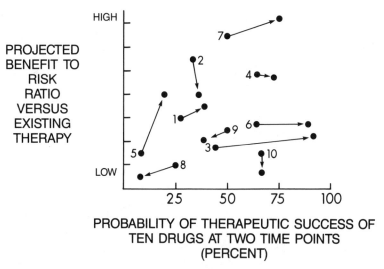

FIG. 1.40. A scattergram showing change in 10 drugs over a specified time period for two variables. Modified from Spilker (1988b) with permission.

Illustrates a scattergram with different size points.

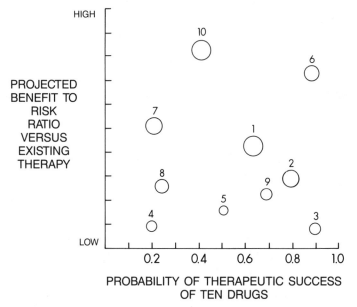

FIG. 1.41. A scattergram showing a third variable expressed in terms of dot size. Modified from Spilker (1988b) with permission.

Points may be shown to move over time using arrows (Fig. 1.40). A third variable may be illustrated by making the dots of different sizes that are proportional to the third variable (Fig. 1.41). Areas may be shaded and reference lines used (Fig. 1.42). A special case of the scattergram is a dot plot or dot diagram. In this graph the abscissa represents discrete categories rather than a continuous scale (e.g., Fig. 8.53). The dot plot is described in detail by Krieg et al. (1988).

Illustrates use of both vertical and horizontal reference lines.

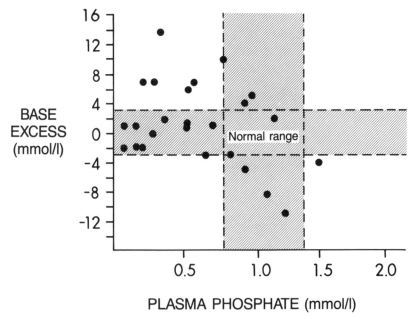

FIG. 1.42. Relation between hypophosphatemia and base excess. Reprinted from Knell et al. (1972) with permission.

Illustrates use of a line to connect each observation measured at discrete time points.

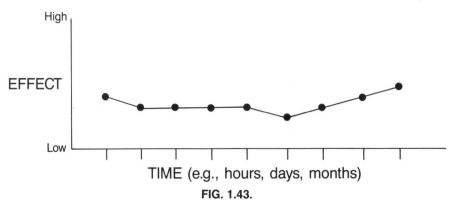

FIG. 1.43.

• All of the area under (or above) a curve may be shaded.

• All of the area under a curve may contain a photograph or drawing related to the subject of the graph.

Line Graphs

A line graph connects values observed over time (Fig. 1.43), over a range of concentrations, dosages, or other parameter. This type of graph is particularly good to illustrate changes in an effect over time. Data points may be each connected (Fig. 1.44, panel A), or approximated (Fig. 1.44, panel B). Individual data points need not be shown (Figs. 1.44, panel C).

Illustrates three methods to present a line graph: points connected, approximated, or not shown.

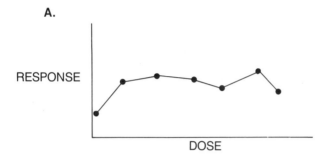

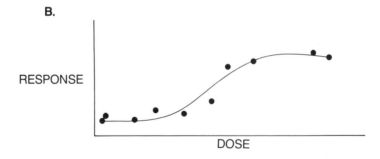

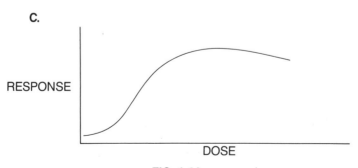

FIG. 1.44.

Variations

1. One may illustrate multiple groups on the same axes, each group with its own line graph (Fig. 1.45, panel E).
2. One or more arrows or other symbols may be used to indicate the point at which one (or more) aspects of the study changed (e.g., drug given, dosage changed, adverse reactions occurred).
3. A cumulative effect may be plotted (Fig. 1.45, panel A).
4. Variability (e.g., SD, SE) in the data may be shown with error bars.
5. One or more hatch marks in an axis may be used to show a discontinuity in the scale. The practice of having a discontinuity is discouraged; however, if a discontinuity is used, the display should indicate it.
6. Both a log scale and arithmetic scale may be used (Fig. 1.46).
7. Moving averages over a specified period may be used (Fig. 1.47).
8. Changes in individual patient values may be shown (Fig. 1.48).
9. Two-dimensional error bars may be shown (Fig. 1.49).
10. Before and after values may be shown (Fig. 1.50).
11. Circular graphs may be used (Figs. 1.51 and 1.52).

Clarity of line graphs must be assured. Figure 1.53 illustrates a common problem and one possible solution. Figure 1.54 illustrates methods to identify specific curves.

Illustrates six methods of obtaining and illustrating dose-response data.

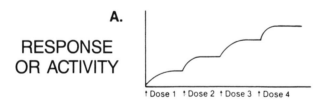

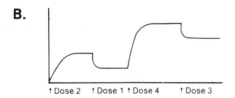

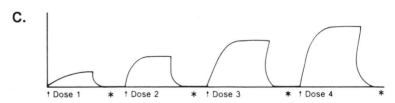

FIG. 1.45. Reprinted from Spilker (1987) with permission.

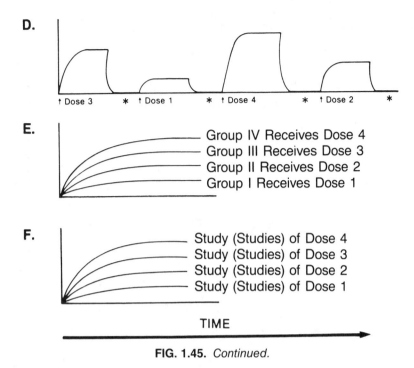

FIG. 1.45. *Continued.*

Illustrates labeling vertical axis with both transformed (logarithmic) scale and untransformed (arithmetic) scale.

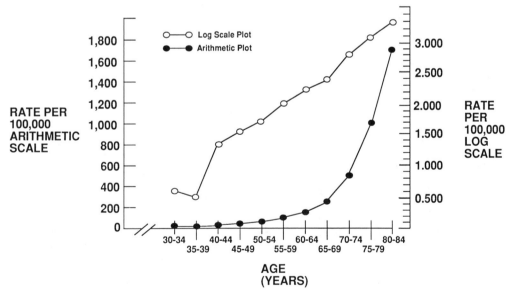

FIG. 1.46. Age-specific hip fracture incidence among white women. Source: National Hospital Discharge Survey 1975 to 1979. Reprinted from Brody (1987) with permission.

• Plotting both transformed and untransformed data on same graph vividly displays the linearizing effect of the logarithmic transformation.

Illustrates use of a moving (rolling) average.

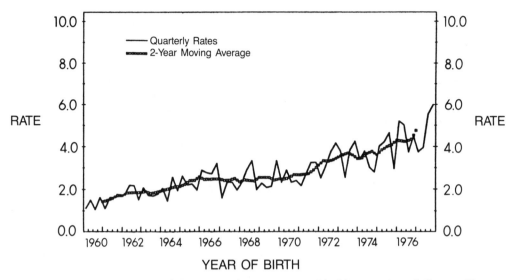

FIG. 1.47. Both quarterly and 2-year moving averages of incidence rates of disease X are shown for cohorts born in different years.

Illustrates a method to show changes in scores for individual patients.

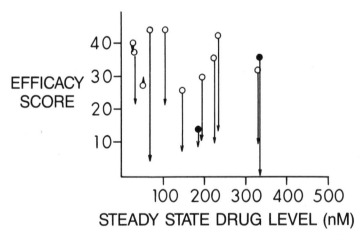

FIG. 1.48. Two or more groups may be identified with different symbols, and changes in an efficacy parameter along the axis may be shown. The x-axis may refer to their steady-state level of drug concentration (shown), to another fixed number, or not to any value.

Illustrates use of error bars in two dimensions and arrows to indicate direction of *43* **change.**

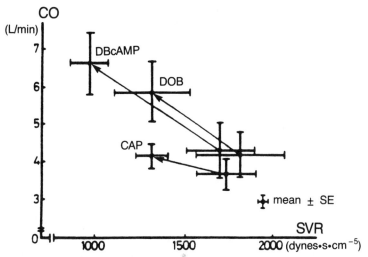

FIG. 1.49. Effect of DBcAMP, dobutamine (DOB), and captopril (CAP) on the relation between cardiac output (CO) and systemic vascular resistance (SVR). Reprinted from Nakanishi et al. (1988) with permission.

Illustrates connecting observations from the same patient.

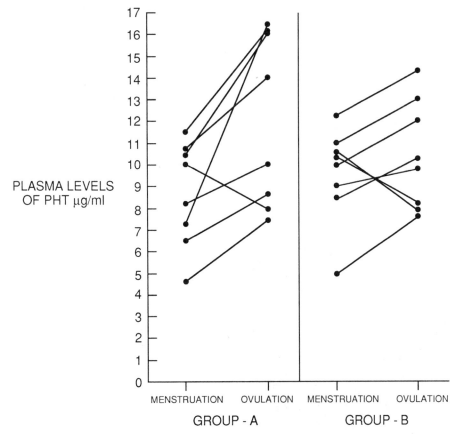

FIG. 1.50. Levels of plasma PHT in catamenial group and controls during menstrual and ovulatory phase. Reprinted from Kumar et al. (1988) with permission.

Illustrates a circular form of a line graph.

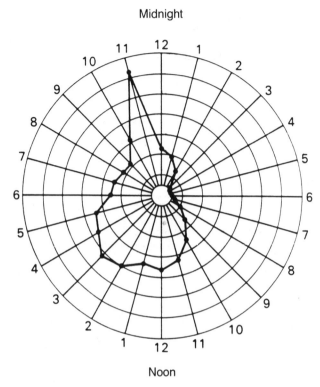

FIG. 1.51. Circular graph showing how one patient's hormonal levels varied throughout a 24-hour period.

• The center of the circle represents 0 on the scale.

• Circular graphs are difficult to read because some of the data appear upside down and rising values may appear to be falling.

Illustrates a circular form of a bar graph.

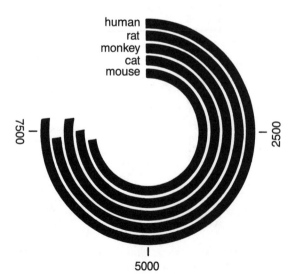

FIG. 1.52. Half life of drug A in five species in terms of heartbeats.

Illustrates methods for clarifying intersecting or adjacent lines.

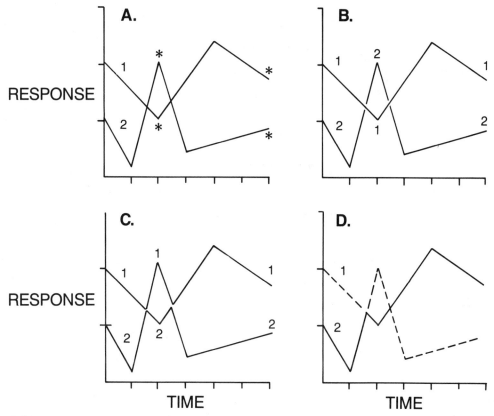

FIG. 1.53. In panel A it is unclear at the "*" whether curve 1 or 2 applies. Panels B, C, and D show three possible interpretations. Panels C and D shows methods of clarifying the curves, but panel C would not be adequate to show data fitting curves in panel D. Modified from Reynolds and Simmonds (1984) with permission.

Illustrates methods of identifying lines on a graph.

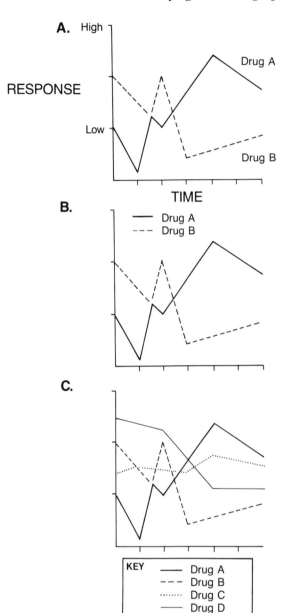

FIG. 1.54. Three methods of identifying the curves in a graph.

• The authors prefer the methodology used in panel A, followed by panel B, and lastly by panel C.

• Several or many curves of widely differing values may be shown by placing sections of a semilogarithmic scale graph above one another using a predetermined order or a random sequence.

Graphs in Three Dimensions

Three-dimensional versions of histograms or line graphs may be created. Examples of three-dimensional histograms have been illustrated. A three-dimensional version of a line graph may be either a two-dimensional graph which uses a third dimension for effect (Figs. 1.55 and 1.56) or alternatively, it may use three axes (Fig. 1.57) and appear as a surface graph (Figs. 1.58 and 1.59). A three-dimensional pie graph is shown later in this chapter.

Illustrates a series of two-dimensional graphs in three dimensions.

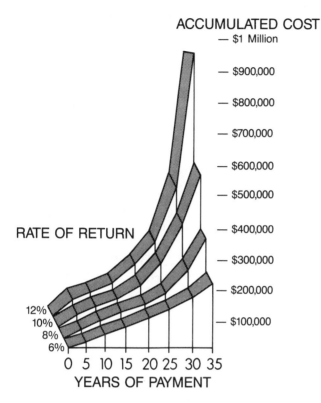

FIG. 1.55. Three-dimensional representation of a series of curves.

Illustrates a series of two-dimensional graphs in three dimensions.

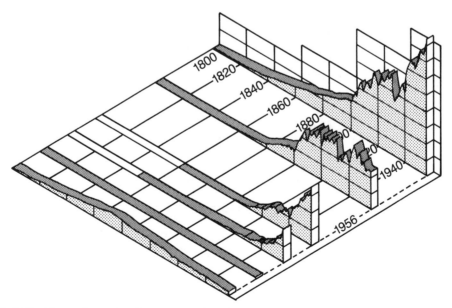

FIG. 1.56. Three-dimensional representation of a series of curves. The y-axis is indicated by horizontal lines. Reprinted from Lockwood (1969) with permission.

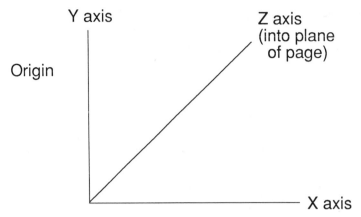

FIG. 1.57. These axes are used in a true three-dimensional graph.

• Three dimensions may also be illustrated with three two-dimensional graphs (i.e., XY, XZ, and YZ planes).

Illustrates a true three-dimensional graph.

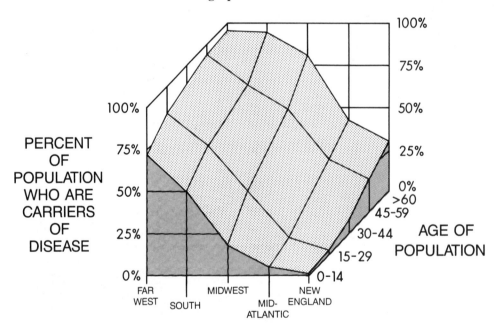

FIG. 1.58. Three-dimensional surface graph.

Illustrates a true three-dimensional graph.

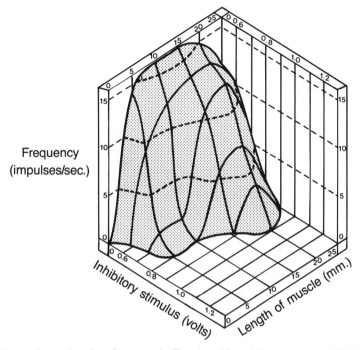

FIG. 1.59. Three-dimensional surface graph. Reprinted from Henneman et al. (1965) with permission.

Presentation of Data Obtained with Visual Analogue Scales

Illustrate the scale used and superimpose responses of (1) the patient, (2) treatment group, (3) all patients at a study site, (4) all patients in a study, (5) all patients across studies, or (6) any defined group of patients. A simple scale to measure three parameters is shown in Fig. 1.60. In this graph, X represents either an individual's marks or the average response of an entire group.

Other forms of visual analogue scales apart from a straight line (e.g., curved lines, circles, lines with numbers, text, anchoring point) are also used (Figs. 1.61 and 1.62). Results of tests using visual analogue scales may also be placed in many types of tables or graphs shown in other sections of this book.

Illustrates a simple visual analogue scale.

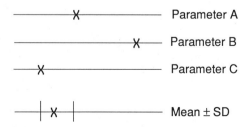

FIG. 1.60. Visual analogue scale marked with an "x" for parameters A, B, and C. A mean for either an individual's scores on a test (or subtest) or for a group's score on a single question (or group of questions) is shown in the lowest line.

Illustrates a variety of visual analogue scales.

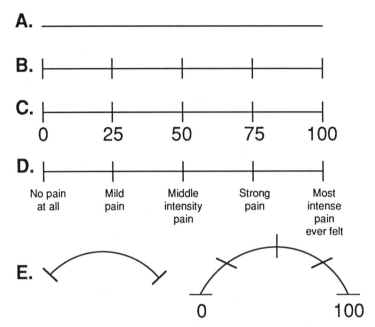

FIG. 1.61. Six examples of visual analogue scales.

Illustrates a variety of visual analogue scales.

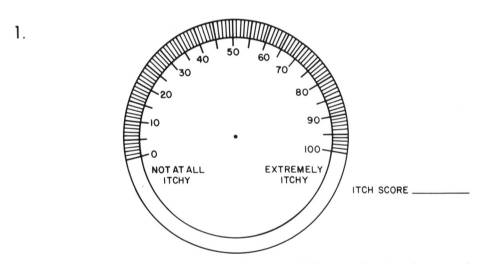

FIG. 1.62. Panels 1 and 2 illustrate round scales and panel 3 is a combination of some scales shown in Fig. 1.61. Reprinted from Spilker (1984) with permission.

2.

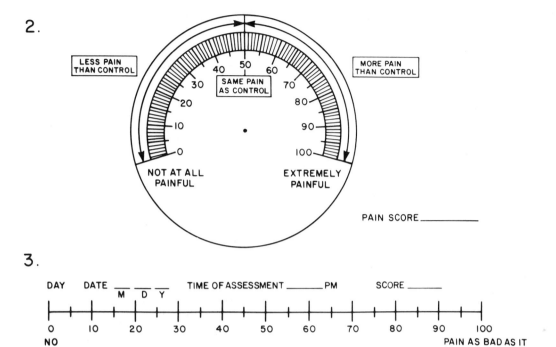

3.

FIG. 1.62. *Continued.*

FIGURES

A great deal of creativity may be spent developing one or many figures to present data. Nonetheless, most figures are examples of a few basic types. These are illustrated below, but for the most part are only infrequently shown in the remaining chapters. Most data sets could be illustrated through use of one or more figures either in addition to or instead of tables and graphs. The illustrator must decide whether figures have advantages over more traditional presentations for the specific data considered.

Representative examples of various figures are illustrated. The overlap between the categorization of figures and graphs is apparent in several examples (e.g., Gantt charts, pie charts, timelines) and a sharp distinction cannot always be made.

Timelines

A timeline is shown in Fig. 1.63.

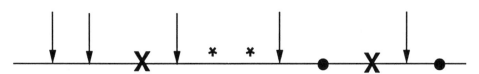

FIG. 1.63. A timeline marked with symbols that would be labeled or identified in the text. Options are given on p. 52.

Options to Use On or Near a Timeline

1. Symbols:	See Fig. 1.63				
2. Text:	Usually in combination with one or more options				
3. Letters:	A	B	C	D	E
4. Numbers:	1	2	3	4	5
5. Dates:	1980	1981	1982	1983	1984
6. Time:	9 AM	10 AM	11 AM	Noon	1 PM
7. Patient initials:	AV	KES	AT	DS	HS

8. Number of patients who . . . (e.g., reacted, did not react, had a specific problem):
9. Two or more of above options:

OTHER FIGURES

A selection of other figures is presented below:

1. Diagrams of a biological process or hypothesis (Figs. 1.64 and 1.65).
2. Diagrams of the human body (Fig. 1.66), part of the body (Fig. 1.67), or specific anatomical structures illustrating a surgical procedure (Fig. 1.68) or other process.
3. Venn diagram (Fig. 1.69). Overlapping circles to figuratively illustrate relationships.
4. Nomograms (Figs. 1.70 and 1.71). Three graduated scales of values that allow a third to be determined when two are known.
5. Pictographs (Fig. 1.72). Pictorial units or symbols in pictographs may each represent a fixed amount or value, or may be drawn in size proportional to the values illustrated. Other uses of pictorial elements include placing a drawing or photograph within the bars of a bar graph or beneath a curve. When each figure represents a fixed quantity the number of similar drawings illustrate the total quantity in the category represented.
6. Flow chart (Fig. 1.73). A series of steps that describe what was or will be done. May involve decision points.
7. Algorithm (Fig. 1.74). A series of answers, usually yes or no, direct one's path through branches to arrive at a final point (e.g., diagnosis, treatment plan, or causal relationship of drug and adverse reaction).
8. Decision trees (Figs. 1.75 to 1.78). Similar to algorithms, but with probabilities assigned to facilitate decision making.
9. PERT chart (Fig. 1.79).
10. Gantt chart (Fig. 1.80). Illustrates time along the x axis and separate (or related) activities are shown as horizontal bars. Each bar may be divided into components to illustrate different aspects (e.g., present status versus planned time to complete the activity).
11. Pie charts in two and three dimensions (Figs. 1.81 to 1.84).
12. Map (Fig. 1.92). Additional maps are shown in Chapter 4.
13. Genealogy chart (Fig. 1.93).
14. Specific diagram to illustrate a hypothesis (Fig. 1.94).

Different types of figures are illustrated in Figs. 1.85–1.91 and other chapters.

Illustrates diagrams of biological processes (Figs. 1.64 and 1.65).

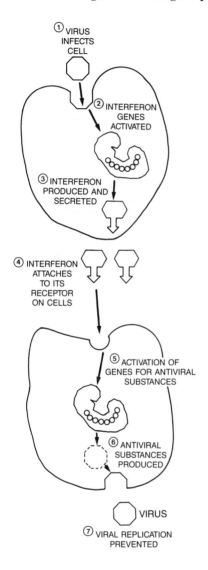

FIG. 1.64. Diagnostic representation of a physiological process which could represent accepted medical views or a hypothesis.

• The number of types of diagrams that may be (and are) used is considerable. Drawings may be representational or abstract (as in the current example). Information to understand the diagram may be placed within the diagram or in the legend. One or multiple panels may be used.

• Schematic diagrams may illustrate anatomical features, biological sounds, diagnostic tests and procedures, pressures, pathological changes, physiological data, clinical findings, and experimental methods.

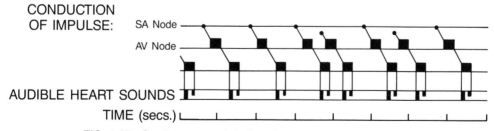

FIG. 1.65. Cardiac rate and rhythm diagram of premature beats.

• This is an abstract representation of conduction patterns and sounds.

Illustrates how a drawing of a human may be used for illustrations.

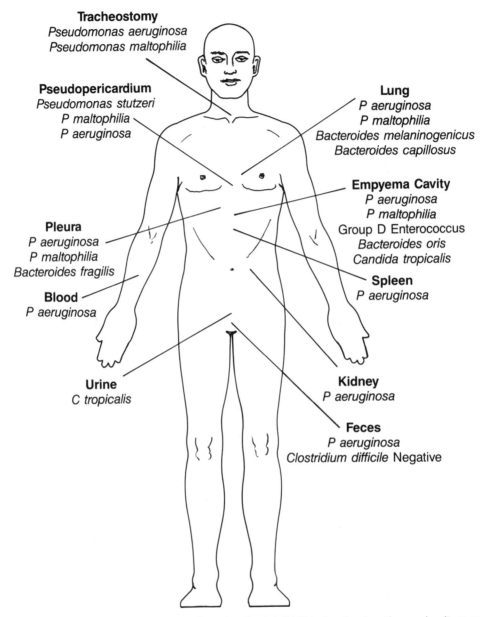

FIG. 1.66. Diagrammatic representation of patient 1 (M.H.) showing location and culture results of autopsy specimens. Reprinted from Dobbins et al. (1988) with permission.

Illustrates how a drawing of part of the human body may be used to present clinical information.

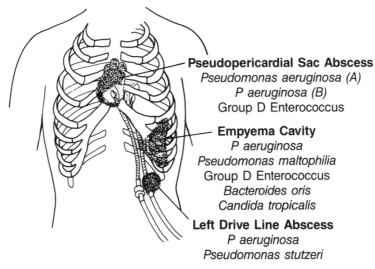

Pseudopericardial Sac Abscess
Pseudomonas aeruginosa (A)
P aeruginosa (B)
Group D Enterococcus

Empyema Cavity
P aeruginosa
Pseudomonas maltophilia
Group D Enterococcus
Bacteroides oris
Candida tropicalis

Left Drive Line Abscess
P aeruginosa
Pseudomonas stutzeri

FIG. 1.67. Schematic diagram of patient 1 (M.H.) showing spatial relationship between total artificial heart, drive lines, and abscesses (shaded areas). Microorganisms isolated from each abscess are listed. A and B indicate the same genus and species but different biotypes. Reprinted from Dobbins et al. (1988) with permission.

Illustrates how a drawing of a medical device may be used.

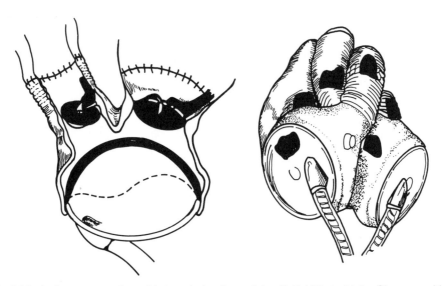

FIG. 1.68. Left, cross section of internal structure of Jarvik-7-100 ventricle. Shows positions of inflated and deflated diaphragm and valves. Shaded patches indicate areas selected for microbial analysis. Right, external view of Jarvik-7-100 artificial heart. Each ventricle is coated with polyurethane polymer (Biomer) and is attached to the other with Velcro. Shaded patches indicate areas selected for microbial analysis. Reprinted from Dobbins et al. (1988) with permission.

Illustrates a Venn diagram.

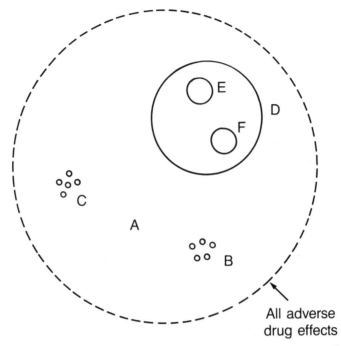

FIG. 1.69. Venn diagram for adverse drug reactions. The areas are not more than semiquantitative. A, cannot be detected or assessed: not notified; methods impracticable; methods unethical. B, individuals in whom method of successive differences can be tried. C, individuals in whom distinctive drug-induced lesions appear. D, cases among which statistically significant associations can be shown. E, successive difference method applicable to groups of cases. F, graded response can be shown in groups of cases. Reprinted from Vere (1976) with permission.

• See Fig. 8.75 for a variation of the Venn diagram. Also, referred to as an Euler diagram.

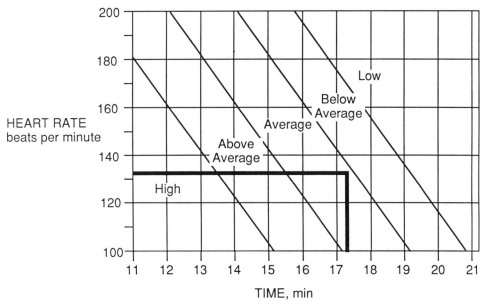

FIG. 1.70. Nomogram that illustrates relative fitness level for 50- to 59-year-old women based on 1-mile walk test used to measure heart rate. Reprinted from Rippe et al. (1988) with permission.

Illustrates a nomogram.

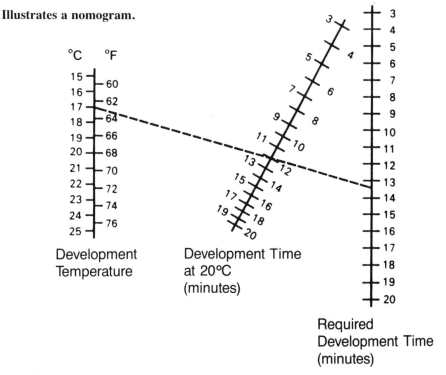

FIG. 1.71. Nomogram for time/temperature. The dotted line is an example of how the three lines are used. When any two numbers are known, the third may be determined simply with a line. Reprinted from Simmonds (1980) with permission.

Illustrates a pictograph.

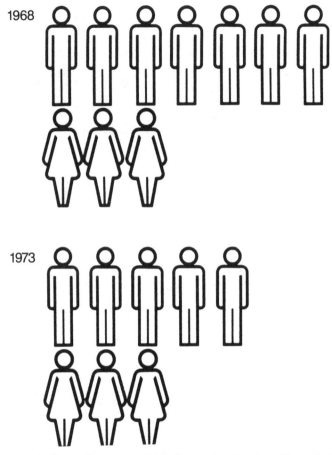

FIG. 1.72. Pictograph. Some illustrators divide figures to show less than whole values. Each symbol is assigned a value and different groups are illustrated with different symbols. Reprinted from Simmonds (1980) with permission.

• Symbols used should be simple, self-explanatory, and represent a fixed value.

• Other types of pictographs are drawn proportional to the amount illustrated (see Chapter 13 for a discussion and example).

Illustrates a flow chart.

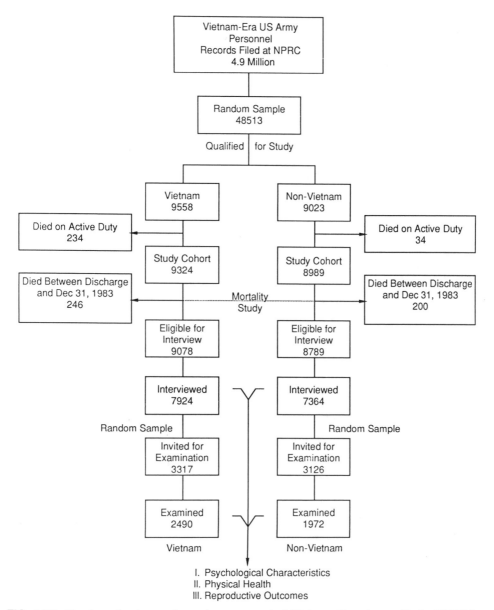

FIG. 1.73. Number of veterans in each component of Vietnam Experience Study. NPRC indicates National Personnel Records Center. Reprinted from Centers for Disease Control Vietnam Experience Study (1988) with permission.

Illustrates an algorithm

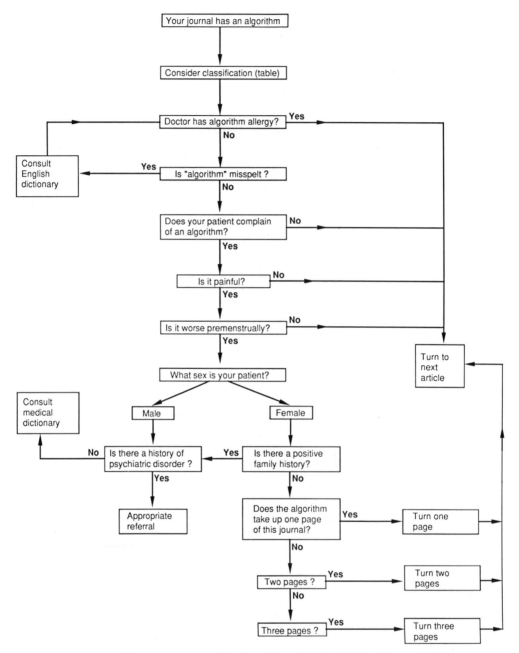

FIG. 1.74. Clinical algorithm. Reprinted from Neville (1985) with permission.

• Probabilities are sometimes given of each outcome.
• Algorithms that aid in reaching a decision are sometimes called decision trees.

Illustrates a simple decision tree.

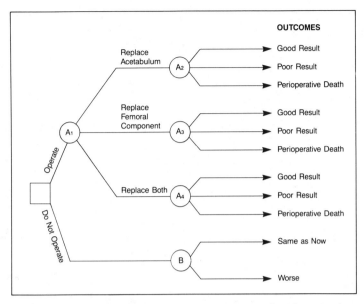

FIG. 1.75. Decision tree for a specific patient with a loose arthroplasty and coronary heart disease. Reprinted from Sackett et al. (1986) with permission.

Illustrates a decision tree with probabilities.

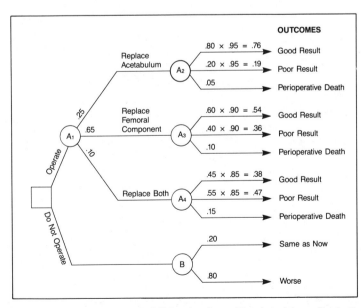

FIG. 1.76. The decision tree with probabilities in place. Reprinted from Sackett et al. (1986) with permission.

Illustrates a completed decision tree with utilities.

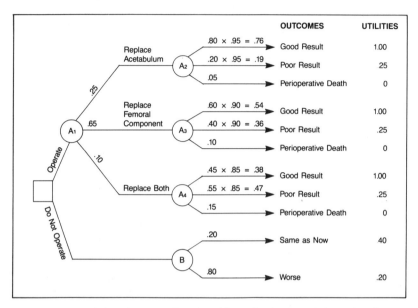

FIG. 1.77. A completed decision tree. Reprinted from Sackett et al. (1986) with permission.

Illustrates how a decision tree may be folded back.

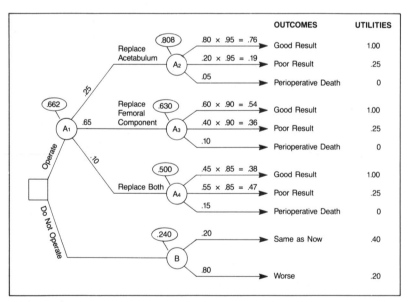

FIG. 1.78. Folding back a decision tree from right to left. If we multiply the utilities by the probabilities of their occurrence and sum them for each chance node, we can assign utilities to chance nodes A₂, A₃, A₁, and B. Reprinted from Sackett et al. (1986) with permission.

Illustrates a PERT chart.

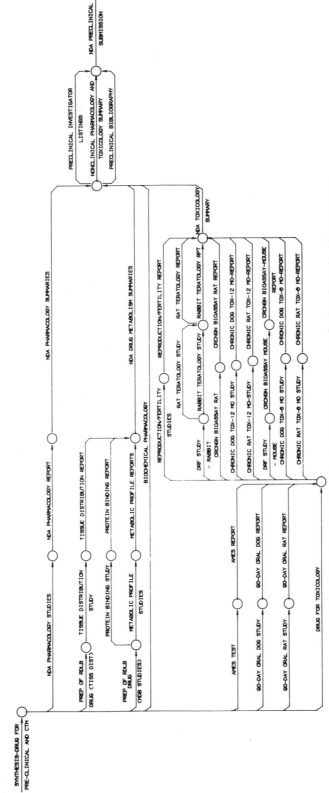

FIG. 1.79. Preclinical NDA network. Reprinted from Spilker (1987) with permission.

Illustrates a Gantt chart.

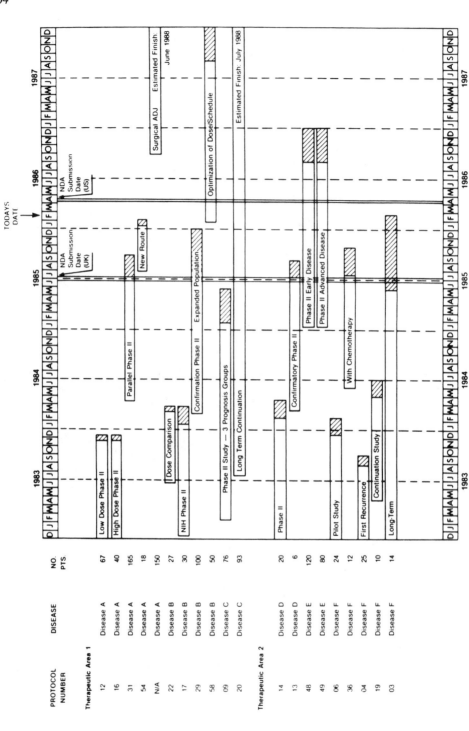

FIG. 1.80. Gantt chart reprinted from Spilker (1987) with permission.

Illustrates a pie chart in two dimensions.

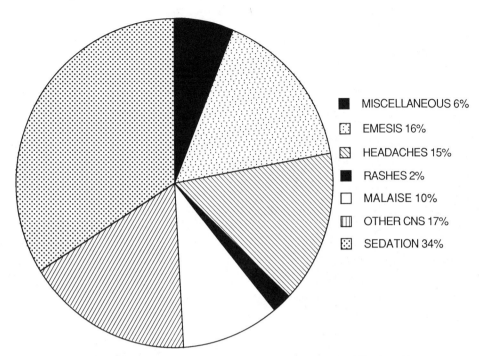

- MISCELLANEOUS 6%
- EMESIS 16%
- HEADACHES 15%
- RASHES 2%
- MALAISE 10%
- OTHER CNS 17%
- SEDATION 34%

FIG. 1.81. Classification of adverse reactions reported for drug X.

• Pie charts are appropriate for nominal categorical data (i.e., categories that have no intrinsic order) only.

• Some pie charts present pieces from largest to smallest.

• Each segment may be plain (i.e., without patterns to visually distinguish it).

• The first line is often drawn to 12 o'clock from the center.

• Three to six segments work best in most cases, but seven to ten may be shown.

• Lines could be used to connect each segment to its key in the legend.

• If multiple pie charts are illustrated the total size of each pie may be proportional to the amount represented, and individual wedges can illustrate percents.

Illustrates a pie chart with one or more slices partially removed for emphasis.

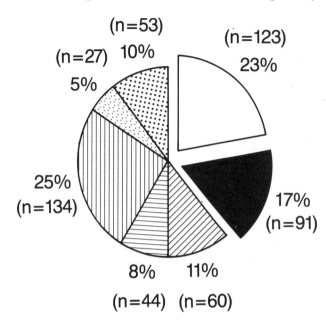

FIG. 1.82. Incidence of various types of adverse reactions emphasizing the relative amounts of those that are dermatological (open slice) and psychiatric (dark slice).

• Each segment is identified by number and percent next to the segment, as opposed to a separate legend.

Illustrates use of sequential diagrams of a pie chart to focus on progressively smaller items.

WEDGE SIZES UNCHANGED

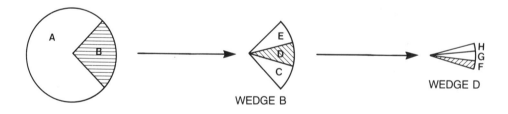

WEDGE SIZES PROGRESSIVELY LARGER

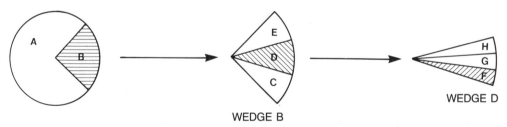

FIG. 1.83. Upper drawings indicate a series of pie wedges where the absolute size of each wedge is unchanged. The lower drawings indicate a series of pie wedges where the absolute size of each wedge becomes progressively greater.

Illustrates a pie chart in three dimensions.

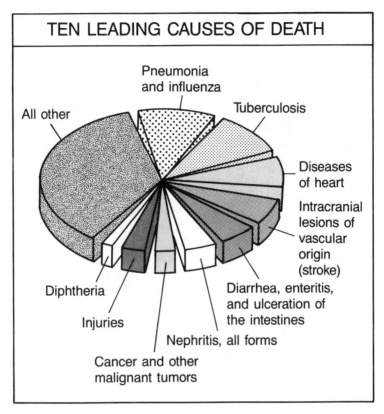

TEN LEADING CAUSES OF DEATH

Pneumonia and influenza

Tuberculosis

All other

Diseases of heart

Intracranial lesions of vascular origin (stroke)

Diphtheria

Injuries

Diarrhea, enteritis, and ulceration of the intestines

Nephritis, all forms

Cancer and other malignant tumors

FIG. 1.84. Leading causes of death in the United States in 1900.

• One or more segments may be separated from the others to add emphasis.

• Each segment could be labeled with a flag placed in the segment.

• The pie could be a photograph or drawing representing an aspect of the material described (e.g., a silver dollar could be divided into segments to illustrate research costs).

Illustrates how events change over time using a circular graph.

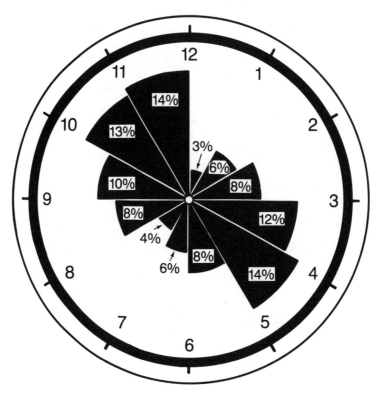

FIG. 1.85. Percent of hospital X's admissions by time between midnight and noon.

• Percents are represented by the linear length of each sector.

• The arcs of each sector are equal, and therefore this presentation is not a pie chart.

• Times could indicate the 12 months of the year or the arcs could be modified to represent seven days of a week or 24 hours in a day.

• Separate bars could be used for values at each hour, month, or other time period depicted.

• Concentric circles of increasing values may be drawn to assist in reading values from the graph.

Illustrates a fan chart to show percent change from one date to another for a category of items.

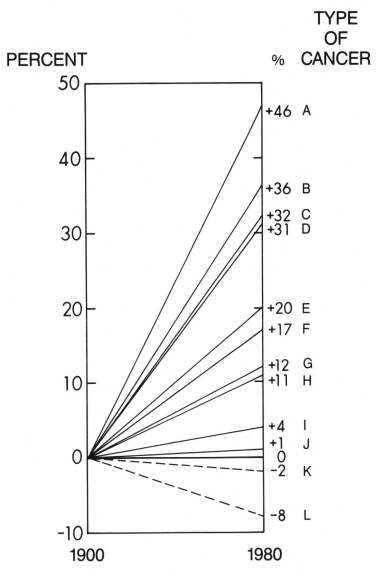

FIG. 1.86. Percent change in incidence rate of 12 cancers from 1900 to 1980.

• Fan charts are not popular because the 2 dates selected may not be appropriate or representative, and no values between the 2 dates are considered. In addition, the use of an index or percent does not present the actual data, which may lead to misinterpretation of the figure.

Illustrates a fan chart to show comparisons of an index for multiple groups.

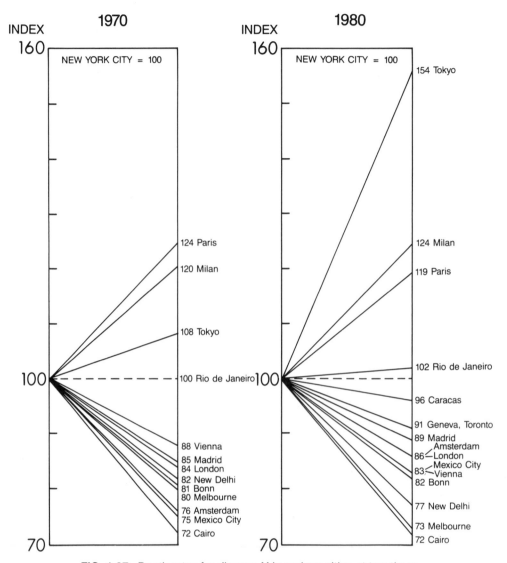

FIG. 1.87. Death rates for disease X in various cities at two times.

• The area of a fan chart below 100 could be shaded.

SELECTED TECHNIQUES TO EMPHASIZE OR ENHANCE A POINT

A few methods to place emphasis on a part of a table, graph, or figure are listed below.

1. Use graphic symbols or elements (e.g., ★, ∗) with more eye appeal than circles or dots. The clarity of such symbols must be evaluated and confirmed.

2. Add contrast or emphasis to specific parts of a figure with shading or other methods. The meaning of the shading must be clarified in a legend, key, or in the text (e.g., to illustrate a normal range, to show ± 2 SD).
3. Compare different formats of the same data (e.g., pie chart, line graph, histogram) to choose the one with the most advantages.
4. Enlarge one section of a figure or graph, either as part of the original or as a separate figure or graph.
5. Enlarge the format to make it more legible.
6. Stretch out or condense one or both axes. Caution must be used to avoid distorting the data and the resulting interpretation.
7. Use colors or various shadings of one color.
8. Add a box around a number, text, or anything else of importance that should be focused on.
9. Use multiple figures that show progressively more (or less) detail (e.g., a map of the United States, then a map of a state, then a map of a city, then a map of a street or neighborhood).
10. Use bold type, italics, or different type for important points.

Illustrates changes in a rank order over time.

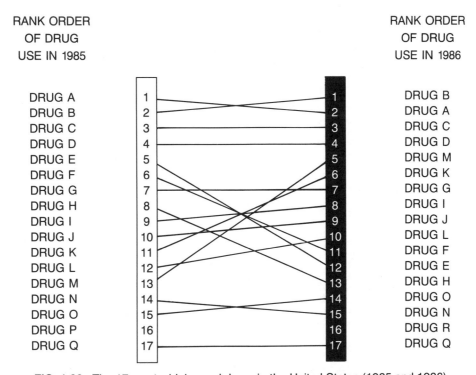

FIG. 1.88. The 17 most widely used drugs in the United States (1985 and 1986).

• Each of the lines used to connect the 2 lists may have different appearances (e.g., dots, dashes, symbols) to facilitate identification. This is especially helpful when numerous lines cross each other.

Illustrates use of circles of various sizes to show relative percents or amounts.

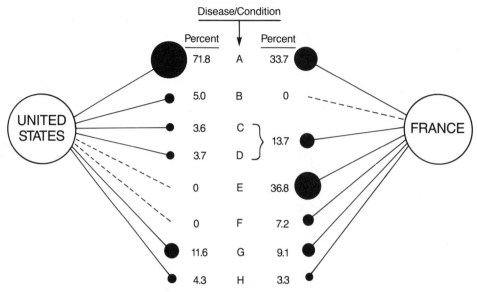

FIG. 1.89. Diagnosed causes of congestive heart failure in United States and France.

Illustrates use of selected symbols to illustrate a pattern of events.

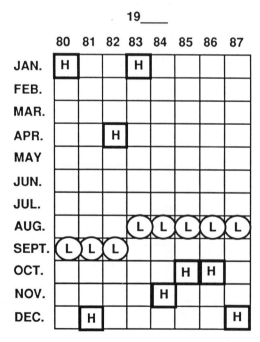

FIG. 1.90. Months in which hospital admissions were highest (H) and lowest (L) over an 8-year period.

Illustrates a step arrangement of bars.

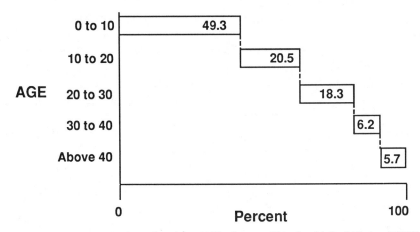

FIG. 1.91. Age distribution of patients with disease X in the United States (1989).

- This type of graph is sometimes referred to as a 100% step-bar chart.
- Bars may be oriented either horizontally or vertically.

Illustrates use of a map to present clinical data.

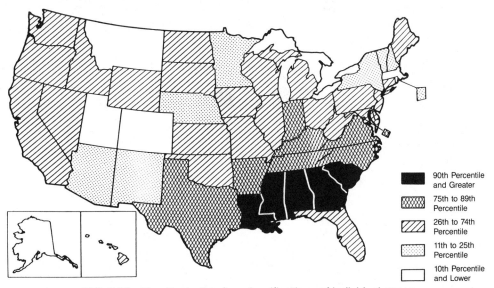

FIG. 1.92. Map illustrating five classifications of individual states.

- Each state could be labeled with its name and exact data.
- Each state could be labeled with a number of symbols (e.g., dots) proportional to the total being represented.
- Each state could be labeled with columns whose height is proportional to a parameter. Shadings could be used on columns to illustrate increases or decreases,

above or below the average United States values. Two columns per state could illustrate data on two separate dates.

• Different sized lines with arrows across maps could illustrate movements of diseases.

• States could be distorted according to any parameter (e.g., number of patients with a certain disease per square mile).

• Each state could be labeled with a pie chart to show various data.

• The entire map could be labeled with dots representing a certain number of events to show density of those events.

• Regions of a map could be demarcated with dark lines and characteristics of the region identified.

Illustrates use of a genealogy chart.

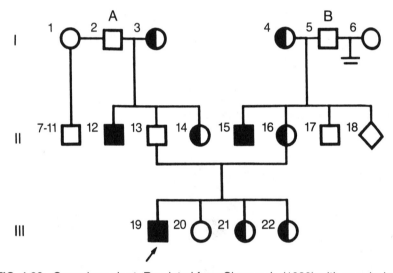

FIG. 1.93. Genealogy chart. Reprinted from Simmonds (1980) with permission.

Illustrates a hypothesis.

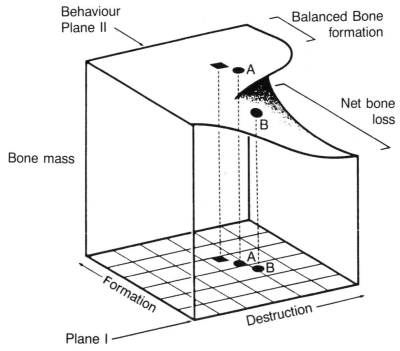

FIG. 1.94. Diagram illustrating a medical theory of how osteoporosis occurs. Reprinted from Simmonds (1980) with permission.

2

Choosing Formats and Preparing Slides

BACKGROUND

The ability of clinical data to convince readers of specific conclusions depends to a large degree on how the data are presented. Whereas poorly presented data may confuse readers, well-presented data encourages accurate and convincing interpretations.

Choosing formats and presenting data may be thought of in terms of three distinct steps. The first step is to determine whether a table, graph, or figure should be used; the second step is to determine how the chosen format will be composed; and the third step is to decide what data and other information to include in the format. The last step involves choosing the contents of the format and is not discussed in this book; however, the material to be presented usually has a major influence on the appearance of the chosen format.

Purpose of a Display and Its Breadth and Depth

A major criterion for choosing tables and figures to present clinical data is the purpose to which the data will be applied. Most purposes are characterized by issues relating to the data's breadth and depth. *Breadth* is considered in terms of the increasing spectrum from a single patient, to a single site study, to a single multiple site study, to multiple studies each consisting of one or more sites, and possibly to evaluations and review of published literature. *Depth* of data presentation varies from a superficial overview to a detailed analysis. Depth may be considered in terms of whether data are intended as (1) informal evaluation(s) of a particular question about a study, (2) formal analyses, (3) summaries for a publication, (4) summaries for a presentation to a professional audience, (5) summaries for a presentation to a lay audience, (6) a formal medical and/or statistical report, or (7) a regulatory submission emphasizing across-study data summaries.

Types of Data to Be Presented

Once the purpose, along with the associated breadth and depth, of the intended display has been identified, one must next categorize the type of data that will be presented. Data displays presented in this book have been grouped into the following 10 categories: (1) study designs; (2) demographics and patient accountability; (3) vital signs; (4) laboratory data; (5) adverse reactions; (6) efficacy; (7) pharmacokinetics; (8) quality of life; (9) compliance, concomitant drugs, and cost-effectiveness; and (10) metaanalyses. Each of these categories is presented in a separate chapter.

Some variables may be defined in either an efficacy or safety category, depending on the context in which they are measured. For example, blood pressure is an efficacy variable when an antihypertensive drug is being evaluated, but is a safety variable when most other types of drugs are being evaluated. Any single display for a particular variable is generally identical whether it is used to evaluate efficacy or safety. Of course, the amount of data presented may easily be controlled according to requirements of a situation.

At What Stage(s) of a Clinical Study Are Formats Chosen?

When an investigator is repeating a previous study design, possibly with a different drug, a different dose of the same drug, or a design modification, the intended formats may be known prior to initiating the study. If a new study design is examined or if an unanticipated type of data are collected, it may be desirable or even necessary to choose formats after the study data are analyzed and interpreted. It is good practice, however, to consider formats prior to initiating a study.

PRINCIPLES OF CHOOSING FORMATS

Although there is no single formula for choosing formats to present data, a number of principles are important.

1. Become familiar with standard formats used in the literature, as well as the advantages, disadvantages, and most appropriate uses of each.
2. Choose formats that present data in the clearest manner possible.
3. When multiple formats are possible, choose those that illustrate the data most convincingly.
4. Proceed in the general order of presenting study design, patient demographics and prognostic indicators, patient accountability, primary efficacy variables or endpoints, secondary efficacy variables or endpoints, safety variables, patient compliance, and other data.
5. Choose multiple formats (whenever possible) to lead readers stepwise from the most specific to the most general data (or vice versa), from one point to others that build on and help develop and support the specific interpretation reached, from one patient to multiple patients, or from primary to secondary objectives. This principle of stepwise presentation may be applied to any type of data (e.g., efficacy, safety, pharmacokinetic, quality of life).
6. Critique one's own choice of formats. Consider whether each table would illustrate the data more clearly if it were a graph (and vice versa). What modifications to the format would make the presentation more clear (e.g., adding or subtracting the amount of data or statistics, modifying the analyses presented)? Are the chosen formats appropriate for the data's use? For example, a large number of tables and figures of vital sign data that might be necessary for a regulatory submission could be replaced by a single sentence in a scientific publication (e.g., drug X had no effect on vital signs).
7. Ask colleagues and friends to critique the formats.

PRACTICAL CONSIDERATIONS IN CHOOSING FORMATS

Basic choices for the individual who wishes to present data include identifying the specific patients whose data are to be presented, the types or categories of data to present, the purpose of presenting the data and other information, and the methodological considerations (e.g., the particular coordinates to choose for the axes, column headings to choose for the tables). After the format is chosen and data are presented in a rough display, enhancements may be added to emphasize certain relationships, trends, numbers, or other points. These enhancements include use of shading, color, arrows or other symbols, bold type, italics, boxes around significant points, and placing two or more graphs next to each other.

Identifying Patients Whose Data Are to Be Presented

Most data sets could be placed in a table or graph for various groupings of patients. Examples include:

1. Single patient in a study. Which of the patient's data are chosen to show and why?
2. Subgroup of patients in a specific treatment group. The subgroup may be determined either before or after a study.
3. All patients at one site in a study on one (or more) treatment.
4. All patients at a subset of sites in a study on one (or more) treatment.
5. All patients in a multicenter study on one (or more) treatment.
6. All patients across a subset of studies (e.g., all studies using a common protocol).
7. All patients of a certain type across all (or a subset) studies (e.g., all patients above 70 years of age who received drug).
8. All patients across all studies who have received drug.
9. All patients with a specific diagnosis (e.g., renal failure) across all studies who have received drug.

Which Types or Categories of Data to Show

Multiple categories are often used to present data from any single clinical study. There should be a logical clinical rationale for the categories chosen. To illustrate this concept, a number of categories of laboratory data are indicated below.

1. Raw data obtained on one particular analyte for one or more patients or groups of patients.
2. Raw data obtained on all analytes for a specific type of test (e.g., liver function).
3. Raw data for patients whose reported values for one or more analytes were outside normal limits.
4. Raw data for analytes in patients with one or more values outside normal limits during testing, but within normal limits at baseline.
5. Raw data which represent notable changes from baseline.
6. Data for analytes where the investigator said the abnormalities were possibly, probably, or definitely drug related.
7. Data for one or more analytes where the investigator said the abnormalities were clinically significant.

8. Data for one or more analytes where the investigator said the abnormalities were clinically significant and either possibly, probably, or definitely drug related.
9. Data for one or more analytes which differed from baseline by some specified percentage (e.g., 10%, 20%, 30%, or X%).
10. Data for one or more analytes which were more than twofold (threefold, X-fold) greater than the top range of normal or less than the lower range of normal.
11. Data for each patient who required treatment because of a laboratory abnormality.
12. Data for each patient who was discontinued from the study because of a laboratory abnormality.

Purposes of Presenting Data and Other Information

Tables are usually preferable to graphs for presenting actual data or statistical results, especially in relatively large quantities. Some questions relating to the actual presentation include:

1. How much data should be included in each table?
2. How much statistical information should be included?
3. How many rows and columns should be shown?
4. Should derived data be shown with raw data?

Graphs and figures are usually preferable to tables for illustrating a trend. Whenever a set of data are amenable to a figure it is usually desirable to use one, unless there are constraints (e.g., numbers of figures permissible).

Other questions to consider are:

1. What formats are possible (e.g., photograph, drawing, map, diagram, flow chart, algorithm), and what are the pros and cons of each?
2. Can two or more formats be combined to make the composite figure more complete and clear?
3. Does a figure present the data more or less clearly than a table or graph?
4. Can a figure's message be enhanced with colors, shading, bold titles, arrows, successive overlays, or other techniques?

Methodological Considerations in Developing Formats

Journals frequently state in their Instructions to Authors that tables, graphs, and figures must stand on their own. This is a touchstone that all authors should use when judging their chosen formats. Other questions to pose about one's choice of format include:

1. How does the table, figure, or graph relate to and support the text and other diagrammatic material?
2. How well does the chosen format present the data and convince the reader of the validity of the interpretation?
3. Would additional data make the conclusion stronger, or would less data make the format more clear?

Occasions When Tables Generally Should Be Used

1. Readers require precise numerical data.
2. Detailed statistical relationships or analyses are to be shown.
3. Detailed results are important to present.

Occasions When Graphs or Figures Generally Should Be Used

1. To emphasize past trends use line graphs.
2. To extrapolate future trends use line graphs.
3. Flow diagrams are often used to illustrate independent, but related activities.
4. To illustrate the relationship between variables, a graph is often best.
5. For static comparisons of data use histograms, especially if the data may be subdivided or viewed in different ways.
6. Line graphs are useful for dynamic comparisons between groups, especially if time is one of the parameters presented.
7. Pie charts are often useful for making three or four comparisons.

Utilizing the above considerations may simplify the choice of a table, graph, or figure, as well as determine its most appropriate makeup.

Development of formats for graphs and figures includes the following technical or methodological considerations:

1. How many axes should be used? If three or four axes are used should the graph be drawn in two or three dimensions?
2. Would a three-dimensional graph be desirable and appropriate?
3. Are there standard graphs that most people in the field use to illustrate data? In pharmacokinetics, for example, there often are.
4. Are there compelling reasons not to use the standard graphs?
5. Should one or both axes be logarithmic or should one use another scale (e.g., probit, square root)? This decision should be justified, since it may greatly alter the visual presentation and interpretation.
6. Should two or more quadrants be used to illustrate data with both positive and negative coordinates?
7. If time is one coordinate of a graph should only past data, future projections, or both be included?
8. Would the graph be improved if two or more of the coordinates were reversed (e.g., should the ordinate and abscissa be interchanged)?
9. What elements would add visual appeal to the graph? These elements can include shading or cross-hatching of bars, putting before and after bars next to each other, simplifying complex graphs, adding color, combining two types of graphs into one, or any of many other variations.
10. If percent changes are described, consider the limitation where decreases may be shown up to 100%, but increases may be shown without limit (e.g., several hundred percent). This is a particular problem when both increases and decreases are combined to create a mean percentage change.

PREPARING SLIDES AND TRANSPARENCIES

Scientists often are provided the opportunity to make verbal presentations of their data. These presentations are usually directed at either scientific peers (e.g., professional meetings) or regulatory bodies (e.g., FDA Advisory Committee). Guidelines on the preparation and delivery of such lectures are beyond the scope of this book, but basic guidelines for selecting and preparing visual aids are discussed below.

The most common visual aids are overhead transparencies and slides. Visual aids should complement, not dominate, the presentation. In particular, a presenter should never copy his talk onto a series of transparencies or slides and then read them to his audience. Furthermore, the presenter must direct his talk to the audience and not to the visual aids. He must be very conscious of maintaining eye contact with his audience without seeming to focus on the slides or transparencies.

When preparing slides or transparencies, simplicity is of utmost importance. Each transparency or slide should reflect only one idea. Care must be taken to insure that each individual slide or transparency will be easily readable by the entire audience (not only those seated in the front rows). Remember that not everybody has perfect eyesight. Printing should be bold and large. Typeset pages should not be photocopied as visual aids—they can never be read. The Center for Professional Advancement (located in East Brunswick, New Jersey) has published suggestions for preparing transparencies and slides. Their suggestions are listed (with permission) later in this chapter.

Minimal typewritten copy and simple, uncrowded graphs and charts are often ideally suited for transparencies. Similarly, slides are most natural when one wants to incorporate figures with small details. Whether using transparencies or slides, one should consider using progressive-disclosure techniques.

Progressive Disclosure or Focus of Information in Slides

Text

Effective slides and efficient transfer of information are often achieved by progressively disclosing more information as one moves from slide to slide within a series. For example, the first slide may present a single statement, and the second slide repeats the first statement but includes an additional statement. This process is repeated any number of times to build up a list of information. This procedure of revealing one or two items at a time reviews and reinforces previously made points.

A similar approach is to show all points on each slide in the series, but to highlight only one line or point on each slide. Thus, the series indicates all points to be made, but each slide focuses on the highlighted material. This approach is often used for introducing parts of a longer presentation. The audience can then follow where in the talk the speaker is.

Tables

The most obvious rule about presenting tables on a slide is to keep it simple. In some cases one or two rows or columns of a table can be shown at a time. When a complex table is to be shown, a couple of techniques can be used to improve audi-

FIG. 2.1.

ence comprehension. The first possibility is to show the column and row headings in the first slide, and add the rows (or columns) in successive slides. Alternatively, it is possible to describe just the headings for the columns in one slide, the headings for the rows in the second slide, and then to add the body of the table in the third slide.

In cases when it is not possible to keep a slide simple, other approaches to progressive disclosure may be used. Two are briefly mentioned here. In the first approach, show a part of a table on a slide. On the second slide show another part of a table in half the slide and reduce the first slide to the other half of the slide. On the third slide show a third part of the table in half the slide and reduce the first two slides to the other half. Continue until the entire table is shown.

In the second approach, show a part of a table on a slide. On the second slide show another part of a table in half the slide and reduce the first slide to the other half. On the third slide show another part of the table in a third of the slide and reduce the first two slides to the other two-thirds. On the fourth slide show the last part in a quarter and reduce the first three slides to three-quarters.

Graphs and Figures

When complex graphs are to be shown there are numerous ways to divide the information into several slides and then to build up to the overall graph. This is often done with overhead transparencies, by laying one on top of another. With graphs it is possible to:

1. Show all "before" states separately from "after" states (e.g., of histograms).
2. Show one curve and then progressively add others.
3. Show points of one group in a scattergram and then progressively add others.

To improve visual distinctions between groups, it is possible to use different colors or different symbols.

Figures may be built up with successive overlays similar to the graphs described above. Different times or comparative groups may be shown successively.

A few additional points follow:

1. For some graphics, black and white slides transmit better than blue and white.
2. Multiple colors generally enhance a slide's eye appeal, but do not enhance communications.

3. Break a long list into two, three, or more slides, each with a smaller number of points.
4. Instruct those who prepare the slide to utilize most or all of the available space on the slide.
5. Use a 3 : 2 ratio of length to height of material to cover the maximum area of a slide (Fig. 2.1). This ratio of length to height allows the camera to get closer and obtain the largest size print, which enables the slide to be read most clearly.

Suggestions for Preparing Transparencies

1. Design each transparency to reflect one idea, expressed in a maximum of six lines, with no more than six words per line.
2. Make sure the printing is large enough. Use Orator typeface, press-on letters, or a Kroy-type lettering system.
3. Use overlays by superimposing additional transparencies on a base transparency to build a concept.
4. Be sure your original design is good quality in order to insure a good quality transparency.
5. Full pages of text do not reproduce well.
6. Do not use the overhead like a reading machine.
7. Cover specific points on a list by sliding a sheet of paper between the transparency and the machine—exposing the points as you are ready.
8. Keep the room lighting as bright as possible while still maintaining image clarity. Where possible, turn off board lights and use room lights.
9. Avoid glare by turning the machine off when there is not a transparency on the light table.

Suggestions for Preparing Slides

A. Format

1. Each slide should communicate a single idea.
2. Excessive data on a chart, graph, or illustration will be difficult to read.
3. Add variety by including some slides that do not emphasize strictly factual information.
4. Slides that illustrate important points of a lecture are generally few in number. Make them simple to stress basic conclusions or points that may be discussed by the lecturer. If many slides are used to complement a lecture, then they should be simple and succinct.
5. Slides prepared for use in a self-taught program must not require an independent teacher to explain or discuss their content. Slides prepared for use in a lecture usually require someone to explain or discuss their content.

B. Preparation

1. When planning a slide, consider using a 3 × 5 inch index card on which to lay out information.
2. Each line of type should be as large as possible.

3. A typical 8½ × 11 inch typewritten page will *not* be legible when projected as a slide.
4. Avoid placing more than six lines on any one slide.
5. Think of the participant in the back row. If you can read a 2 × 2 inch slide without a magnifier, people in the rear seats can probably read it on the screen.
6. Titles should be at the top of slides and generally on the left rather than the center.
7. Do not label the vertical axis of a graph (i.e., ordinate) so that the audience must turn their heads to read it. This is a particularly annoying practice that many people don't consider when preparing slides.

C. Presentation

1. Consider an introductory slide that either lists all of the major topics to be discussed or states the issue(s) to be addressed.
2. Consider a final slide (or slides) that summarizes the conclusions and also helps the audience to remember major points.
3. If the same slide is to be used more than once in a talk, use duplicates.
4. Rehearse the talk with slides in front of an audience. Their feedback will indicate whether the slides are effective and well prepared.

Illustrating Study Designs

GENERAL CONSIDERATIONS

Presentation of schematics or other representations of a study design facilitates discussion of and communications about a study. These formats present information on one or more of the following elements:

1. Overall study design (e.g., parallel or crossover study, single entity or combination drug).
2. Treatment groups in the study.
3. Periods of a study (e.g., screen, baseline, treatment, dose taper).
4. Parts of a study (e.g., initial open-label part, double-blind part).
5. Duration of each period or part of a study.
6. Type of blind used in each period or part of a study.
7. Dosing schedule(s) used in each period or part of a study.
8. Projected or obtained sample size.
9. Time points at which specific evaluations are scheduled to be made.
10. Time point at which patients are randomized to treatment.
11. Other details (e.g., dosage forms, routes of administration).

Each of these 11 items is briefly discussed below.

1. *Overall study design* A presentation of the overall study design usually includes the identity of the treatment groups (e.g., placebo, active drug, test drug at dose A, test drug at dose B) and, therefore, implicitly indicates the type of control(s) used. Historical controls may also be indicated in a schematic of the overall study design.

Illustrative types of *parallel studies* are shown in Fig. 3.1, *crossover studies* in Fig. 3.2, *sequential studies* in Figs. 3.3 and 3.4, and *combination drug studies* in Fig. 3.5.

2. *Treatment groups in the study* This information is usually displayed as part of the overall study design, but may be displayed separately.

3. *Periods of a study* Some or all of the following periods may be indicated: screen, baseline, dose ascension, maintenance phase of treatment, dose taper, and follow-up periods. These may be indicated in a schematic or in a time and events presentation. Periods may be identified as pilot phase, treatment period, double-blind controlled period, or with other notations. Study results may be shown separately for each study period.

4. *Parts of a study* Parts of a study may differ from periods of a study (see above). Parts refer to different blinds, treatment drugs, or drug doses for a specific

group or groups. Two examples are given in Fig. 3.6. In each of these examples only the treatment period of the study is illustrated.

If doses 2 and 3 in example B are not given to all patients, but only to those who require more or less drug, then the study would generally be considered as having one part.

5. *Duration of each period or part of a study*　This is usually indicated by a simple notation (e.g., 4 weeks, 2 to 4 months) next to the schematic diagram of the overall study design. Alternatively a separate list of each period or part of a study could be listed with its duration given as specific times, ranges of times, or criteria used to define its duration (e.g., until patients' values of X decrease by 10 percent).

6. *Type of blind used in each period or part of a study*　This is usually indicated by a notation (e.g., single-blind period, double-blind period) in the schematic of the overall study design.

7. *Dosing schedule(s) used in each period or part of a study*　These are often presented in tables, apart from a schematic of the overall study design, especially when the dosing schedule is complex. Numerous examples are presented later in this chapter.

8. *Projected or obtained sample size*　This category of information may relate to the number of projected, currently enrolled, or completed patients. Patient accountability information, which is discussed further in Chapter 4, is not presented under this category. Numbers for each group in the study may be given in a table or schematic.

9. *Time points at which specific evaluations are scheduled to be made*　This category involves one aspect of a time and events chart, i.e., the time of day or days (weeks, months) at which specific evaluations are to be conducted (listed in a protocol) or were conducted (described in a publication).

10. *Time point at which patients are randomized to treatment*　This notation may accompany a schematic or may be assumed based on a description of the protocol in the text. In a few studies this event may occur on two (or more) separate occasions for each patient.

11. *Other details*　This category includes aspects such as dosage forms (e.g., capsules, tablets, solutions) and routes of administration. Dosage forms are discussed later in this chapter.

The above elements may be presented in a simple or elaborate manner using one or more of the following formats:

1. A schematic diagram.
2. A timeline.
3. A table.
4. A written description.
5. A combination of two or more of these formats.

It should be noted that presentations of study designs do not always illustrate the *overall* study design, but often illustrate only selected aspects.

The most common presentations of study design elements in the published literature are:

1. Overall study design schematic with or without additional descriptive comments as an overlay.
2. Overall study design combined with a time and events table.

3. A timeline, illustrating major events.
4. A table of the dosing regimen.
5. A table of the time and events.
6. A graph of study results plus schematic of part or all of the study design. This is usually accomplished by superimposing the study design onto a display of the results. Thus, the primary purpose of the schematic is to help interpret efficacy or safety data.

Author's note: Some tables and figures in this chapter (e.g., Figs. 3.7 to 3.9 and 3.11 to 3.13) were not primarily created to present elements of the study design. Those displays indicate how inclusion of study design elements in a table presenting efficacy or safety results may facilitate the interpretation of the data.

DOSAGE SCHEDULES

Other terms for dosage schedules are dosage regimen, titration-schedule, treatment doses, allowable dosage levels, dosage assignment, maximum dosage, dosing paradigms, dosing schedules, and infusion regimen. Although some of these terms are restricted to parenteral drugs (e.g., infusion regimen) or to maximal levels permitted by the protocol, most terms may be interchanged.

A single complete dosing schedule should include and specify the (1) different groups being dosed, (2) times at which doses are to be given, and (3) makeup of each dose in terms of the number and size of specific dosages to be given. Additional information should clarify details about the (1) dose to be given (e.g., rate of infusion); (2) number of tablets or total dose to be taken each day, week, month, or other time; (3) drug packaging; (4) basis on which treatment groups are defined (e.g., patient weights, creatinine clearance values); and (5) number of patients in each group. Dosing schedules may only include some of these elements or may include others. The remaining tables in this chapter (Tables 3.4 to 3.28) illustrate common formats for displaying dosing information.

Illustrates a presentation of sample size information.

TABLE 3.1. Number of Completed Patients in a Study

	Number of completed patients		
	Baseline	Treatment	Follow-up
Treatment A	85	78	77
Treatment B	82	77	75

Illustrates one means of identifying which days of a study are in different phases.

TABLE 3.2. Identifying Phases of a Study, Including Five Dosing Periods

Group	Screen phase[b]	Days of treatment phase[a]					Follow-up phase
		Dosing period number					
		1	2	3	4	5[c]	
I	−20 to −6	1–3	8–10	15–17	22–24	29–31	36–38
II	−13 to +1	8–10	15–17	22–24	29–31	36–38	43–45

[a]Numbers indicate study days for drug administration and observations in each dosing period.
[b]Inclusive days for admission to the screen phase. This table is particularly appropriate for a Phase I or Phase IIa dose ranging study.
[c]Following completion of the study, a decision will be made whether to amend the protocol and proceed to a higher dose in order to adequately assess the safety and dose tolerance of the drug.

Illustrates the treatment assignment for each patient per study day.

TABLE 3.3. Treatment Assignment Codes[a]

Patient number	Study day			
	1	2	3	4
2, 5	B	D	A	C
6, 1	C	A	D	B
3, 7	D	C	B	A
4, 8	A	B	C	D

[a]This table illustrates a latin-square type design. For example, patients numbered 2 and 5 receive drug B on day 1, drug D on day 2, etc.

TABLE 3.4. Dosing Schedule According to Creatinine Clearance

Creatinine clearance (ml/min/1.73m^2)	Dose	Sampling times (hours postdose)
0–5	800 mg qd	pre-oral, 1, 2, 4, 6, 8, 24
5–10	800 mg bid	pre-oral, 1, 2, 3, 4, 6, 12
10–25	800 mg tid	pre-oral, 1, 2, 3, 4, 5, 8
25–50	800 mg qid	pre-oral, 1, 2, 3, 6
>50	800 mg qid	pre-oral, 1, 2, 3, 6

• A separate dosing schedule could be prepared according to different categories (e.g., patient weight, body surface area).

TABLE 3.5. Dosing Schedule

Dose level	Days	Drug A		Drug B	
		Total daily dose	Regimen[b]	Total daily dose	Regimen
A	1–3	150 mg	75 mg bid	75 mg	25 mg qam, 2 × 25 mg qhs
B	4–6	300 mg	100 mg tid	150 mg	2 × 25 mg tid
C	7–13 (14–21)	450 mg	2 × 75 mg tid	225 mg	3 × 25 mg tid
D[a]	14–21	600 mg	2 × 100 mg tid	300 mg	4 × 25 mg tid

[a]Dose level D may be used at the investigator's discretion if lack of clinical efficacy has been demonstrated at dose level C during treatment days 7–13.
[b]A separate dosage regimen may be given for the washout phase.

• The total number of capsules administered per dose or per day could be added in a separate column.

TABLE 3.6. Dosing Schedule[a]

Group number	Mg/dose	Total daily dose (mg)
1	2	6
2	4	12
3	8	24
4	12	36
5	16	48
6	24	72
7	32	96

[a]A column for route of administration may be added if two or more routes are used.

TABLE 3.7. Dosing Schedule

Group	Treatment day 1		Treatment day 2		Total dose	Number of volunteers
	Drug	Unit dose[a]	Drug	Unit dose[a]		
1. Treated–low dose	Placebo	4 caps	Placebo & drug	4 caps	5 mg	6
2. Control–low dose	Placebo	4 caps	Placebo	4 caps	0 mg	3
3. Treated–high dose	Placebo	4 caps	Placebo & drug	4 caps	10 mg	6
4. Control–high dose	Placebo	4 caps	Placebo	4 caps	0 mg	3

[a] Given only once.

TABLE 3.8. Dosing Schedule

Group	No. of vols.	Screen/ baseline	Dosing period[a]								Follow-up period
			1	2	3	4	5	6	7	8	
I	9	−13 to −2[b]	100 mg[c]	200 mg	300 mg	600 mg	900 mg	1200 mg	1500 mg		d
II	9	−13 to −2[b]		200 mg	300 mg	600 mg	900 mg	1200 mg	1500 mg	1800 mg	d

[a] Dosing periods must occur sequentially; a minimum of 1 day must separate adjacent periods and a minimum of 1 week must separate the dosing period within each group.
[b] Inclusive days for admission to screening phase. Day 1 is defined as the first treatment day for that group.
[c] Dose of drug or matching placebo.
[d] One week after the last treatment day for the group.

TABLE 3.9. Dosing Schedule

Drug (mg/m²)[a]			Day 1 375 →						Day 2 375 →						Day 3 375 →			
Approximate time	7 am	8 am	9 am	10 am	2 pm	6 pm	10 pm	2 am[b]	6 am	10 am	2 pm	6 pm	10 pm	2 am[b]	6 am	10 am	2 pm	6 pm	10 pm
Tablets	4	4	4	4	4	4	4	4	4	4	4	4	4	4	4	4	4	4	4

Drug (mg/m²)			Day 8 375 →						Day 15 400 →						
Approximate time	7 am	8 am	9 am	10 am	2 pm	6 pm	10 pm	2 am	6 am	10 am	2 pm	6 pm	10 pm	2 am[b]	6 am	10 am
Tablets	4	4	4	4	4	4	4	4	4	4	4	4	4	4	4	4

[a] Escalate 50 mg/m² each week until toxicity is encountered, then continue weekly maintenance at nontoxic dose level.

[b] ± 2 hours.

TABLE 3.10. Dosing Schedule

Treatment group	Placebo baseline phase (6 weeks)[a]	Active treatment phase (6 weeks)			Total daily dose
		Morning	Midday	Evening	
A Placebo (N = 16–20)	Placebo tid[b]	Placebo	Placebo	Placebo	0
B Active bid (N = 16–20)	Placebo tid	900 mg	Placebo	900 mg	1800 mg
C Active tid (N = 16–20)	Placebo tid	600 mg	600 mg	600 mg	1800 mg

[a]A maximum of two additional 2-week periods of placebo therapy may be given during the baseline phase if deemed necessary (i.e., maximum of 10 weeks total on placebo).

[b]Patients will be instructed to take the entire contents of one bottle of medication (three capsules) before breakfast (7–9 am), before the midday meal (11 am–1 pm), and before the evening meal (5–7 pm).

TABLE 3.11. Dosing Schedule

Treatment group	Baseline phase 6 weeks[a]	Treatment phase 6 weeks	Withdrawal phase 6 weeks
A (6 patients)	Placebo bid[b]	Placebo bid	Placebo bid
B (6 patients)	Placebo bid	100 mg bid	Placebo bid
C (6 patients)	Placebo bid	300 mg bid	Placebo bid
D (6 patients)	Placebo bid	600 mg bid	Placebo bid
E (6 patients)	Placebo bid	900 mg bid	Placebo bid

[a]A maximum of two additional 2-week periods of placebo therapy may be given during the placebo baseline phase if deemed necessary (i.e., maximum of 10 weeks total on placebo).

[b]Patients will be instructed to take the entire contents of one bottle of medication (three capsules) before breakfast and before the evening meal.

TABLE 3.12. Dosing Schedule

Treatment group	Treatment phase I infusion (0–1 hr)		Treatment phase II infusion (1–10 hrs)		
	Dose (mg)	Infusion rate (ml/hr)	Total dose (mg)	Infusion rate (ml/hr) (1–2 hr)	Infusion rate (ml/hr) (2–10 hr)
A	40	100	100	50	25
B	60	100	100	50	25
C	80	100	100	50	25
D	100	100	100	50	25
E	120	100	100	50	25

TABLE 3.13. Dosing Schedule

Infusion regimen	Total time	Total dose	Infusion bag number	Infusion rate[a]
0.1 mg/kg bolus	60 sec	0.1 mg/kg	1	5.5 ml[b]
0.9 mg/kg/hr	1 hr	0.9 mg/kg	1	50 ml/hr
0.2 mg/kg/hr	1 hr	0.2 mg/kg	2	44 ml/hr
0.075 mg/kg/hr	4 hr	0.3 mg/kg	2	17 ml/hr

[a]Rate adjusted for 10 percent overfill of infusion bags.

[b]Bolus volume.

TABLE 3.14. Maximum Dosages of Drug X

Solution	Use	Concentration	Maximum, infusion rate[c] (ml/kg/min)	Maximum dose (ng/kg/min)	Maximum duration of infusion (minutes)	Maximum total dose (µg/kg)
P[a]	Infused into patient	4.0 µg/ml	0.002	8	30	0.24
D[b]	Infused into dialyzer	4.0 µg/ml	0.004	16	240	3.84

[a]Solution P will be infused intravenously at a rate of up to 0.002 ml/kg/min (8 ng/kg/min) directly into the patient beginning 15 min prior to starting dialysis. This infusion should be discontinued approximately 5 min before starting the dialysis procedure. If dialysis cannot be started within 5 min after the patient has received solution P for 10 min, the infusion may be continued for up to an additional 20 min.

[b]At the start of dialysis, solution D will be infused directly into the arterial side of the dialyzer. This infusion will last throughout the dialysis period at a rate of up to 0.004 ml/kg/min (16 ng/kg/min) until all blood in the dialyzer has been recycled to the patient by the conclusion of dialysis.

[c]Infusion rate (ml/kg/min) of drug will be based on *actual* body weight (kg) measured prior to dialysis.

TABLE 3.15. Dosages in a Two-Part Study

Part A: Placebo phase

Placebo dosage	Day	Morning	Midday	Evening
0 mg/day	−6 to 0	1		1

Part B: Double-blind treatment phase

Dosage[a]	Day	Morning	Midday	Evening
225 mg/day	1–3	1	1	1
300 mg/day	4–7	2	1	1
450 mg/day	8–42	2	2	2

[a]75 mg tablets or matched placebo.

TABLE 3.16. Dosing Schedule

Subgroup	Patient number	Priming iv bolus dose (mg/kg)	Initial iv bolus blocking dose (mg/kg)	Time[a] of initial iv bolus blocking dose (min)
A1	1–9	—	0.20	—
A2	11–19	0.03	0.17	3
A3	21–29	0.03	0.17	6
A4	31–39	0.03	0.22	3
A5	41–49	0.03	0.22	6

[a]Relative to priming iv bolus dose.

TABLE 3.17. Variable Dosage Regimens

Dosing frequency			Total daily dose (mg/day)
bid	tid	qid	
4 mg			8
	4 mg		12
8 mg		4 mg	16
12 mg	8 mg		24
16 mg		8 mg	32
24 mg	16 mg	12 mg	48

TABLE 3.18. Daily Dosage Regimen for Treatment Days 1–28

Study day, elapsed time	Time (Military)	Actual time	Placebo group	Drug group	
				4 mg/capsule	8 mg/capsule
0 hours	0800–1000	8–10 am	1	1	1
4 hours	1200–1400	12–2 pm	2	2	2
8 hours	1600–1800	4–6 pm	1	1	1
12 hours	2000–2200	8–10 pm	2	2	2

TABLE 3.19. Study Design

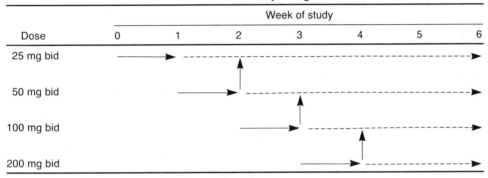

$\longrightarrow$ = Patients treated with the dose indicated.

- - - - $\blacktriangleright$ = Patients may continue dose based on response.

$\uparrow$ = Patients' dose may be decreased one level based on response.

• In this design all patients are progressively increased until they reach the 200 mg bid dose level, unless there is a reason not to.

TABLE 3.20. Dosing Schedule

Treatment period	Study days	Dose level[a]	Bottle number	Treatment Drug (no. and strength of caps) am	pm	Placebo (P) (no. of caps) am	pm
1	1	200 mg/day	2	1 × 100 mg	1 × 100 mg	1P	1P
2	2–5	100 mg/day	1	1 × 50 mg	1 × 50 mg	1P	1P
3	6–12	200 mg/day	2	1 × 100 mg	1 × 100 mg	1P	1P
4	13–25	300 mg/day	3	1 × 150 mg	1 × 150 mg	1P	1P
5	26–27	100 mg/day	1	1 × 50 mg	1 × 50 mg	1P	1P
6	28–30	Placebo	4	1P	1P	1P	1P

[a]If intolerable adverse experiences develop, the dosage may be decreased in multiples of 100 mg/day down to a minimum of 100 mg/day.

TABLE 3.21. Suggested Titration Schedule

Prescription for start of week	Number of 250 mg tablets prescribed			Total daily dose, mg	Total tablets each day	Total tablets each week
	am	noon	pm			
0	1		1	500	2	14
1	1	1	1	750	3	21
2	1	1	2	1000 (1g)	4	28
3	2	1	2	1250	5	35
4	2	2	2	1500	6	42
5	2	2	3	1750	7	49
6	3	2	3	2000 (2g)	8	56
7	3	3	3	2250	9	63
8	3	3	4	2500	10	70
9	4	3	4	2750	11	77
10	4	4	4	3000 (3g)	12	84

TABLE 3.22. Dosing Schedule

Study day	Dose level	Low dose regimen[a]	High dose regimen[a]	Placebo (P) regimen[a]	Total number of capsules per day
1–3	A	300 mg = 1 × 100 and 1 × 50 mg	300 mg (1 × 100 and 1 × 50 mg)	0 mg = 2 × P	4
4–7	B	600 mg = 1 × 200 and 1 × 100 mg	600 mg (1 × 200 and 1 × 100 mg)	0 mg = 2 × P	4
8–11	C	600 mg = 1 × 200 and 1 × 100 mg	800 mg (2 × 200 mg)	0 mg = 2 × P	4
12–28	D	600 mg = 3 × 100 mg	1200 mg (3 × 200 mg)	0 mg = 3 × P	6

[a]All regimens are given bid at _____ am and at _____ pm, or at 12-hr intervals.

TABLE 3.23. Dosing Schedule

Dosing period	Group	Number of patients	Dose (mg)	Prepackaged medication	Added by investigator
1	I	4	100	1 × 100 mg or 1P[a]	5P
2	II	6	200	2 × 100 or 2P	4P
3	I	4	300	1 × 300 or 1P	5P
4	II	6	600	2 × 300 or 2P	4P
5	I	4	900	3 × 300 or 3P	3P
6	II	6	1200	4 × 300 or 4P	2P
7	I	4	1500	5 × 300 or 5P	1P
8	II	6	1800	6 × 300 or 6P	0

[a]P, placebo capsule.

TABLE 3.24. Dosing Schedule

	Number and size of active capsules[a]	Number of placebo capsules	Total number of capsules/dose
Treatment group A			
Morning dose	0	3	3
Midday dose	0	3	3
Evening dose	0	3	3
Treatment group B			
Morning dose	3 × 300 mg	0	3
Midday dose	0	3	3
Evening dose	3 × 300 mg	0	3
Treatment group C			
Morning dose	2 × 300 mg	1	3
Midday dose	2 × 300 mg	1	3
Evening dose	2 × 300 mg	1	3

[a]During the placebo baseline phase, patients in each treatment group will take three capsules of placebo three times daily.

TABLE 3.25. Dosing Schedule

Subgroup	Patient number	N	Initial bolus dose	Estimated dose[a] (mg/kg)	Type of maintenance	Reversal to occur in patients
A1	1–9	9	ED_{25}	0.03	bolus	—
A2	11–19	9	ED_{50}	0.05	bolus	—
A3	21–29	9	ED_{75}	0.07	bolus	—
A4	31–39	9	ED_{95}	0.10	infusion	32,34,36,38
A5	41–49	9	1.5 ED_{95}	0.15	infusion	42,44,46,48
A6	51–59	9	2.0 ED_{95}	0.20	infusion	52,54,56,58
A7	61–69	9	2.5 ED_{95}	0.25	infusion	62,64,66,68
A8	71–79	9	2.5 ED_{95}	0.25	fixed bolus	72,74,76,78
A9	81–89	9	3.0 ED_{95}	0.30	infusion	82,84,86,88

[a]Actual doses estimated from Study Z.

Illustrates a method of adding aspects of study design to presentation of efficacy data.

TABLE 3.26. Schedule for Reversing Different Dosages of a Neuromuscular Blocking Drug (NMB) with Neostigmine in Patients Receiving Various Anesthetics

Subgroups	Anesthesia type	N	NMB, initial dose (μg/kg)	Reversal with neostigmine dose (μg/kg)	Percent recovery from NMB at time of reversal
Part 1					
A1	Narcotic	9	10[b]	45	25
B1	Isoflurane	9	5[b]	45	25
C1	Halothane	9	5[b]	45	25
Part 2					
A2	Narcotic	9	ED_{95}	[a]	—
A5	Narcotic	9	ED_{95}	[a]	—
B2	Isoflurane	9	ED_{95}	[a]	—
C2	Halothane	9	ED_{95}	[a]	—
Part 3					
A3	Narcotic	9	$1.5–2 \times ED_{95}$	45	10
B3	Isoflurane	9	$1.5–2 \times ED_{95}$	45	10
C3	Halothane	9	$1.5–2 \times ED_{95}$	45	10
D1	Narcotic	9	(100 μg/kg) Pancuronium	45	10
Part 4					
A4	Narcotic	9	$1.5–2 \times ED_{95}$	[a]	—
B4	Isoflurane	9	$1.5–2 \times ED_{95}$	[a]	—
C4	Halothane	9	$1.5–2 \times ED_{95}$	[a]	—

[a] Spontaneous recovery to 95% recovery.
[b] Initial dose. Additional doses may be given.

TABLE 3.27. Sample Tables of Dosage Regimens for Acute Single-Dose Drug Studies

Study day	Patient group code[a]	Dosing period no.[b]	Medication capsules		Total active dose (mg)
			Active group (N = 12)	Placebo (P) group (N = 6)	
1	A	1	1 × 200 mg + 5 P	6 P	200
4	B	2	2 × 200 mg + 4 P	6 P	400
8	A	3	3 × 200 mg + 3 P	6 P	600
11	B	4	4 × 200 mg + 2 P	6 P	800
15	A	5	5 × 200 mg + 1 P	6 P	1000
18	B	6	6 × 200 mg + 0 P	6 P	1200

Dose period	Placebo group (N = 6), no. of placebo capsules	Number of study drug capsules				Active drug group (N = 12)	
		0.5 mg	1.0 mg	4.0 mg	8.0 mg	Placebo capsules (no.)	Total dose (mg)
1	4	1	0	0	0	3	0.5
2	4	0	1	0	0	3	1.0
3	4	0	2	0	0	2	2.0
4	4	0	0	1	0	3	4.0
5	4	0	0	2	0	2	8.0
6	4	0	0	0	2	2	16.0

[a] A and B are two separate groups of patients.
[b] The time between dosing periods may be specified in terms of a fixed time, the minimum or maximum time allowed, or a range of times.

TABLE 3.28. Sample Tables of Dosage Regimens for Multidose Drug Studies

Day of study	Low-dose group						High-dose group				
	Placebo group (tablets)	75-mg tablets	150-mg tablets	P[a]	Total (mg/dose)	Total (mg/day)	75-mg tablets	150-mg tablets	P[a]	Total (mg/dose)	Total (mg/day)
1	3	1	0	2	75	300	0	1	2	150	600
2–5	3	0	1	2	150	600	0	2	1	300	1200
6–10	3	1	1	1	225	900	0	3	0	450	1800

Daily time of dosing (days 1–21)

No. of capsules to be taken

Elapsed time (hr)	Actual time (hr)	Placebo (P) group (N = 6)	Active drug		Total (mg/day)	
			Low dose (N = 12)	High dose (N = 12)	Low dose	High dose
0	8–10 am	2 P	1–5 mg + 1 P	2–5 mg	20	40
4	12–2 pm	2 P	1–5 mg + 1 P	2–5 mg		
8	4–6 pm	2 P	1–5 mg + 1 P	2–5 mg		
12	8–10 pm	2 P	1–5 mg + 1 P	2–5 mg		

Weight of patient (kg)	Total dose of study drug (mg) for three groups of patients in each of the 9 weeks of study[b]								
	1	2	3	4	5	6	7	8	9
10–19.9	50 (50)	100 (100)	100 (100)	150 (50, 100)	150 (50, 100)	200 (200)	200 (200)	100 (100)	0
20–39.9	100 (100)	150 (50, 100)	150 (50, 100)	200 (200)	200 (200)	300 (300)	300 (300)	150 (50, 100)	0
40–60	150 (50, 100)	200 (100, 100)	200 (100, 100)	300 (100, 200)	300 (100, 200)	400 (200, 200)	400 (200, 200)	200 (200)	0

[a] P, placebo.
[b] The tablet sizes required for each dose are in parentheses (tablets are assumed to be available in 50, 100, and 200 mg). Placebos are used to make up two tablets per dose.

1. COMMON PARALLEL DESIGNS

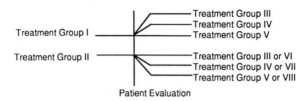

2. TWO PART PARALLEL STUDY

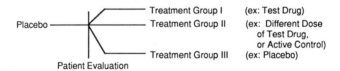

3. PARALLEL DESIGN WITH PLACEBO INITIATION

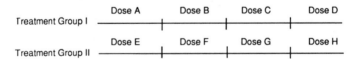

4. INTRODUCTION OF PLACEBO DURING TREATMENT

Treatment Group I	Placebo	Treatment Group I
Treatment Group II	Placebo	Treatment Group II
Treatment Group III	Placebo	Treatment Group III

5. MULTIPLE DOSES WITHIN EACH TREATMENT GROUP

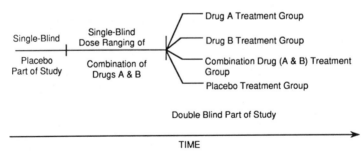

6. PARALLEL EVALUATION OF A COMBINATION DRUG

FIG. 3.1. Selected schemata for treatment periods of parallel studies. Baselines are not illustrated, and time is along the abscissa.

• Unless indicated, each part may be conducted in either a single-blind or double-blind manner.

• In schemata 1 to 4, each treatment group may constitute a different dose or drug.

• In schema 3, the placebo trial may be conducted at the end of the study.

• In schema 4, the placebo trial may be conducted at an announced or unannounced time during the treatment and for a specified or unspecified duration.

• In schema 5, each dose is of a fixed or variable length, and doses may be given in a systematic or random order.

• One or more of the doses in each treatment group may be a placebo, or each of the two treatment groups could be subdivided into two or more subgroups (e.g., drug and placebo) at each dose period. Reprinted from Spilker (1984) with permission.

1. SINGLE CROSSOVER WITH NO INTERVENING BASELINE

2. SINGLE CROSSOVER WITH INTERVENING BASELINE

3. DOUBLE CROSSOVER WITHOUT INTERVENING BASELINES

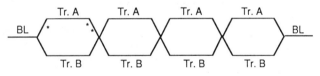

Continued

FIG. 3.2. Selected schemata for crossover studies.

• Schemata 1 to 5 may be open-label, single-blind, or double-blind.

• All baselines that occur after treatment has been initiated include washout of drug.

• In schema 1, there is usually a brief washout period between treatments A and B.

• Although the change from one treatment to another in all schemata is shown as being time dependent, it is possible that this change may be dependent on the condition of the patient's disease state. Reprinted from Spilker (1984) with permission.

BL, baseline; Tr.A, treatment A; Tr. B, treatment B.
*, dose ascension part of each period; **, dose taper part of each period.

4. DOUBLE CROSSOVER WITH INTERVENING BASELINES

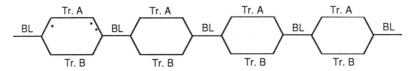

5. EXTRA PERIOD CROSSOVER

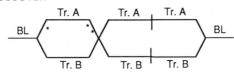

6. OPEN-LABEL CROSSOVER WITHOUT RANDOMIZATION

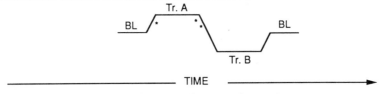

TIME

FIG. 3.2. *Continued.*

Illustrates boundaries for closed sequential design.

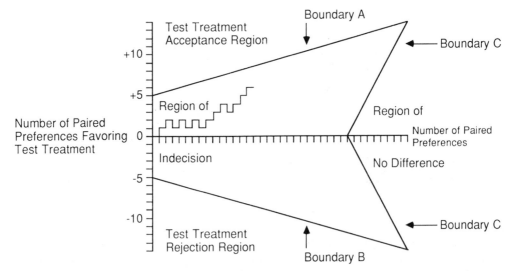

FIG. 3.3. Trial continues until observed number of preferences (ignoring ties) crosses a boundary line. The test treatment is considered superior to the control treatment if boundary line A is crossed, inferior to the control treatment if boundary line B is crossed, and equal to the control treatment if boundary line C is crossed. Reprinted from Meinert and Tonascia (1986) with permission.

Illustrates sequential design procedure.

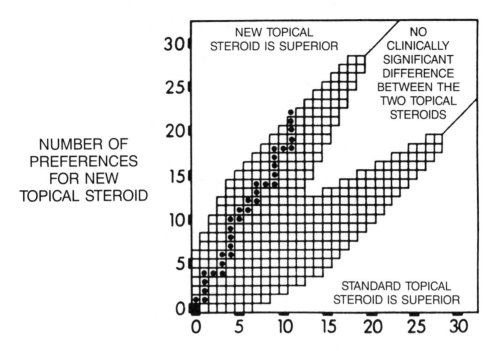

FIG. 3.4. Reprinted from Rodda (1974) with permission.

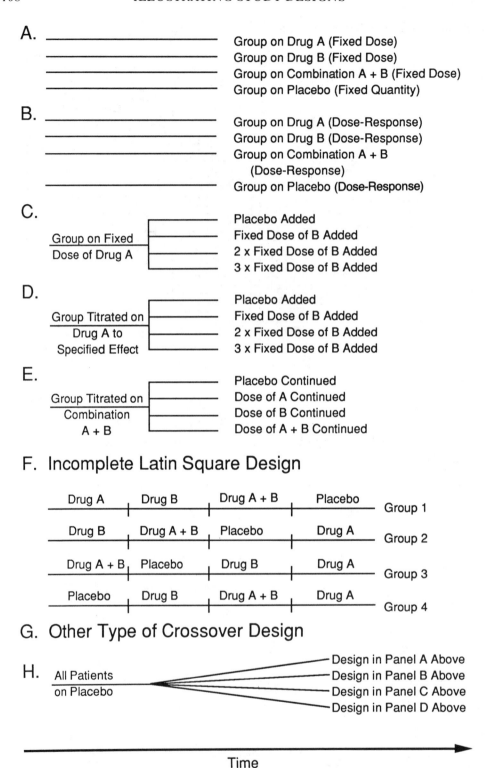

FIG. 3.5. Selected study designs to evaluate combination drugs. Many variations on these study designs are possible. Reprinted from Spilker (1987) with permission.

A.

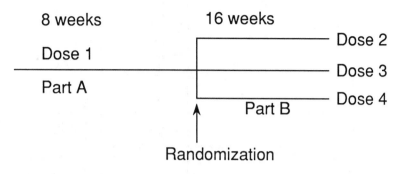

B.

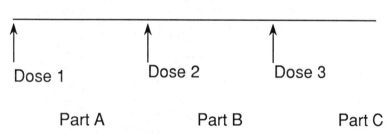

FIG. 3.6. Schematic diagrams illustrating parts of a study. In panel A the parts are defined as before and after randomization. In panel B the parts are defined as occurring during different dosing periods.

Illustrates using dosing information to annotate a display of efficacy data.

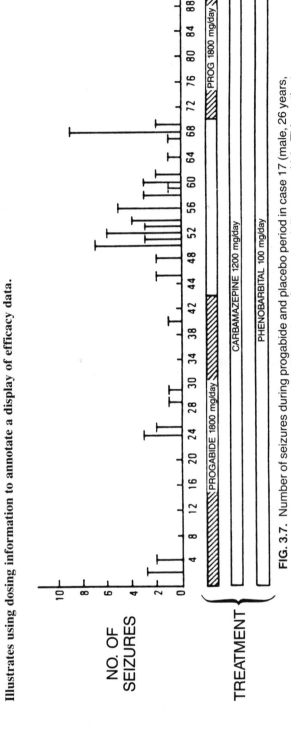

FIG. 3.7. Number of seizures during progabide and placebo period in case 17 (male, 26 years, 55 kg, complex partial seizures, pretrial seizures frequency daily to weekly). This patient dropped out of the study because of increased seizure frequency during the placebo period. The readministration of progabide (PROG) led to a complete control of attacks. Reprinted from Loiseau et al. (1983) with permission.

Illustrates incorporating study phase (treatment or no treatment) into a display of efficacy data.

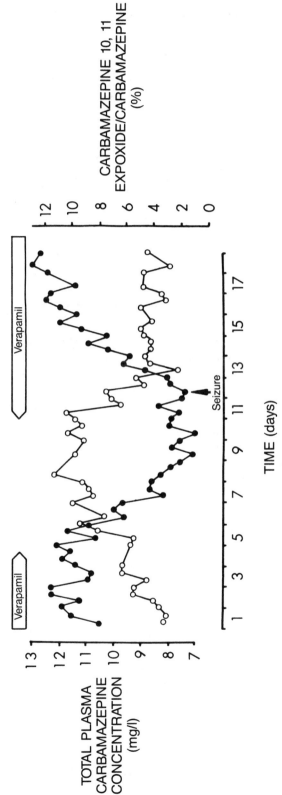

FIG. 3.8. Serial plasma carbamazepine concentrations (●) and carbamazepine-10,11 epoxide : carbamazepine ratios (○) in a patient with refractory epilepsy during verapamil withdrawal and restoration. Reprinted from Macphee et al. (1986) as presented by Brodie and Feely (1988), with permission.

• An arrow indicating the start of treatment may be used in this or many other figures.

Illustrates using dosing information to annotate a display of efficacy data.

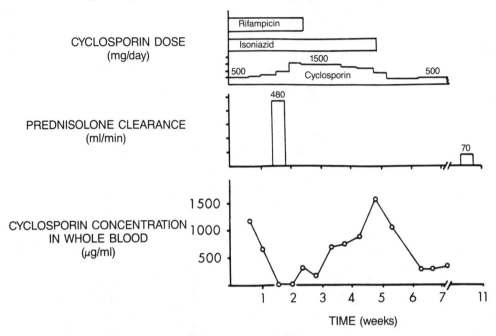

FIG. 3.9. Effect of treatment with rifampicin on prednisolone metabolism and circulating cyclosporin concentrations in a patient with a transplanted kidney. Reprinted from Langhoff and Madsen (1983) as presented by Brodie and Feely (1988), with permission.

Illustrates the different parts of a study.

113

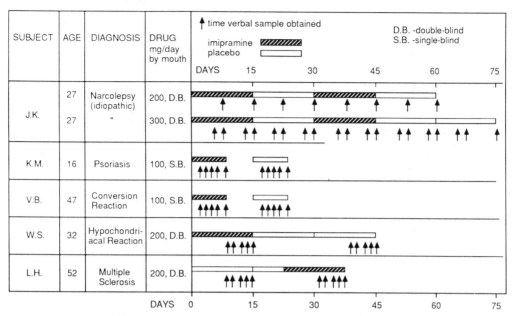

FIG. 3.10. Summary of subjects, drug dosage, and order. Reprinted from Gottschalk et al. (1965) with permission.

Illustrates a dosing schedule.

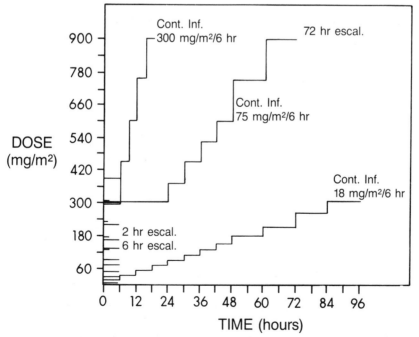

FIG. 3.11. Projected time course of five schedules of dose escalations to reach the maximally tolerated dose (MTD).

• Months of study may be plotted on the abscissa to show projected time to reach the MTD. The number of escalations and estimated MTD may be shown.

Illustrates how changing drugs or dosages in individual patients affects an efficacy parameter.

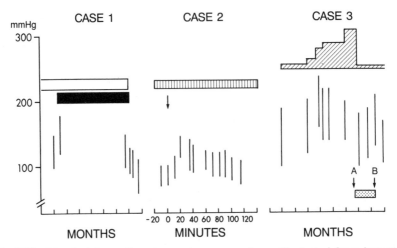

FIG. 3.12. Difficulties in interpreting drug adverse reactions, illustrated from hypertension. **Case 1**, hypertension unresponsive to clonidine (solid bar), but relieved by withdrawing oral contraceptive (open bar). **Case 2**, interaction in a normal subject given small doses of debrisoquin continuously, with a single 50 mg oral dose of phenylephrine (↓). **Case 3**, a patient-doctor interaction: up to A the patient was not taking the bethanidine tablets (dosage, prescribed from hospital, 40 mg/day rising to 300 mg/day, diagonal hatch lines). At A an admonition was given. At B the general practitioner agreed to withdraw diethylpropion (horizontal hatch lines); bethanidine now 30 mg/day. Reprinted from Vere (1976) with permission.

Illustrates the distinct parts of a study on a graph of efficacy data.

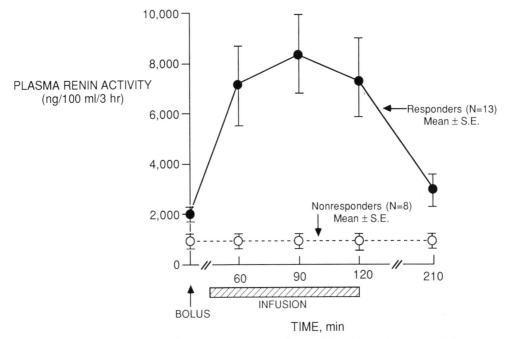

FIG. 3.13. Plasma renin activity in response to drug X in 21 hypertensive patients.

Illustrates a means of enhancing a display of efficacy data with details of the overall study design.

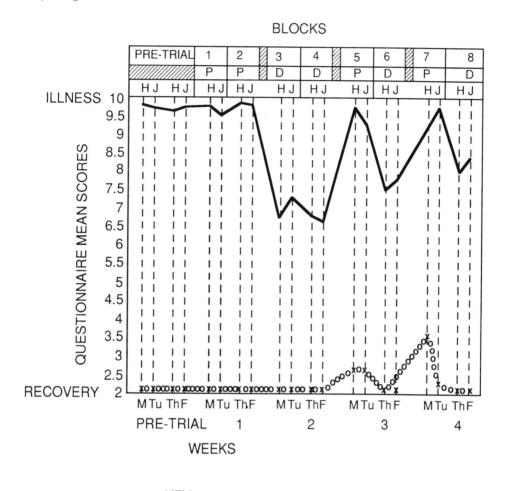

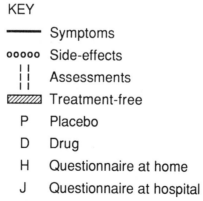

FIG. 3.14. Mean symptom scores on each trial. Reprinted from McPherson and Le Gassicke (1965) with permission.

- All eight drug scores were lower than all eight placebo scores.

Illustrates dosing schedule and study phases.

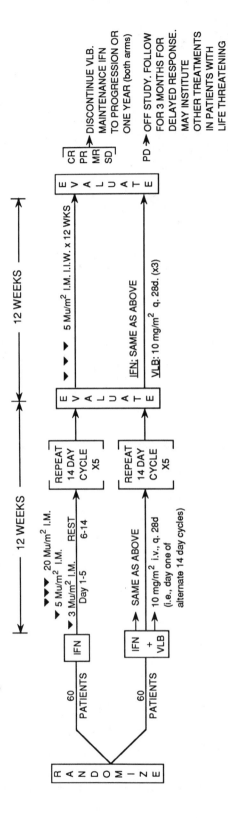

FIG. 3.15. Schematic diagram of a drug being evaluated in patients with advanced renal adenocarcinoma.

Illustrates a relatively complete display of study information.

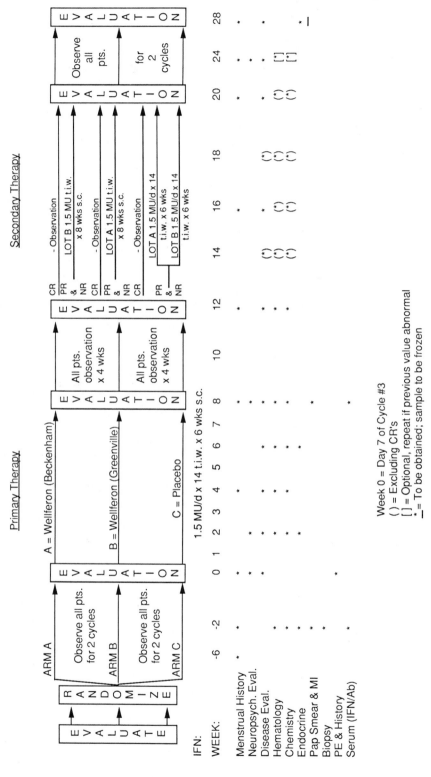

FIG. 3.16. Schematic diagram of a clinical study in patients with condylomata acuminata.

Illustrates a schematic diagram of a clinical study plus time and events chart.

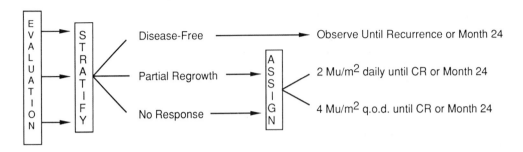

Month	12		13	14	15	16	17	18	19	20	21	22	23	24
Evaluation	⋆			⋆				⋆						⋆
Hematology	⋆		⋆	⋆ ⋆ ⋆		⋆	⋆	⋆	⋆	⋆	⋆	⋆	⋆	⋆
Chemistries	⋆		⋆	⋆ ⋆ ⋆		⋆	⋆	⋆	⋆	⋆	⋆	⋆	⋆	⋆
Physical Exam	⋆			⋆		⋆		⋆		⋆		⋆		⋆
Chest X-Ray	⋆							⋆						⋆

FIG. 3.17.

Illustrates a schematic of study design showing three-dimensional expansion of part of the design.

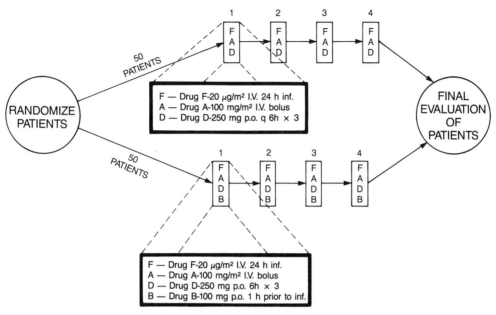

FIG. 3.18. Monthly treatment cycle.

Illustrates a schematic diagram of a clinical study.

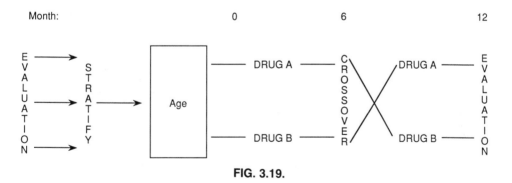

FIG. 3.19.

Illustrates annotating a study schematic with a display of scheduled evaluations.

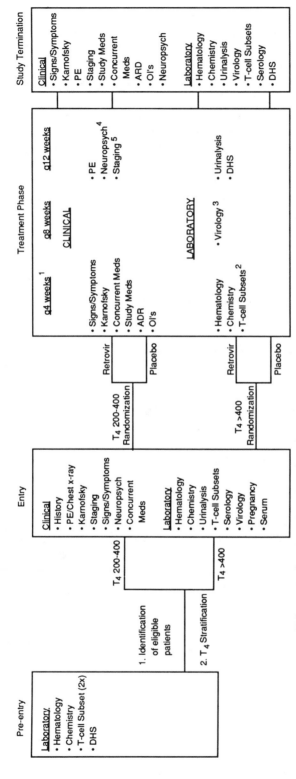

FIG. 3.20. Combination of study schematic plus time and events chart.

[1]These will be done biweekly for the first 8 weeks then every 4 weeks thereafter.

[2]T-cell subsets will be determined every 4 weeks for the first 12 weeks then every 12 weeks thereafter.

[3]Serum p24 antigen levels will be determined every 4 weeks for the first 12 weeks then every 12 weeks thereafter. Viral cultures will be done every 24 weeks.

[4]The RCPM will be administered every 12 weeks and supplemented with the WAIS-R at 24 and 48 weeks.

[5]Assessment of disease stage will be done every 12 weeks during treatment as appropriate.

Illustrates time when tests are administered to patients.

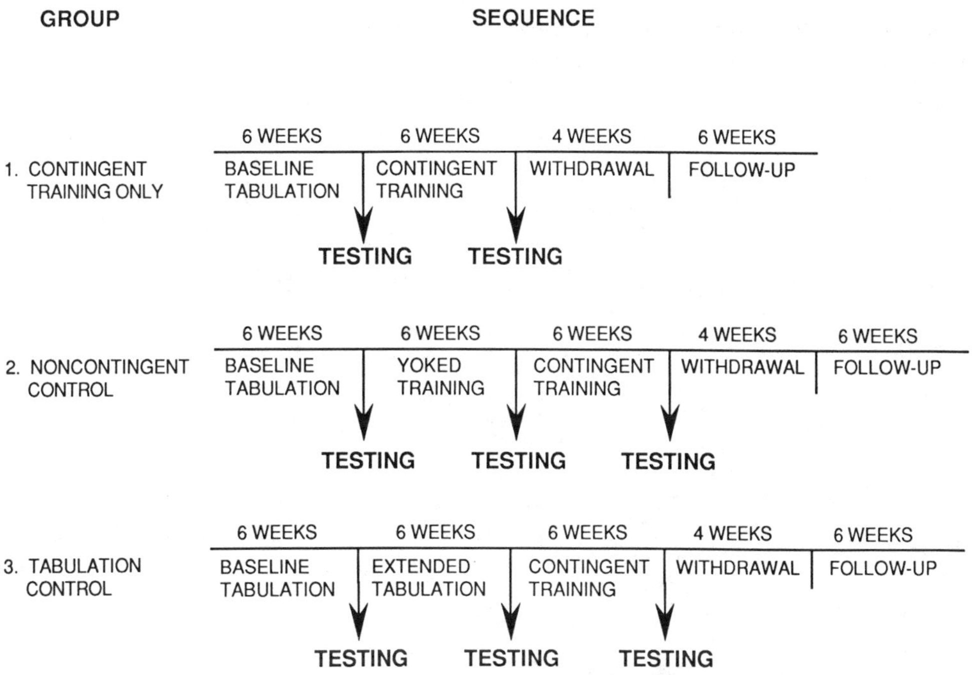

GROUP   SEQUENCE

	6 WEEKS	6 WEEKS	4 WEEKS	6 WEEKS
1. CONTINGENT TRAINING ONLY	BASELINE TABULATION	CONTINGENT TRAINING	WITHDRAWAL	FOLLOW-UP

           TESTING   **TESTING**

	6 WEEKS	6 WEEKS	6 WEEKS	4 WEEKS	6 WEEKS
2. NONCONTINGENT CONTROL	BASELINE TABULATION	YOKED TRAINING	CONTINGENT TRAINING	WITHDRAWAL	FOLLOW-UP

         TESTING   **TESTING**   **TESTING**

	6 WEEKS	6 WEEKS	6 WEEKS	4 WEEKS	6 WEEKS
3. TABULATION CONTROL	BASELINE TABULATION	EXTENDED TABULATION	CONTINGENT TRAINING	WITHDRAWAL	FOLLOW-UP

         TESTING   **TESTING**   **TESTING**

FIG. 3.21. Experimental design, indicating when test battery was administered to each group. Reprinted from Lantz and Sterman (1988) with permission.

Illustrates a flow chart of events leading up to the point of patient randomization.

1. Suspected metastatic, previously untreated colon or rectal cancer.

2. Diagnostic studies done to confirm, to give baseline measurements and to verify patient eligibility.

3. Patient and physician elect to enroll in this study.

4. Register patient by calling, 1-800-334-9796, extension 4893 or 4626. Patient number will be assigned.

ASYMPTOMATIC　　　　　　　**SYMPTOMATIC**

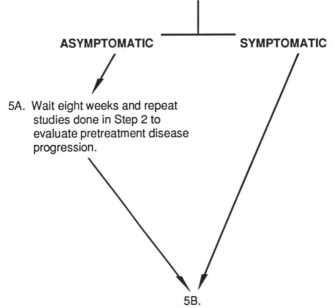

5A. Wait eight weeks and repeat studies done in Step 2 to evaluate pretreatment disease progression.

5B.
Randomize with code provided by the Burroughs Wellcome Co. and begin treatment.

FIG. 3.22. A Phase III, randomized, double-blind, placebo-controlled trial of 5-fluorouracil, with or without large doses of Wellcovorin® (leucovorin tablets), in measurable metastatic colon and rectal carcinoma.

Illustrates a schematic of multiple clinical studies indicating a few elements (e.g., dose, duration of study, N, status of final medical report).

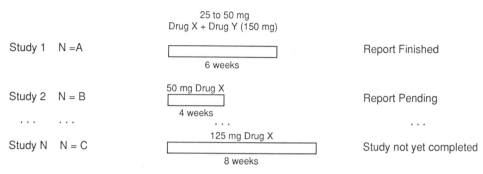

FIG. 3.23. Schematics of many studies (abbreviated).

Illustrates a photograph of medical equipment used in a study.

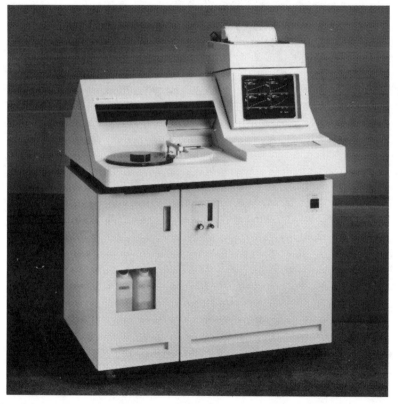

FIG. 3.24. Spectrophotometer, Model Z-9000 GFAAS by Hitachi. Photograph provided by Hitachi Instruments Inc. of Danbury, CT.

• Photographs of medical devices may also be illustrated.

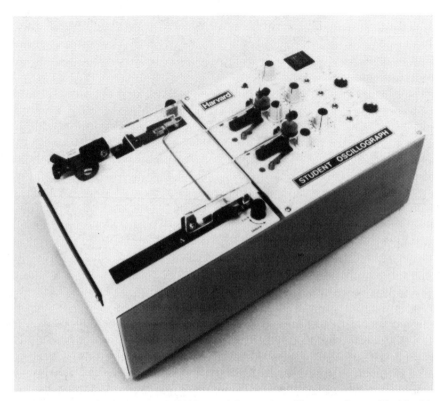

FIG. 3.25. Two channel oscillograph of Harvard Apparatus. Photograph provided by Harvard Apparatus Inc. of South Natick, MA.

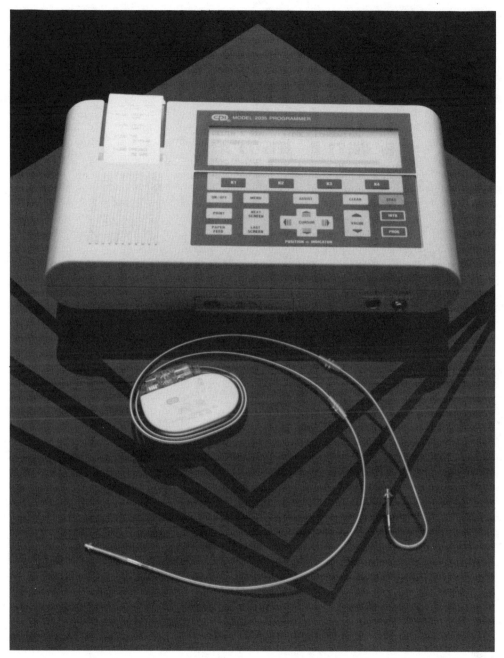

FIG. 3.26. Cardiac pacemaker (Vista™ Series Single Chamber Pacemaker System). Photograph provided by Cardiac Pacemakers Inc. of St. Paul, MN.

4

Demographics and Patient Accountability

DEMOGRAPHICS

Whenever inexperienced players get the ball in basketball or American football they usually have a strong desire to go directly to the basket or attempt to score a touchdown. But it is usually necessary to make certain that everyone on the team is properly positioned and aware of the overall strategy. Likewise, after a clinical study is completed one should first look over the demographic and prognostic characteristics to insure that the groups being compared are similar in important aspects.

The next step in presenting and interpreting data involves patient accountability. In this step the investigator determines which data may legitimately be ignored and how missing data will be handled. Data should be analyzed and interpreted only after these important steps have been completed.

The presentation of demographic variables usually involves tables rather than figures. Nonetheless, demographic data may be easily illustrated with pie charts, histograms, or other formats if desired; these are straightforward to create, and are not shown here. Demographic presentations are shown in Tables 4.1 to 4.6. Prognostic variables and pertinent patient characteristics may be shown with demographic data or separately (Tables 4.7 and 4.8). Combining data from multiple sites or studies becomes more complex and the type of presentation may vary; representative presentations are given in Tables 4.9 to 4.11.

Presentation of patient accountability is highly variable from study to study. The best presentations often cannot be determined prior to a study because considerations such as the precise problems encountered and types of patient dropouts and discontinuations cannot be known in advance. On the other hand, there are certain standard approaches for presenting duration of treatment, number of complete patients, number of patients with evaluable data, and other aspects of patient accountability. Tables 4.12 to 4.30 depict basic formats for presenting accountability data. The final tables in this chapter (Tables 4.31 to 4.35) present formats for displaying selected study characteristics.

Various pictorial displays (e.g., maps, flow diagrams) are often used to present data on study characteristics and patient accountability. Figures 4.1 to 4.7 provide prototypes for the presentation of study characteristics, and Figs. 4.8 to 4.12 of patient accountability.

After the demographic and patient accountability data have been presented, the safety and efficacy data may be evaluated with greater understanding of the nature, makeup, and amount of data from each treatment group.

Demographics of a Multiple Center Study

1. A complete presentation will include one table for each site, and another table for all sites combined. In many medical reports the combined table is included in the body of the paper and the individual site tables are included in an appendix.
2. Each table has the same format as a single site study.
3. Discussion of these tables should mention intersite differences between the individual sites. In most situations, however, the sites are not statistically compared.
4. Sometimes a brief table giving site-specific summaries, may suffice (e.g., see Table 4.9). Table 4.9 is really more appropriate, for multiple-study presentation, but the principle being presented is the same.

STUDY CHARACTERISTICS

In addition to presenting characteristics of patients included in a study, it is often important to present characteristics of the study. Methods of presenting study design characteristics are described in Chapter 3. Other aspects to consider include characteristics of study sites, investigators, or procedures used in conducting the study. This could relate to almost any aspect of a study, including those discussed in the methods section of a published article. A few examples are shown in Tables 4.31 to 4.35.

Illustrates listing demographic data from a single patient study.

TABLE 4.1. Demographics for a Single Patient Study

Characteristic	Value
Age (yrs)	
Sex	
Race	
Height (cm)	(Normal, Abnormal)
Weight (kg)	
Blood pressure (mm Hg)	
Medical history	

• Information on important demographic characteristics (e.g., age, sex, race) in a single patient study may be given in the text rather than in a table.

• If appropriate to study objectives, baseline values of relevant variables (e.g., disease symptoms) may be included in the demographic listing.

• In a crossover study, some information (e.g., blood pressure, temperature, baseline symptoms) is recorded at the beginning of each period. The data listing must be modified accordingly.

• Some demographic characteristics affect a patient's prognosis. Those demographics should be identified in the text and discussed.

Illustrates listing of demographic data from individual patients in a "small" study.

TABLE 4.2. Clinical and Demographic Data on 10 Patients with Allergic Rhinitis[a]

No.	Initials	Age	Sex	Diagnostic pattern	Allergens tested intracutaneously
1	SM	22	F	Seasonal/Perennial	Elm, June grass
2	SS	20	F	" "	Cottonwood, common sage
3	BMcK	39	M	" "	Prairie sage, Russian thistle
4	NB	20	F	" "	June and rye grass
5	JK	18	F	" "	Red top and timothy grass
6	DM	35	M	" "	Timothy grass, giant ragweed
7	AV	38	F	" "	Lamb's quarters, Western waterhemp
8	MS	33	F	" "	Rye grass, Russian thistle
9	JM	30	M	" "	June grass, Russian thistle
10	EJ	32	M	" "	Oak, common sage

[a]Reprinted from Falliers et al. (1978) with permission.

• When only a few patients are in the study, demographic data are often listed instead of summarized.

• If this study compared two treatment groups, then the above listing should be ordered by treatment group.

• This is a horizontal listing of the data (i.e., each row indicates a different patient). This layout is usually used when few patients are enrolled. If the number of relevant baseline variables is large with respect to the number of patients, then a vertical listing (i.e., each column representing a different patient) may be more appropriate. See Table 4.3 for an example.

Illustrates listing of demographic data from individual patients in a "small" study.

TABLE 4.3. Characteristics of Six Male Anxious Chronic Schizophrenic Patients Who Completed the Study[a]

Patient no.	2	3	4	6	7	9
Age (years)	53	34	32	24	46	44
Marital status	Married	Single	Single	Single	Single	Married
Race	Black	White	White	White	White	White
Occupation	None, former clerk	None, former college student	None, former college student	None, former scholar	Taxi driver	None, former cement mixer
Duration since onset of symptoms (years)	3	10	9	10	5	4
No. of previous psychiatric hospital admissions	1	25	13	Inpatient for large part of time	2	1
Diagnosis (DSM II)	Paranoid type (during study: residual type)	Chronic, undifferentiated	Chronic, undifferentiated	Chronic, undifferentiated	Paranoid type	Acute schizophrenic episode (during study: residual type)
Classification (see text)	?Process; Schneider-positive; paranoid	Process; Schneider-positive; nonparanoid	Process; Schneider-positive; paranoid	Process; ?Schneider, nonparanoid	?Process; ?Schneider-positive paranoid	Reactive; Schneider-negative paranoid
Premorbid adjustment	Good	Fair	Poor	Good	Fair	Good
Personality deterioration	Moderate	Severe	Severe	Very severe	Doubtful	Moderate
Antipsychotic medication, daily dose	Trifluoperazine hydrochloride, 15 mg	Thioridazine, 800 mg	Thioridazine, 300 mg	Thioridazine, 400 mg	Thioridazine, 200 mg	Thioridazine, 400 mg
Final daily dose of chlordiazepoxide during study	150 mg	300 mg	225 mg	200 mg	200 mg	225 mg
Conspicuous schizophrenic symptoms during study	No	Yes	Yes	Yes	Yes	No

[a]Reprinted from Kellner et al. (1975) with permission.

Illustrates baseline data of two treatment groups plus use of footnotes to annotate data.

TABLE 4.4. Detailed Presentation of Patients Baseline Status[a]

Patient	Pretrial seizure frequency	Age at onset (years)	Associated pathology	Associated AEDs[b] (mg/day)	Progabide (mg/day)
Group I (placebo/verum)					
1	Daily to weekly	27	—	PB (150), CBZ (600), clobazam (30)	1,800
3	Clusters every 3 weeks	14	Anxiety	PB (100), CBZ (400), PHT (100), VPA (600)	2,400
5	Weekly	12	Behavioral	PHT (200)	1,200
8	Weekly to monthly	14	—	PB (100), CBZ (800), clobazam (60)	1,800
10 (ter)	Monthly	≤1	—	PB (200), clobazam (120)	2,100
11	Daily to weekly	5	—	PB (100), PHT (250)	1,500
14	Daily to weekly	11	Psychiatric disturbances	PB (200), CBZ (800), clobazam (40)	2,100
15	Weekly to monthly	18	Mental retardation, left pyramidal syndrome	PB (130), CBZ (600), PHT (80), pheneturide (400)	1,800
101	Weekly	5	Mental retardation, behavioral disturbances	PB (75), VPA (1,000), ESM (500)	600
102	Weekly	16	Psychiatric disturbances	PB (200), CPZ (6)	2,100
Mean ± SE	—	12.3 ± 2.37	—	—	1,740 ± 166
Group II (verum/placebo)					
2	Monthly	10	—	PB (122.5), CBZ (600), PHT (60), pheneturide (300)	1,800
4	Monthly	13	Anxiety, depression	CBZ (600)	1,800
6 (bis)	Weekly to monthly	29	Mental retardation, Addison's disorder, embolic disease	CPZ (6)	2,700
					2,400

Continued

TABLE 4.4. (*Continued*)

Patient	Pretrial seizure frequency	Age at onset (years)	Associated pathology	Associated AEDs[b] (mg/day)	Progabide (mg/day)
7	Monthly	7	Mental retardation, athetosis	PB (200), CBZ (600)	1,200
9	Daily	4	Mental retardation	PB (80), CBZ (500)	900
12	Daily to weekly	11	Mental retardation, cerebral palsy	PB (150), PHT (300), clobazam (30), CPZ (2)	1,500 1,200
13	Weekly	3	Behavioral disturbances	CBZ (800), PRM (750)	2,100
16	Weekly	40	Anxiety	PB (100), CBZ (600)	1,800
103	Monthly	10	Mental retardation	PB (200), VPA (2000)	2,100
104	Weekly	10	—	PB (200), PHT (400), VPA (2,000)	2,400
Mean ± SE	—	13.7 ± 3.69	—	—	1,830 ± 170

[a]Patients 1–16 had partial seizures, patients 101–104 generalized seizures (double randomizations). Dropouts were replaced by other patients with the same code number. Reprinted from Loiseau et al. (1983) with permission.
[b]AED, antiepileptic drug; CPS, complex partial seizures; GM, grand mal; CBZ, carbamazepine; PB, phenobarbital; PHT, phenytoin; VPA, valproic acid; ESM, ethosuximide; PRM, primidone.

• Since some patients' data require two rows in the table, clarity would be improved if a blank line were inserted between patients.

• Types of seizures could be presented as a separate column. This could refer to all seizure types or only to those that were uncontrolled at the start of the study.

Illustrates summary of demographic data from multiple treatment groups.

TABLE 4.5. Demographics for a Controlled Study

Characteristic	Treatment A (N =)	Treatment B (N =)	. . .[b]	Treatment Z (N =)	All patients (N =)
Sex					
Female					
Male					
Race					
Caucasian					
Black					
Other[a]					
Age (years)					
Mean					
Median					
SD					
Range					
Height (cm)					
Mean					
Median					
SD					
Range					

[a]This footnote explicitly identifies the "other" category of race.
[b]. . . , indicates that more columns may be added.

• This table often has references to an appendix which lists individual patient data. However, for small studies this listing may replace the summary table (e.g., Table 4.2).

• A final column of all treatments combined is optional and is not often included in the presentation.

• Numerical variables such as age may be summarized in a categorical form (e.g., 0 to 10 yr, 10 to 20 yr, 20 to 30 yr, etc.).

• A similar table should be prepared for each center in a multicenter study.

• When summarizing numerical variables, it is helpful to include both mean and median as this gives evidence of the "shape" of the distribution.

• This table often includes baseline values of all variables that might interact with or otherwise affect the study treatments.

• This table should include all variables that could affect the interpretation of the results of the study (e.g., the last two columns of Table 4.2).

• For crossover studies, some information (e.g., blood pressure) should be summarized at the start of each period.

• There is disagreement within the scientific community whether to statistically compare the treatment groups with respect to baseline variables. If they are compared, results could be included in the table by adding a column reporting the p-values.

Illustrates demographics, prognostic variables, and pertinent patient characteristics.

TABLE 4.6. Characteristics of Study Population—"Baseline"[a]

Characteristic[b]	Intervention (N = 92)	Control (N = 89)
Mean age (years ± SD)	80.9 (± 5.8)	82.0 (± 5.8)
Sex (% male)	96	96
Race (% white)	74	73
Marital status (% married)	52	57
Living arrangements (% home)	77	84
Admission service (%)		
Surgery	52	53
Medicine	41	41
Psychiatry	7	6
No. of medical problems (mean ± SD)	6.4 (± 2.5)	6.0 (± 2.4)
Mean length of stay in days (± SD)	18.3 (± 16.1)	16.6 (± 14.9)
Functional status[c] (%)		
Independent	41	37
Semidependent	51	61
Dependent	8	2
Mental status score, No. of errors (± SD)	2.0 (± 2.8)	1.9 (± 2.5)

[a]Reprinted from Becker et al. (1987) with permission.
[b]There were no significant differences between groups for any characteristics (p > .10).
[c]Based on activities of daily living. Independent, includes all seven activities; semidependent, requires assistance with some activities; and dependent, requires assistance with all activities.

• Any relevant patient characteristics (e.g., vital signs, laboratory values) may be included in this type of table.

Illustrates prognostic variables without demographic characteristics.

TABLE 4.7. Prognostic Variables at Baseline

Prognostic variables at baseline	Drug (N = 945)	Placebo (N = 939)
Age (median years)[a]	63.0	65.0[b]
Number of risk factors (mean)	1.5	1.6
Standing diastolic blood pressure at entry (mean)	85.7	86.3
Sick leave prior to study	29(3)[c]	46(5)[b]
Prior use of diuretics	174(18)	214(23)[b]
Ventricular tachycardia during course	77(8)	105(11)[b]
Exertional chest pain at less than maximum effort	378(40)	406(43)
Duration of chest pain greater than 30 min at onset	888(94)	887(94)
Maximal SGOT greater than four times upper limit of normal	482(51)	492(52)
Sinus, atrial, supraventricular, tachycardia during course	150(16)	174(18)

[a]In this study, age is considered a prognostic variable as well as a demographic characteristic.
[b]$p < 0.05$.
[c]Number in parenthesis equals percent.
SGOT, serum glutamic-oxaloacetic transaminase.

Illustrates how prior therapy variables may be summarized.

TABLE 4.8. Summary of Prior Therapy

Patients with the following therapy	Number of patients in placebo group[a] N(%)	Number of patients in drug group[a] N(%)
Hydralazine	2 (1.2)	
Hygroton	1 (0.6)	
Low sodium diet		1 (0.6)
Isoniazid	1 (0.6)	
Alpha-methyldopa	2 (1.2)	1 (0.6)
Hydroflumethiazide		1 (0.6)
Lomotil		1 (0.6)

[a]Total number of patients at start of study were 168 in placebo group and 176 in the drug group.

• This type of table is often used to introduce the efficacy data.

Illustrates how demographic data may be grouped under general categories from multiple studies or multiple sites from one study.

TABLE 4.9. Basic Demographic Summary of Multiple Studies

Study category	N	Sex		Race			Age (years)					
		Male	Female	White	Black	Other	<18	18–29	30–39	40–49	50–59	60–69
Pharmacokinetic and dose-ranging												
15-01	12	7	5	•	•	•	0	1	0	2	5	4
01-01	4	4	0	4	0	0	0	2	2	0	0	0
Major dose-response by study number												
02-01	70	42	28	66	3	1	0	28	17	16	9	0
03-01	25	14	11	21	2	2	0	6	4	10	4	1
03-02	26	24	2	20	3	3	1	17	7	1	0	0
05-01	40	36	4	39	0	1	0	20	14	5	1	0
06-01	20	11	9	20	0	0	0	5	4	5	5	1
06-02	22	20	2	16	5	1	1	14	3	4	0	0
07-01	31	26	5	25	2	4	0	6	8	11	4	2
	26	20	6	23	2	1	0	9	8	6	2	1
08-01	63	24	39	27	24	12	0	7	18	15	13	10
	34	12	22	20	8	6	0	7	6	9	9	3
09-01	25	16	9	18	7	0	0	12	8	2	3	0
	40	19	21	34	6	0	0	7	13	14	6	0
10-01	25	17	8	24	0	1	0	15	3	1	6	0
	40	36	4	35	3	2	0	23	10	5	2	0
Totals (Studies 02–10)	487	317	170	388	65	34	2	176	123	104	64	18
Major dose-response by type of anesthesia												
Balanced anesthesia	265	163	102	201	41	23	1	91	65	56	39	13
Halothane anesthesia	82	67	15	75	5	2	1	39	21	14	6	1
Enflurane anesthesia	74	31	43	54	14	6	0	14	19	23	15	3
Isoflurane anesthesia	66	56	10	58	5	3	0	32	18	11	4	1
Totals (Studies 02–10)	487	317	170	388	65	34	2	176	123	104	64	18

• Instead of demographic variables along the top, categories based on cumulative doses given could be listed to portray exposure to study drugs.

Illustrates summary of demographic variables in individual study sites and combined.

TABLE 4.10. Demographic Characteristics—Combined Patients Across Multiple Centers

Parameter	Center 1[a]				Center 2				Combined centers			
	Drug A (N =)	Drug B (N =)	Placebo (N =)	Total (N =)	Drug A (N =)	Drug B (N =)	Placebo (N =)	Total (N =)	Drug A (N =)	Drug B (N =)	Placebo (N =)	Total (N =)
Age[b]												
Mean												
SD[c]												
Range												
Sex												
Male												
Female												
Race												
White												
Black												
Oriental												
Other[d]												
Height (cm)[e]												
Mean												
SD												
Range												
Weight (kg)[e]												
Mean												
SD												
Range												

[a]Instead of individual centers, data could be combined by groups of centers, age group of patient (e.g., 2–11 years, 12–18 years, and above 18 years), type of study, or other categories.

[b]Age could be divided into decades or broad groups (e.g., below 18, 18–65, above 65). Age is given based on the date treatment was initiated.

[c]SD, standard deviation.

[d]Specify the identity of "other" in a footnote.

[e]Height and weight percentiles could be used instead of raw data. Alternatively, the median percentiles could be given in this table.

Illustrates demographics of multiple studies grouped according to type of study.

TABLE 4.11. Demographic Characteristics

Study category[a]	Study number	Total no. of patients	Sex		Race				Age		
			Male	Female	White	Black	Asian	Other[b]	Below 18	18–65	Above 65
Pharmacokinetic											
1.											
2.											
Dose-ranging											
1.											
2.											
Double-blind											
1.											
2.											
Open-label											
1.											
2.											
Long-term treatment											
1.											
2.											

[a]Multiple studies are generally listed within each category.
[b]Specify "other".

- For best presentation, study categories should be mutually exclusive.

PATIENT ACCOUNTABILITY

Illustrates tracking patients at various study milestones.

TABLE 4.12. Patient Accountability Tracking to Help Evaluate Selection

Number of patients					
Originally sought (N)	Interviewed (N)	Signed informed consents (N)	Passed screen (N)	Entered study (N)	Finished study (N)

- See Chapter 19 of *Guide to Planning and Managing Multiple Clinical Studies* (Spilker, 1987) for variations of this table.
- The percent decrease from left to right may suggest "investigator effort" at selling the concept of and need for the study.
- It would be useful to know how many of the patients who met eligibility criteria were actually sought.
- Although this table is not an accountability tool, it aids in extrapolating results.

Illustrates specific attendance of patients at scheduled evaluations in a study.

TABLE 4.13. Participation of Patients in a Study[a]

Patient number	Weekly visit appointments kept					
	1	2	3	4	5	6
1	+	○	+	+	+	+
2	○	+	+	+	○	+
3	+	+	+	+	+	+
4	+	○	○	○	+	+
5	+	+	+	○	○	○
6	+	+	+	+	+	+
7	+	+	○	○	+	+
8	+	+	+	+	○	+
9	+	+	+	+	+	○
10	+	+	+	+	+	+
11	○	○	+	+	+	+
12	+	+	○	+	○	+
Total	10	9	9	9	8	10

[a]If all patients were treated on the exact same dates, then specific dates could be given in the heading.

- Compliance with other aspects of a study could be identified (e.g., pill counts at each visit graded as percent of pills expected, maintenance of diary, satisfactory compliance—yes or no).
- Footnotes of acceptable excuses could be listed.
- Makeup sessions (if part of the study) could be indicated.

Illustrates from which analyses patients were excluded and the reasons.

TABLE 4.14. Patient Data Excluded from Efficacy Analyses

Patient number	Exclusions	Reason
1003	TAF[a] day 15	No hour 0 data for day 15
1008	all analyses	TAF > 500 at baseline
1020	day 15 weekly global	Took prohibited medications days 6–13
	posttreatment global	Took prohibited medications days 16–posttreatment
1025	TAF day 15	No hour 0 data for day 15
1041	all analyses	TAF > 500 at baseline
1070	all analyses	TAF > 500 at baseline
2016	all analyses	TAF > 500 at baseline
2018	all analyses	TAF > 500 at baseline
2020	all analyses	TAF > 500 at baseline
2053	all analyses	TAF > 500 at baseline
2066	all analyses	TAF > 500 at baseline
2070	all analyses	TAF > 500 at baseline
2073	all analyses	TAF > 500 at baseline
2076	day 1 on-site	Only had hour 0 data for day 1
	diary	Only had day 0 data for diary
3015	day 15 on-site	Only had hour 0 data for day 15
4032	day 15 on-site	Took Comtrex (prohibited medication) < 24 hr before day 15
	day 15 weekly global	Took prohibited medications days 12–15

[a]TAF, total air flow.

Illustrates identification of the basic "efficacy" and "safety" population.

TABLE 4.15. A General Accountability Table of Patients in a Study

Treatment group	Number enrolled	Number evaluatable for efficacy	Number evaluatable for safety
Drug A	50	48	50
Drug B	47	47	47
Drug C	50	49	49
Total	147	144	146

• For multiple-site study, the above summary should be provided for each center.

• Many studies have more than one efficacy analysis (due to multiple variables and/or multiple assessments). In this type of accountability presentation, a patient is considered to be evaluatable for efficacy if he or she is evaluatable for at least one of those analyses. By this convention, some patients may be evaluatable for efficacy even if they are prematurely discontinued from the study.

• Except for rare instances, the number of patients evaluatable for safety is the same as the total number of patients enrolled. Exceptions include (1) patients entered more than once in the same study (only first exposure is formally analyzed), (2) patients who have no observations following administration of study drug, and (3) patients discontinued or dropped out before receiving any doses.

• This summary is often accompanied by one or more tables listing nonevaluatable patients and stating why they are not evaluatable (e.g., Tables 4.14, 4.16, and 4.17).

Illustrates summary of reasons for exclusion from efficacy analyses by treatment groups.

TABLE 4.16. Exclusions from Analysis of Effectiveness Because of Protocol Violations

	Drug A			Drug B	
Protocol violation	40 hs	20 bid	40 bid	150 bid	Total
Concomitant drug	7	2	5	5	19
Initial endoscopy or ulcer size out of range	5	6	3	4	18
Prior surgery	1	0	1	0	2
Uncooperative patient off drug	2	4	2	4	12
Total	15	12	11	13	51

- This table is a more detailed summary of the efficacy portion of a table like 4.15.

Illustrates specific identification and data of nonevaluatable patients.

TABLE 4.17. Identification of Nonevaluatable Patients

	Drug	Patient number	Reason
Efficacy analyses	A	14	Inappropriately entered study
		25	Noncompliance
	B	10	Dropped out before receiving sufficient drug exposure
	C	23	Previously entered as patient number 2
		18	No observations postdrug
Safety analyses	C	23	Previously entered as patient number 2
		18	No observations postdrug

Illustrates summary of patients who prematurely withdrew from a study.

TABLE 4.18. Reasons Why Patients Dropped Out of a Study on Their Own[a]

Reason for withdrawal	Number withdrawn[b]
1. Adverse drug reactions	1
2. Disease worsened	2
3. Disease improved on therapy	5
4. Personal reasons unrelated to study (e.g., moved, married)	1
5. Other—specify	1

[a]Multiple studies may be combined or presented individually in the same table.
[b]May be grouped separately for two or more treatments.

- If multiple studies are presented it may be useful to present also the percent of patients who withdrew in each category.

Illustrates summary of patients prematurely discontinued from a study.

TABLE 4.19. Reasons Why Patients Were Prematurely Discontinued from a Study

Reason	Number
1. Poor compliance with drug	
2. Poor compliance with study	
3. Adverse drug reactions	
4. Disease worsened	
5. Other—specify	

- Reasons for withdrawal are dichotomized by source—patient (Table 4.18) or investigator (Table 4.19).

Illustrates reasons for discontinuation according to study group and whether patients received drug.

TABLE 4.20. Summarization of Premature Discontinuations

	Number of patients receiving					
	Study drug		Placebo		Total	
A. *Patients who received drug* Reason	Number	Percent	Number	Percent	Number	Percent
Died						
Moved out of area						
Adverse reaction						
Concomitant illness						
Deterioration of disease						
Protocol violation by patient						
Protocol violation by staff						
Improvement of disease						
Laboratory abnormality						
Personal reasons unrelated to study						
Reason(s) not stated						
Other (list)						
Total						

B. *Patients who did not receive drug* Reason	Number of patients
Each reason is listed	
Total	

• Issue of premature discontinuations is usually of sufficient importance to also rate its own individual patient listing (Table 4.21).

• Some studies would also have a table identifying the withdrawn patients (Tables 4.21 and 4.22).

• Adverse reaction as a reason for discontinuation is important enough to be always individually identified (Tables 4.22 and 4.24).

Illustrates identification of individual reasons for premature discontinuation and duration of treatment at the time of discontinuation.

TABLE 4.21. Listing of Patients Prematurely Discontinued from Study

Patient	Highest full dosing day completed	Reason for terminating early
		Treatment = Placebo
1001	8	Did not return for treatment
2076	0	Withdrew from study
3015	14	Severe cold symptoms developed and was unable to complete study due to symptoms
3061	14	Had car trouble and could not return for treatment
		Treatment = Drug X
1002	11	Unable to continue due to new employment
1026	17	Deterioration of allergic condition
2065	8	Did not return for treatment
2055	14	Had evidence of bronchospasm and increased nasal congestion and decided to withdraw
3032	14	Intercurrent illness and/or significant personal event external to treatment situation and did not return
3043	1	Did not return for treatment
3050	16	Intercurrent illness and/or significant personal event external to treatment situation
		Treatment = Drug Y
1003	1	Did not return for treatment
3053	7	Intercurrent illness and/or significant personal event external to treatment situation

Illustrates identification of patients prematurely discontinued due to adverse reactions.

TABLE 4.22. Patients Discontinued Due to Adverse Reactions

Drug	Patient number	Age	Sex	Other relevant variable(s)	Adverse reaction	Intensity of reaction

• Other relevant variables could include: race, treatment used, and eventual outcome of adverse reaction.

• For studies being reported to the FDA, the agency is extremely interested in all premature discontinuations due to adverse reactions. These additional data, as presented in this table, are necessary for this subset of patients. The summary of Table 4.20 and the list of Table 4.21 are not sufficient by themselves.

• The clinical importance of the adverse reaction may be listed.

Illustrates study characteristics of dosing.

TABLE 4.23. Number of Unique Patients/Volunteers by Maximum Daily Dose and Treatment Duration[a]

Type	Maximum dose (mg/day)	Duration of treatment (weeks or years)							
		<1	1–4	5–8	9–12	13–26	27–52	1 yr–1.5 yr	1.5 yr–2 yr
Patient	<150	22	27	8	6	2	3	0	0
	150–299	44	235	125	32	38	14	7	3
	300–449	80	363	288	96	131	88	59	28
	450–599	13	324	317	189	362	155	123	72
	600–749	2	132	94	37	56	41	29	19
	≥750	3	79	52	28	18	6	6	4
	Total	164	1,160	884	388	607	307	224	126
Volunteer	<150	64	1	0	0	0	0	0	0
	150–299	78	0	0	0	0	0	0	0
	300–449	17	0	0	0	0	0	0	0
	450–599	0	0	1	0	0	0	0	0
	600–749	0	0	0	0	0	0	0	0
	≥750	0	0	4	0	0	0	0	0
	Total	159	1	5	0	0	0	0	0

Type	Maximum dose (mg/day)	Duration of treatment (years)							
		2–2.5	2.5–3	3–3.5	3.5–4	4–4.5	4.5–5	Over 5	Total
Patient	<150	0	0	0	0	0	0	0	68
	150–299	0	0	1	1	0	0	0	500
	300–449	12	14	12	7	10	0	1	1,189
	450–599	47	30	12	9	6	3	2	1,664
	600–749	11	19	11	6	7	4	5	473
	≥750	4	1	2	1	0	0	0	204
	Total	74	64	38	24	23	7	8	4,098
Volunteer	<150	0	0	0	0	0	0	0	65
	150–299	0	0	0	0	0	0	0	78
	300–449	0	0	0	0	0	0	0	17
	450–599	0	0	0	0	0	0	0	1
	600–749	0	0	0	0	0	0	0	0
	≥750	0	0	0	0	0	0	0	4
	Total	0	0	0	0	0	0	0	165

[a]Treatment duration indicates the total period of treatment at any dose level.

• Duration of exposure data could be presented separately for any two or more groups based on gender, concomitant drugs, severity of illness, type of study, or other factors.

Illustrates use of codes to describe data about discontinued patients.

TABLE 4.24. Patients Discontinued Because of Adverse Reactions in the Double-Blind Treatment Period

Investigator	Drug group	Patient number	Adverse finding	Onset (Day)	Severity[a]	Relationship to test drug[a]	Patient outcome[a]
Nash	Active	1	Arrhythmia	42	2	4	1
			Headache	42	2	3	1
			Paresthesia	42	3	4	1
		5	Bradycardia	15	1	4	1
		13	Bradycardia	90	4	4	1
		35	Bradycardia	58	3	4	1
	Placebo	40	Bradycardia	70	3	4	1

[a]If space permits, it is better to write out values instead of using codes. If codes are necessary, a footnote must include definitions used.

Illustrates a classification of patients across numerous studies.

TABLE 4.25. Classification of Surgical Procedures

Type of surgical procedure[a]	Number of patients (by study number)										Total	Percent of total
	02-01	03-01	03-02	05-01	06-01	06-02	07-01	08-01	09-01	10-01		
Abdominal	2	0	2	0	0	2	2	18	7	13	46	9
Abdominal gynecological	19	3	0	4	2	0	1	22	5	3	59	12
Vaginal gynecological	4	1	2	0	1	0	1	11	13	7	40	8
Neurological	2	0	0	1	0	0	10	1	1	0	15	3
Orthopedic	36	8	17	29	6	15	17	17	26	21	192	39
Proctological	0	1	0	0	0	1	0	3	0	3	8	2
Urological	1	4	1	0	3	1	7	13	3	12	45	9
Vascular	0	0	0	0	1	0	0	0	0	1	2	1
Other[b]	6	8	4	6	7	3	19	15	10	5	83	17
Total	70	25	26	40	20	22	57	100	65	65	490	100

[a]Other categorizations could be used to characterize patients treated.
[b]This footnote would specify the surgeries comprising the "other" category.

Illustrates duration of dosing in different treatment groups.

TABLE 4.26. Summary Statistics for Duration of Dosing

Daily dosing frequency (Number doses/day)			Duration (days) of dosing				
Drug X	Drug Y	Number of patients	Median	Mean	SD	Min	Max
0		9	5	12	17	2	56
1 (qd)		1	1	1		1	1
2 (bid)		4	9	9	5	2	14
3 (tid)		174	121	131	89	2	303
4 (qid)		58	89	94	71	3	288
	0	4	7	7	2	4	8
	2 (bid)	5	3	6	9	1	22
	3 (tid)	89	138	135	86	2	301
	4 (qid)	30	114	123	72	12	300

Illustrates numbers of individual patients dosed for different lengths of time.

TABLE 4.27. Duration of Exposure to Clinical Trial Materials

Double-blind segment

	Number of patients	
Weeks in segment	Drug X	Drug Y
≥ 0	179	92
≥ 4[a]	163	85
≥ 16[b]	140	79
28 to 52[c]	78	44

Drug X exposure in open-label and double-blind segments

	Number of patients	
Weeks receiving drug X	Open label	Both segments
≥ 0	41	192
≥ 4[a]	34	182
≥ 16[b]	29	165
28 to 52[c]	13	98

[a]Includes all patients in indicated segment for at least 24 days.
[b]Includes all patients in indicated segment for at least 99 days.
[c]Includes all patients in indicated segment for at least 172 days.

Illustrates drug utilization by a population of patients (group data, single or multiple sites, observational data).

TABLE 4.28. Use of a Drug in a Population

Number of prescriptions dispensed[a]	Number of users	Percent of users	Cumulative percent
1			
2			
3			
4 to 6			
7 to 10			
11 to 15			
Above 15			

[a]The quantity of drug dispensed to users could be shown.

Illustrates fate of patients in a study.

TABLE 4.29. Summary Account of Patients—Combined Centers Double-Blind and Open-Label Segments

A. Double-blind segment Status	Number (%) of patients			
	Drug X			Drug Y
Total enrolled		179 (100)		92 (100)
Discontinued from study during double-blind segment		23 (13)		7 (8)
Failed to return to clinic	13 (7)[a]		1 (1)[a]	
Adverse reactions	5 (3)		3 (3)	
Intercurrent illness	2 (1)		0 (0)	
Protocol violation	2 (1)		1 (1)	
Treatment failure	1 (1)		2 (2)	
Entered open-label segment		28 (16)		13 (14)
Insufficient symptom relief	15 (9)[a]		5 (5)[a]	
Adverse reactions	9 (5)		6 (6)	
Both adverse reaction and insufficient relief	4 (2)		2 (2)	
Continued in double-blind segment		128 (72)		72 (78)

B. Open-label segment Status	Number (%) of patients	
	Open-label drug X	
Total entered		41 (100)
Discontinued from study during open-label segment		9 (22)
Adverse reaction	6 (15)[b]	
Failed to return to clinic	2 (5)	
Physical abnormality	1 (2)	
Continued in open-label segment		32 (78)

[a]Percentages based upon 179 drug X and 92 drug Y recipients, respectively.
[b]Percentages based upon 41 patients in the open-label segment.

• The use of two columns where one would suffice for each drug may be confusing to the reader. A single column per drug in parts A and B would be more clear.

Illustrates doses administered throughout a study.

TABLE 4.30. Dose Administered by Treatment Week—Combined Centers[a]

Week[b]	Study drug			Placebo		
	Mean	Median	Range	Mean	Median	Range
6						
7						
8						
9						
10						
11						
12						
13						
14						
15						
16						
17						
18						
19						
20						
21						
22						
23						
24						
25						
26						

[a]Values are expressed in mg/kg per day.
[b]Weeks 1 to 5 are baseline, 6 to 11 are dose ascension, 12 to 22 treatment, and 23 to 26 taper and posttreatment.

• Separate tables for each of the individual centers could be constructed.

Illustrates three entries in what could be a long list.

TABLE 4.31. Investigators Who Evaluated Drug X in a Specific Large Study or in Many Separate Studies

Country	Name of investigator	Title	Affiliation	Location	Type of practice
A	Smith, A.	Professor, Department Head, Gastroenterology	Big Deal U.	Megacity	Tertiary care
B	Jones, T	Gastroenterologist	Doppler Hospital	Village	Community hospital
B	Brown, C.	Internist	—	Village	Private practice

- Potential table headings include study number and number of patients enrolled on each treatment.

Illustrates relevant contributions of patients from different sites in a study.

TABLE 4.32. Table to Illustrate the Proportion of Patients from Centers Who Contributed the Most or Least Number of Patients

	Patients eligible and randomized	Patients eligible but not randomized[a]
X number of centers that contributed the most patients to a study		
Y number of centers that contributed the least number of patients to a study		

[a]Patients refused to sign the informed consent form or the physician did not offer them an option to enroll in the study.

- X and Y may be the same numbers. Specific centers may be identified.
- Other parameters may be used to qualify the numbers of patients (e.g., patients who were most ill, patients who were above 70 years of age, patients who had creatinine clearances above 1.5).

Illustrates overall characteristics of a group of studies.

TABLE 4.33. Summary of Completed Randomized, Double-Blind, Placebo-Controlled Clinical Studies Evaluating Drug X

| Study number | Patients (N)/ centers (N) | Drug dosage | | | | Results |
		Amount (mg)	Frequency (daily)	Interval (hours)	Duration (days)	
06	272/4	1, 4, 8	3	3	1	Efficacy (p<0.01 vs. placebo) demonstrated for all dosages; dose-response relationship established.
08	119/2	16	1		1	Efficacy (p<0.05 vs. placebo) demonstrated; duration of effect was 8–10 hrs.
13	60/1	8, 16	2	12	15	Efficacy (p<0.05 vs. placebo) demonstrated for both dosages; dose-response relationship apparent on Treatment Day 1; duration of effect was 8–10 hrs.
04	33/1	2	3	6	2	Support for efficacy obtained.
05	57/1	4	3	3	1	Support for efficacy obtained.
07	76/1	4	3	6	2	Support for efficacy obtained.

Illustrates characteristics of investigators who participated in a large study.

TABLE 4.34. Characteristics of General Practitioners Who Participated in a Study

	Age group (years)			Total Number (%)
	25–34	35–49	≥50	
Sex				
Male	292 (65.8)[a]	54 (12.2)	50 (11.3)	396 (89.2)
Female	42 (9.5)	5 (1.1)	1 (0.2)	48 (10.8)
Specialization				
No	206 (46.4)	23 (5.2)	19 (4.3)	248 (55.9)
Yes	128 (28.8)	36 (8.1)	32 (7.2)	196 (44.1)
Also working in hospital				
No	287 (64.6)	53 (11.9)	48 (10.8)	388 (87.4)
Yes	47 (10.6)	6 (1.4)	3 (0.7)	56 (12.6)
No. of health service practitioners[b]				
≤500	89 (20.4)	5 (1.1)	1 (0.2)	95 (21.8)
501–1000	84 (19.3)	12 (2.8)	4 (0.9)	100 (22.9)
1001–1500	89 (20.4)	15 (3.4)	4 (0.9)	108 (24.8)
≥1500	65 (14.9)	26 (6.0)	42 (9.6)	133 (30.5)
Total	334 (75.2)	59 (13.3)	51 (11.5)	444 (100)

[a]Percentages in parentheses.
[b]Missing data for eight practitioners.

- Many other characteristics could be presented.
- Decimal points of percents may also be aligned vertically to enhance clarity.

Illustrates quality of data obtained in a study.

TABLE 4.35. Quality of the Completed Forms Used in a Study (Percentages in Parentheses)

	Start	Months of study			
		3	6	9	12
Forms with:					
Serious errors	363 (9.2)	53 (1.4)	51 (1.5)	32 (1.0)	49 (1.5)
Minor errors only	915 (23.1)	646 (17.4)	485 (13.8)	326 (9.8)	314 (9.7)
No. of errors	2681 (67.7)	3023 (81.2)	2970 (84.7)	2959 (89.2)	2875 (88.8)
Total no. of forms	3959 (100)	3722 (100)	3506 (100)	3317 (100)	3238 (100)

Illustrates a method for presenting a historical perspective of various characteristics of the study population (single or multiple studies).

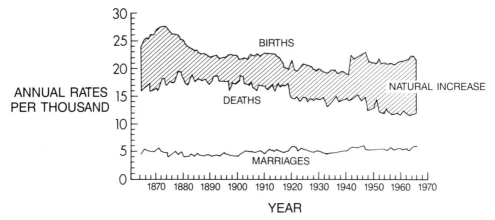

FIG. 4.1. The demographic transition in Ireland, 1864–1966. From Kosinski (1970) with permission. Based on data from the Statistical Abstract of Ireland, 1967.

• Shading between the "birth" and "death" lines emphasizes the magnitude of the population growth and allows the reader to immediately focus on the variability of that increase.

Illustrates a general pictorial presentation of data source (multiple sites).

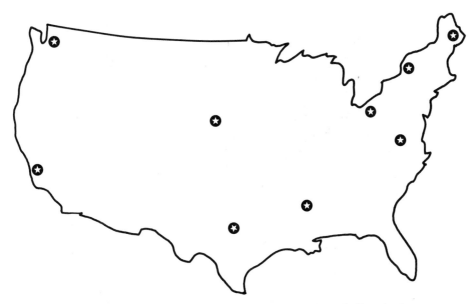

FIG. 4.2. Map of United States indicating location of all study sites.

• A map indicating the location of each study site in a multisite study may be helpful in interpretation, especially if a geographic effect is likely (e.g., in allergy studies where the type of pollen may be geographically specific).

• Different symbols (e.g., circles, stars, triangles) or colors may be used to indicate the geographic location of different patients or demographic characteristics (e.g., infants, elderly, blacks, females) of patients enrolled at each site.

• Different symbols or colors may be used to indicate different types of studies (e.g., pharmacokinetics, efficacy), phase of studies, patient populations, dosages, or other characteristics at each study site.

• Different states or counties may be marked with different hatch marks or colors to indicate different frequencies, incidences, or prevalences.

Illustrates a detailed presentation of data source (single or multiple studies).

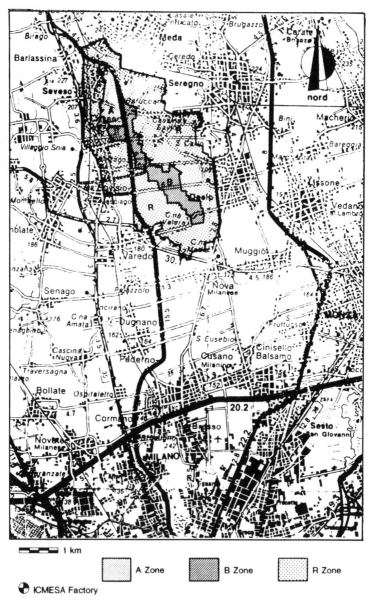

FIG. 4.3. Map shows ICMESA factory, zones contaminated by 2, 3, 7, 8-tetrachlorodibenzo-p-dioxin (TCDD) after accident on July 10, 1976, and surrounding urban areas, including Milan and Monza, Italy. A, B, and R zones refer to different TCDD concentrations in soil. Reprinted from Mocarelli et al. (1986) with permission.

• In addition to indicating "physical" location of study population, map contains additional information such as background exposure to environmental influences.

Illustrates the prevalence and location of the disease under investigation (single or multiple studies).

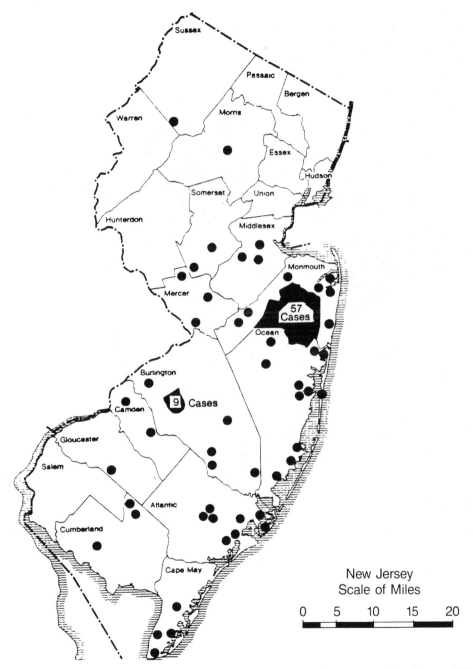

FIG. 4.4. Geographic distribution of Lyme disease by location of exposure, New Jersey, 1978 to 1982. Reprinted from Bowen et al. (1984) with permission.

• Map showing geographical distribution of condition being studied may help reader to place the results of study in proper context.

Illustrates using a grid to add more detailed information to a map.

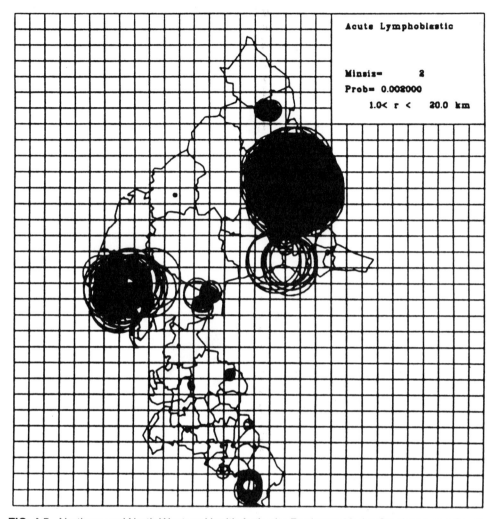

FIG. 4.5. Northern and North Western Health Authority Regions with the Southport and South Sefton Health Districts divided by local authority areas. The squares are the National Grid reference system. The circles are the 1,792 that are significant at the $p < 0.002$ level. Reprinted from Openshaw et al. (1988) with permission.

• Shows how efficacy data may be imposed on pictorial representation of study area.

Illustrates using a progressive series of maps to localize the presentation and provide a geographical perspective.

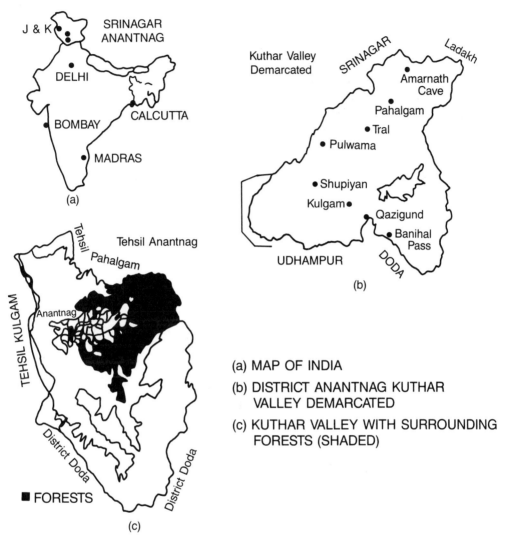

(a) MAP OF INDIA

(b) DISTRICT ANANTNAG KUTHAR VALLEY DEMARCATED

(c) KUTHAR VALLEY WITH SURROUNDING FORESTS (SHADED)

FIG. 4.6. (**a**) Map of India showing states of Jammu and Kashmir; (**b**) District Anantnag and Kuthar Valley; (**c**) Kuthar Valley with shaded area denoting forests and mountains. Reprinted from Koul et al. (1988) with permission.

Illustrates using differential shading to indicate characteristics of study population (single or multiple studies).

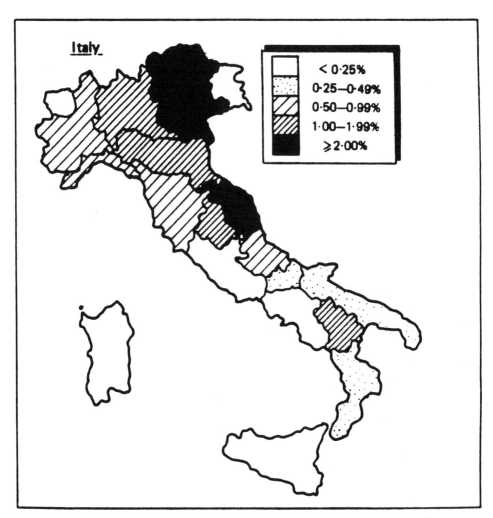

FIG. 4.7. Map of Italy showing the proportion of general practitioners in each region who participated in study. Reprinted from Avanzini et al. (1987) with permission.

• This display may be used to evaluate the representativeness of the sample.

Illustrates a method for evaluating rate of patient accrual (single or multiple sites).

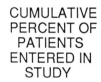
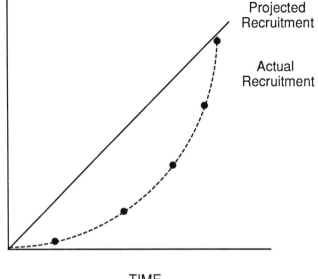

TIME

- Can calculate ratios of

$$\frac{\text{Actual time for recruitment}}{\text{Planned time for recruitment}}$$

  after study is completed

- Can calculate percent of $\quad\dfrac{\text{Actual recruitment}}{\text{Projected recruitment}}\quad$ at any time point

  during the study

FIG. 4.8. A comparison of actual and predicted patient accrual rates.

Illustrates the flow of patients through a clinical study (single or multiple sites).

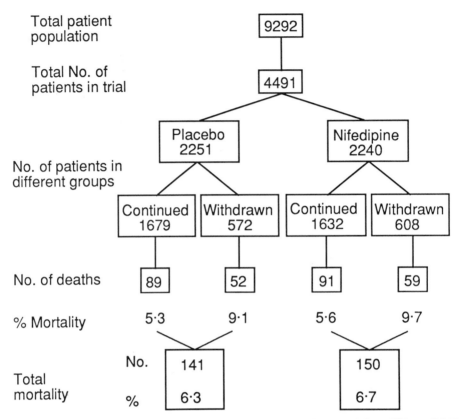

FIG. 4.9. Outcome at 28 days in patients entered for study. Reprinted from Wilcox (1986a) with permission.

- This traces the flow of patients through study.
- By reporting mortality data for withdrawn patients, this presentation helps the reader to assess the representativeness of sample.
- Reasons for death could be incorporated into this figure (e.g., cardiac or non-cardiac).
- Deaths could be divided into those in patients entered appropriately or inappropriately into the study.

Illustrates general accountability for all patients entered in a study.

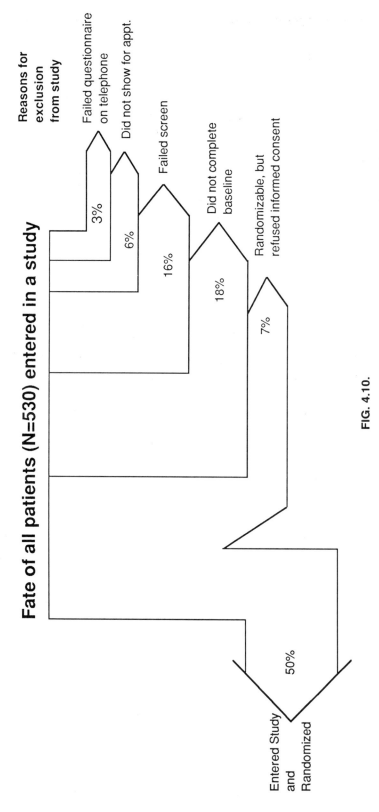

Fate of all patients (N=530) entered in a study

Reasons for exclusion from study

Failed questionnaire on telephone — 3%

Did not show for appt. — 6%

Failed screen — 16%

Did not complete baseline — 18%

Randomizable, but refused informed consent — 7%

Entered Study and Randomized — 50%

FIG. 4.10.

• For multiple site studies, a similar display should be provided for each site, and the results compared in tables, text, or figures.

Illustrates number of exposures for cases and controls for a case control study.

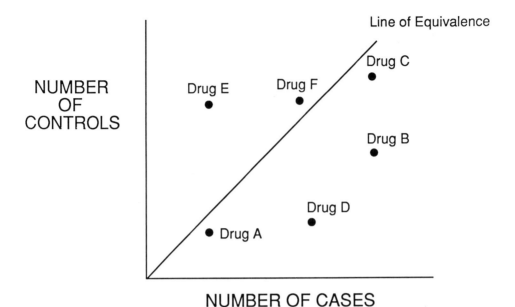

FIG. 4.11. Drug exposures of patients taking six different beta receptor antagonists.

• If the mark representing a drug lies to the right of the line of equivalence, there were more cases than controls treated with the indicated drug, and vice versa.

• Patients taking two or more drugs could be shown separately.

• Exposures to nondrugs may be illustrated.

• Adverse reactions may be illustrated, where each point is a different adverse reaction.

• Percents of cases and controls may be illustrated.

Illustrates clinic visits missed by patients in a study.

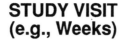

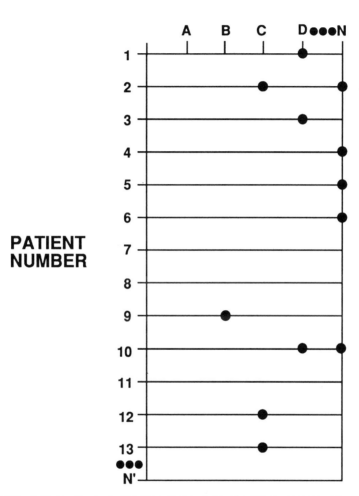

FIG. 4.12. A grid to illustrate the time that individual patients remained in a study.

• This could be easily modified to illustrate clinic visits attended.

• Time points A to N would represent specific days, weeks, or months in which patients made clinic visits.

5

Vital Signs

The universe of safety data has been divided into three chapters for ease of presentation. This chapter and the next present tables and figures used for more quantitative numerical data (e.g., vital signs, laboratory data) plus results of physical examinations and physiological tests (e.g., electrocardiograms). Chapter 7 has displays for presentation of data describing adverse reactions, which are usually obtained in terms of a patient's signs and symptoms, and are thus more subjective.

A list of commonly measured safety parameters is presented in Table 17.17 of *Guide to Clinical Studies and Developing Protocols* (Spilker, 1984). There is not always a clear distinction between safety and efficacy data, i.e., some data may be collected to assess both safety and efficacy. In addition, a number of parameters may be measured as safety data in one study and as efficacy data in another study. Blood pressure is an excellent example of this, but most safety parameters could be viewed as efficacy parameters in certain contexts.

VITAL SIGNS

Most tables of vital sign data in this chapter present blood pressure or heart rate data. Data on respiration rate or temperature could be similarly presented. Table 5.1 provides a sample listing that is appropriate for small studies and Tables 5.2 to 5.7 address mean effects. Tables 5.8 to 5.17 focus on individual values. Tables 5.18 to 5.25 display electrocardiographic data and the final two tables (Tables 5.26 and 5.27) present physical examination data. The eight figures depict ways of presenting vital sign data.

Illustrates listing of blood pressure values appropriate for small studies (individual patient data, single site or study).

TABLE 5.1. Diastolic Blood Pressure Values

Patient no.	Sex	Age	Days 25 to 34			Days 35 to 48		
			Baseline value	Period value	Diff.	Baseline value	Period value	Diff.
1	F	63	103	106	3	103	102	−1
4	F	33	96	86	−10	96	90	−6
5	M	63						
6	F	40	96	84	−12	96	76	−20
8	F	62	103	94	−9	103	98	−5
11	M	28	102	92	−10	102	92	−10
12	F	38	100	103	3	100	97	−3
13	M	50	101	96	−5	101	94	−7
15	M	43	96	92	−4	96	85	−11
19	M	29	95	91	−4	95	94	−1
21	M	48	99	90	−9	99	80	−19
24	M	35	101	108	7			
23	F	53	101	98	−3	101	90	−11
26	F	57	101	86	−15	101	82	−19
32	F	49	112	108	−4	112	100	−12
35	M	30						
36	M	49	109	104	−5	109	94	−15
37	F	57	103	110	7	103	78	−25
40	M	49						
82	M	30						
83	F	34	103	86	−17	103	98	−5
85	F	54	96	85	−11	96	100	4

• Note: blood pressure data are used for efficacy.

• A small number of patients allows for complete listing. A bottom row giving mean values would be helpful.

• Within and/or between treatment tests could be made.

• Note that the "Baseline" column is the same for both days 25 to 34 and days 35 to 48. A better presentation might be to include the column once.

• These data are from a crossover study—patients received a different drug on days 25 to 34 than on days 35 to 48.

Illustrates summary data and statistics of vital sign data (group data, single site or study).

TABLE 5.2. Summary of Blood Pressure Data, Combined Centers[a]

	Study week[b]	Study drug			Placebo		
		N	Mean ± SE	Range	N	Mean ± SE	Range
Systolic blood pressure (mm Hg)	0						
	2						
	4						
	6						
	8						
	10						
	12						
	15						
	18						
	21						
	24						
	25						
	26						
Diastolic blood pressure (mm Hg)	0						
	2						
	4						
	6						
	8						
	10						
	12						
	15						
	18						
	21						
	24						
	25						
	26						

[a]A similar table would be constructed for pulse rate, respiration rate, temperature, and body weight. Body weights are often presented separately for patients 2 to 11 years and 12 to 18 years (ages are determined at week 0). Separate tables for each of the individual centers could be constructed.
[b]Weeks 0 to 5 are baseline, 6 to 22 are drug treatment, 23 to 26 are taper and posttreatment.

• Presentation would be improved if median values were also included.

Illustrates a method for presenting within-treatment analyses of vital sign data (group data, single site or study).

TABLE 5.3. Blood Pressure—Within-Treatment Group Changes—Combined Centers[a]

| | | Study drug | | | | Placebo | | | | |
| | | | | Change score ANOVA[e] | | | | | Change score ANOVA[e] | |
Study week[b]	N[c]	Treatment mean ± SE	Baseline mean ± SE[d]	Estimated difference[f]	p value[g]	N	Treatment mean ± SE	Baseline mean ± SE	Estimated difference[f]	p value[g]
Systolic blood pressure (mm Hg)										
6										
7										
8										
9										
10										
11										
12										
13										
15										
18										
21										
24										
Diastolic blood pressure (mm Hg)										
6										
7										
8										
9										
10										
11										
12										
13										
15										
18										
21										
24										

[a]A similar table could be prepared for each vital sign and body weight group. Separate tables for each center in a multicenter study could be constructed.

[b]In other studies this column could represent hours postdose or other time measurements.

[c]N, number of patients evaluated each week in the study drug (or placebo) group.

[d]Baseline mean ± SE is based on the baseline measurement at week 5 or last baseline visit. For each study week, baseline summary is calculated using only the patients who are present at that week.

[e]ANOVA, Analysis of Variance.

[f]Treatment week 7 or 8, etc. minus baseline.

[g]Two-sided test.

Illustrates method for presenting between-treatment analyses of vital sign data (group data, single site or study).

TABLE 5.4. Blood Pressure—Between-Treatment Group Changes—Combined Centers[a]

		Treatment minus baseline[b]				Between treatment analysis[c]	
		Study drug		Placebo			
	Study week	N	Mean ± SE	N	Mean ± SE	Mean diff. ± SE	p value[d]
Systolic blood pressure	6						
	7						
	8						
	9						
	10						
	11						
	12						
	13						
	15						
	18						
	21						
	24						
Diastolic blood pressure	6						
	7						
	8						
	9						
	10						
	11						
	12						
	13						
	15						
	18						
	21						
	24						

[a]A similar table could be constructed for each vital sign and body weight group. Separate tables for each site in the multicentered study could be constructed.

[b]These data could also be presented as baseline *minus* treatment.

[c]Between treatment = (mean treatment *minus* baseline for study drug group) minus (mean treatment *minus* baseline, for placebo group).

[d]Two-sided test.

• Choice of presenting treatment minus baseline or baseline minus treatment is usually made so that entries in the table's body are positive.

Illustrates within-treatment changes of vital sign data presented in a format amenable to also presenting results of between-treatment comparisons (group data, multiple sites or studies).

TABLE 5.5. Pretreatment and Treatment Summary Statistics for Week 4 (Days 25–33) Blood Pressure (Diastolic Values in Recumbent Position)

Investigator	Treatment group	Number of patients	Pretreatment		Treatment		Change from pretreatment	
			Mean	Median	Mean	Median	Mean	Median
Allwood, Charles	Drug	17	100.8	99.0	91.4	95.0	−9.4	−7.0
	Placebo	16	103.2	102.5	102.1	100.5	−1.1	−2.5
	Diff.		− 2.4		− 10.7		− 8.3	
Kaplan, Norman, etc.	Drug	7	99.1	100.0	94.6	95.0	−4.5	−6.0
	Placebo	11	99.4	100.0	98.6	98.0	−0.8	−2.0
	Diff.		− 0.3		− 4.0		− 3.7	

- A final row consisting of all investigators combined would be helpful.
- p-Values for both within-treatment and between-treatment changes could be added.

Illustrates maximum changes of vital signs during a prespecified interval (group data, single site or study).

TABLE 5.6. Summary of Mean Arterial Pressure and Heart Rate at Time of Maximum Change During the First 5 Minutes After Rapid, Medium, or Slow Bolus Administration of Drug During Stable Narcotic Anesthesia

Dose (mg/kg)	Speed of drug administration[a]	N	Mean arterial pressure (% baseline)			Heart rate (% baseline)		
			Mean	SE	Range	Mean	SE	Range
0.03	Rapid	8	99.9	3.1	93–115	94.2	5.0	77–114
0.05	Rapid	9	99.3	2.8	86–111	92.7	1.3	85–98
0.07	Rapid	7	91.9	2.3	82–98	94.5	1.9	88–103
0.10	Rapid	8	94.9	2.3	88–105	87.9	4.7	72–113
0.15	Rapid	9	102.4	2.9	86–114	95.2	1.8	86–104
0.20	Rapid	9	82.2	8.8	46–120	103.7	6.1	86–141
0.25	Rapid	9	86.1	6.1	66–112	106.0	4.5	89–127
0.20	Medium	9	98.1	7.5	73–138	102.1	4.2	89–123
0.25	Medium	9	91.8	7.6	64–138	97.4	4.0	81–115
0.25	Slow	9	99.7	2.6	92–116	96.7	2.0	90–111

[a]Rapid, 5–15 sec; medium, 30 sec; slow, 60 sec.

• The reader needs to know how often the mean arterial pressure was measured during the specified 5 min period. Also, it is important that the same number of measurements be made for each patient.

• Note the presentation uses percent baseline rather than mm Hg.

• The presentation might also include median change.

Illustrates statistical analysis of blood pressure values at time of maximum change during a prespecified interval (group data, multiple sites or studies).

TABLE 5.7. Statistical Analysis of Maximum Changes in Mean Blood Pressure (BP) and Heart Rate (HR) From Preinjection (Control) Values During the First 5 Minutes After the Initial Drug X or Drug Y Bolus Dose

Drug dose (mg/kg)	Variable	N	Preinjection value			Postinjection value at time of maximum change			Paired t-test	
			Mean	SE	Range	Mean	SE	Range	Mean difference	p value[a]
Study 02										
Drug X										
0.03	BP[b]	8	74.6	4.2	61–94	70.8	4.5	55–91	− 3.8	0.2821
	HR[c]	8	76.1	4.7	62–102	70.4	4.7	56–96	− 5.8	0.0001[d]
0.04	BP	24	72.1	2.5	48–98	69.4	2.0	50–90	− 2.7	0.1094
	HR	25	67.8	2.4	57–118	65.1	2.2	51–110	− 2.8	0.0001[d]
0.05	BP	9	76.5	4.0	63–99	76.3	4.2	60–96	− 0.3	0.9105
	HR	9	65.2	1.7	56–73	64.2	1.7	57–74	1.0	0.4117
0.08	BP	9	79.8	3.1	65–93	78.3	2.9	66–91	− 1.6	0.3849
	HR	8	68.5	3.0	60–84	69.4	3.3	58–82	0.9	0.7318
Active control										
0.10	BP	8	74.6	3.9	61–95	87.7	4.5	66–110	13.1	0.0001[d]
	HR	8	66.9	3.3	58–85	75.9	4.7	56–95	9.0	0.0444[d]

Study 03	Drug X										
	0.023	BP	7	80.1	4.9	71–107	74.7	4.4	62–99	− 5.5	0.0242[d]
		HR	7	71.4	4.3	58–87	69.9	4.6	53–85	− 1.6	0.6360
	0.04	BP	26	73.9	2.4	57–110	67.9	1.8	53–96	− 5.9	0.0001[d]
		HR	26	71.9	3.1	52–130	66.8	2.8	49–119	− 5.1	0.0077[d]
	0.05	BP	9	81.5	5.8	60–114	79.3	5.5	54–109	− 2.1	0.5189
		HR	9	63.3	5.2	39–85	58.0	4.7	38–81	− 5.3	0.1402
	0.06	BP	9	77.5	3.9	57–100	71.8	5.2	53–109	− 5.7	0.0220[d]
		HR	9	78.6	6.2	52–104	69.3	7.1	38–103	− 9.2	0.0043[d]
Active control											
	0.08	BP	12	73.7	4.3	59–103	82.4	3.4	69–104	8.8	0.0269[b]
		HR	12	70.2	4.8	51–105	83.8	6.1	51–126	13.7	0.0002[b]

[a]Two-sided tests.
[b]BP, mean blood pressure, expressed as mm Hg.
[c]HR, heart rate, expressed as beats/min.
[d]p<0.05.

• The paired t-test is questionable for the groups where N = 7,8,9 but probably is acceptable for N = 12 and is definitely acceptable for N = 24,25,26. A sign test may be used throughout small and large sized groups in order to always have a valid test.

Illustrates identification of patients with subjectively defined noteworthy values of vital signs (individual patient data, multiple sites or studies).

TABLE 5.8. Patients with Clinically Significant Abnormal
Blood Pressure Values During Treatment[a]

Treatment group	Patient no.	Site no.	Blood pressure value (mm Hg)	Observed at (weeks)	Related to study drug (Y, N, P, U)[b]	Action taken	Outcome
Drug	321	3	150/80	8	U	None	Improved
			140/75	22	P	Increased surveillance	Improved
	482	4	170/80	24	N	None	Improved
Placebo	214	2	100/50	10	N	None	Improved
	220	2					
	244	2					

  [a]A similar table would be constructed for each vital sign plus each body weight group. Patients' age, sex, and race could be added.
  [b]Y, definite; N, not related; P, possible; U, unknown.

• Table or text should indicate who determined clinical significance (investigator or sponsor).

Illustrates summary of patients with objectively defined noteworthy changes in vital signs (group data, multiple sites or studies).

TABLE 5.9. Incidence[a] of ≥20% Changes in Heart Rate or Mean Blood Pressure Following Bolus Doses of Drug X or Active Control

Study 02	Drug X (mg/kg)				Active control (mg/kg) 0.10
	0.03	0.04	0.05	0.08	
Heart rate					
≥ 20% Increase	0/8	0/25	0/9	1/8	4/8
≥ 20% Decrease	0/8	0/25	0/9	0/8	0/8
Mean blood pressure					
≥ 20% Increase	1/8	0/24	0/9	0/9	2/8
≥ 20% Decrease	0/8	2/24	0/9	0/9	0/8

Study 03	Drug X (mg/kg)				Active control (mg/kg) 0.10
	0.023	0.04	0.05	0.06	
Heart rate					
≥ 20% Increase	0/7	2/26	0/9	0/9	5/12
≥ 20% Decrease	0/7	2/26	1/9	3/9	0/12
Mean blood pressure					
≥ 20% Increase	1/7	0/26	0/9	0/9	5/12
≥ 20% Decrease	0/7	0/26	0/9	0/9	1/9

  [a]Ratio expresses number of patients exhibiting the indicated change/number of patients in the treatment group.

• This presentation identifies the incidence of alarming or notable changes.

• This table may be followed with a table looking at a ≥ 30% change and another ≥ 40% change, or all these changes may be combined (see next table).

Illustrates summary of objectively defined noteworthy changes of vital signs, using several definitions of noteworthy (group data, multiple sites or studies).

TABLE 5.10. Increases in Cardiovascular Parameters[a]

Parameter	Change from baseline	Total		Study A1				Study A2				Study A3			
		N^b	$\%^c$	Dose 1		Dose 2		Dose 1		Dose 2		Dose 1		Dose 2	
				N	%	N	%	N	%	N	%	N	%	N	%
Heart rate	>20%														
	>30%														
	>40%														
Systolic blood pressure	>20%														
	>30%														
	>40%														
Diastolic blood pressure	>20%														
	>30%														
	>40%														
Cardiac output	>20%														
	>30%														
	>40%														
Stroke volume	>20%														
	>30%														
	>40%														

[a]Changes for increases and decreases could be expressed in separate tables.
[b]N, number of patients with specified increases.
[c]Percentages may be based on the number of patients given that dose, or on the total number of patients exposed. The presentation should clearly indicate which denominator was used.

Illustrates a variation of Table 5.10 (group data, single site or study).

TABLE 5.11. Changes in Mean Arterial Pressure at Site 1[a]

A. Increases in mean arterial pressure

| | Total | | Initial dose (mg/kg) | | | | | | | | | |
| | | | 0.00–0.30 | | 0.36–0.40 | | 0.50 | | 0.60 | | 1.30 | |
	N[b]	%	N	%	N	%	N	%	N	%	N	%
Change ≥20%	42/560	(7.5)	31/394	(7.9)	10/125	(8.0)	1/20	(5.0)	0/20	(0)	0/1	(0)
Change ≥30%	13/560	(2.3)	9/394	(2.3)	4/125	(3.2)	0/20	(0)	0/20	(0)	0/1	(0)
Change ≥40%	7/560	(1.3)	5/394	(1.3)	2/125	(1.6)	0/20	(0)	0/20	(0)	0/1	(0)

B. Decreases in mean arterial pressure

| | Total | | 0.00–0.30 | | 0.36–0.40 | | 0.50 | | 0.60 | | 1.30 | |
	N	%	N	%	N	%	N	%	N	%	N	%
Change ≥20%	21/560	(3.8)	9/394	(2.3)	3/125	(2.4)	3/20	(15.0)	6/20	(30.0)	0/1	(0)
Change ≥30%	10/560	(1.8)	4/394	(1.0)	0/125	(0)	3/20	(15.0)	3/20	(15.0)	0/1	(0)
Change ≥40%	4/560	(0.7)	1/394	(0.3)	0/125	(0)	2/20	(10.0)	1/20	(5.0)	0/1	(0)

[a]A separate table for all sites combined could be constructed as well as tables for specific subgroups of patients. Separate tables could be constructed for changes in heart rate.

[b]N is the ratio of the number of patients with the indicated change divided by the number of patients who received the individual dose, or all doses.

Illustrates relating dose to frequency of noteworthy changes (group data, multiple sites or studies).

TABLE 5.12. Increases in Mean Arterial Pressure Above 20 Percent[a]

Study (by inhalation agent)	N	Initial dose (mg/kg)									
		0.00–0.05	0.06–0.10	0.11–0.15	0.16–0.20	0.21–0.25	0.26–0.30	0.36–0.40	0.50	0.60	1.30
02-01 (Balanced)	0/70		0/20		0/10		0/10	0/10	0/10	0/10	
03-01 (Balanced)	0/25	0/5		0/5		0/5		0/5		0/5	
03-02 (Balanced)	0/26	0/1		0/5		0/5		0/5		0/5	0/1
05-01 (Halothane)	0/39		0/4		0/10			0/9			
06-01 (Halothane)	1/20		0/20	0/5	1/5			0/5			
06-02 (Halothane)	0/22		0/5	0/6	0/5			0/6			
07-01 (Balanced)	4/30		3/20			1/5					
(Isoflurane)	5/26	1/5	2/16			2/5			0/5		
08-01 (Balanced)	1/42		0/13	1/12	0/10			0/7			
(Enflurane)	2/23		0/8	2/15							
09-01 (Balanced)	3/25		0/5	1/5		0/5		1/5	1/5		
(Enflurane)	6/40		3/21		1/10			2/9			
10-01 (Balanced)	4/25	1/10	1/10		1/5		1/5	1/5			
(Isoflurane)	4/20		3/2				0/10				
Totals	3/453	2/21	12/167	4/53	3/55	3/25	1/25	4/66	1/20	0/20	0/1

[a] A separate table could be constructed for decreases greater than 20 percent or 30, 40, or increases (decreases) greater than another percent. Changes in vital signs can be related to dose of drug.

Illustrates a listing of all vital sign values for patients with noteworthy changes in heart rate (single patient data, multiple sites or studies).

TABLE 5.13. Vital Signs for Patients with Heart Rate Changes Above 40 Percent[a]

Patient	Age	Sex	Study	Drug dose (mg/kg)	Preinjection values[b]				Postinjection values			
					Systolic pressure (mm Hg)	Diastolic pressure (mm Hg)	Mean arterial pressure (mm Hg)	Heart rate (beats/min)	Systolic pressure (mm Hg)	Diastolic pressure (mm Hg)	Mean arterial pressure (mm Hg)	Heart rate (beats/min)
32	45	Male	19-02	4	90	66	74	66	104	52	69	94
06	63	Male	18-02	7	141	90	107	100	150	90	110	60
42	38	Female	19-02	10	90	60	70	76	105	70	82	114
21	65	Female	18-02	12	131	80	97	60	120	60	80	90
55	34	Male	19-02	16	85	64	71	69	110	80	90	100

[a]Similar tables could be created for patients with heart rate changes above other specified percents or for patients with mean blood pressure changes above a specified percent.
[b]Other vital signs or parameters could also be listed.

Illustrates a listing of all data associated with changes that required treatment (individual patient data, multiple sites or studies).

TABLE 5.14. Blood Pressure Changes that Required Treatment[a]

Study no.	Patient no.	Patient age	Drug dose (mg/kg)	Patient sex[b]	Vital sign	Control value	Value at time of maximum change	Percent of control value[c]	Time from drug injection to onset of change[d] (min)	Approximate duration of maximum change[e] (min)	Action taken
02-01	18	49	0.2	M	BP: Systolic (mm Hg)	115	65	56	1.5	14	iv fluids administered
					Diastolic (mm Hg)	75	40	53	1.5	14	
					Mean (mm Hg)	88	48	55	1.5	14	
					Heart rate (No./min)	80	92	115	1.5	5.5	
09-01	51	36	0.18	F	BP: Systolic (mm Hg)	94	65	69	4.5	1.0	discontinuation of enflurane and administration of 10 mg ephedrine to increase BP
					Diastolic (mm Hg)	62	40	64	3.5	1.0	
					Mean (mm Hg)	73	48	66	3.5	1.0	
						62	58	94	2.5	0.5	
22-01	3	71	0.4	M	BP: Systolic (mm Hg)	110	80		2	8	infusion of iv fluids and discontinuation of N$_2$O
					Diastolic (mm Hg)	60	45				
					Mean (mm Hg)	77	55				
					Heart rate (No./min)	68	64				
22-01	5	77	0.4	M	BP: Systolic (mm Hg)	120	70		2	8	infusion of iv fluids, discontinuation of N$_2$O and administration of iv phenylephrine
					Diastolic (mm Hg)	55	30				
					Mean (mm Hg)	75	40				
					Heart rate (No./min)	55	50				

[a] Other vital signs or changes in other parameters that required treatment could be listed in separate tables.
[b] Other demographics could be listed in addition to or instead of age and sex.
[c] The difference could be listed.
[d] The time to maximal change could be listed in addition to or instead of this value.
[e] The approximate time to full recovery could be listed in addition to or instead of this value.

• The presentation focuses directly on effects that required intervention.
• If vital signs are measured sequentially throughout a study, one will become concerned if these types of changes appeared predominantly later on in the study (indicating a possible accumulation of drug).
• A definition of onset of change must be given.

Illustrates a method of categorizing blood pressure response as an efficacy variable (group data, multiple sites or studies).

TABLE 5.15. Patterns of Blood Pressure Response by Investigator

Investigator/ study number	Treatment	Response categories		Total number of patients
		A & B	C, D, E, F	
Allwood (7)	Drug	11	4	15
	Placebo	1	13	14
Kaplan (6)	Drug	0	3	3
	Placebo	1	8	9
Nasher (1)	Drug	9	6	15
	Placebo	2	7	9
Belts (5)	Drug	10	4	14
	Placebo	3	10	13

- The table must have a definition of the response categories.
- An "across all studies" summary would be desirable.

Illustrates a summary of blood pressure values in a study when measured as an efficacy variable (group data, single site or study).

TABLE 5.16. Antihypertensive Efficacy

Supine diastolic blood pressure responses by pretreatment values
Week: 4 (Days 25–34)
Treatment: _____
Daily dose: _____

| Supine diastolic BP (mm Hg) | Pretreatment supine diastolic response categories | | | | | Mean (standard deviation) diastolic values | | |
| | Normalized (reaching 90 mm Hg or less) | Decrease not reaching normotension | | | Total patients | Pretreatment | Treatment period | Change from pretreatment |
		10 mm Hg or more	5 to 9 mm Hg	4 mm Hg or less (or incr.)		Mean (std dev)	Mean (std dev)	Mean (std dev)
0 to 94	1	0	0	0	1	94.0 (0.00)	82.0 (0.00)	−12.0 (0.0)
95 to 105	28	3	6	14	51	99.2 (3.06)	89.5 (9.32)	− 9.7 (8.50)
106 to 115	4	1	1	3	9	110.1 (2.03)	95.4 (12.20)	−14.7 (10.66)
116 and above	0	0	0	0	0	0.0 (0.00)	0.0 (0.00)	0.0 (0.00)
Total patients	33	4	7	17	61	100.8 (4.92)	90.2 (9.89)	−10.6 (8.86)

- Blood pressure is illustrated as an efficacy variable.
- The lower limit of diastolic BP (0) in column 1 is unrealistic. It is especially "funny" since 94 mm Hg is both the lowest observed value and the upper bound of the lower range.
- Column for mean labeled "Treatment period" may be replaced by the last week on treatment or may be the mean of the entire treatment period. The heading should be appropriate.
- Statistical comparison comparing number normalized to number not normalized would be appropriate for row 2, and possibly row 3, and for total.
- This particular table is confusing and not recommended.

Illustrates the number of patients who achieved prespecified falls in blood pressure with different dosing regimens (group data, single site or study).

TABLE 5.17. Number of Patients with Diastolic Pressure Changes of Various Sizes During Constant Rate and Titrated Infusions of Drug X

Diastolic pressure change (mm Hg)	Constant rate AV 10–15	Titrated infusion rates		
		.05	5.0	10.0
+41 to +50	0	0	0	0
+31 to +40	1	1	0	0
+21 to +30	6	2	3	1
+11 to +20	47	20	57	15
+ 1 to +10	100	294	268	81
0	0	73	47	11
− 1 to −10	100	137	142	66
−11 to −20	56	6	12	16
−21 to −30	22	1	2	5
−31 to −40	4	0	0	1
−41 to −50	2	0	1	0
−51 to −60	1	0	0	0
−61 to −70	2	0	0	0
−71 to −80	0	0	0	0
−81 to −90	1	1	0	0
Totals	342	535	532	196

ELECTROCARDIOGRAMS

Illustrates a summary of quantitative electrocardiogram data (group data, single site or study).

TABLE 5.18. Summary of Electrocardiographic Data

EKG characteristic	Assessment	N	Baseline[a] mean	Week mean	Median	SD	Range
PR interval	Baseline						
	Week 1						
	Week 2						
	Posttreatment						
QRS interval[b]							
QR interval[b]							
Heart rate[b]							

[a]Baseline mean for patients evaluated at each specific time point.
[b]All time assessments would be listed for each EKG characteristic.

• Summary statistics can be expanded to include change from baseline values. An appropriate within-treatment comparison could then be made (paired t-test for large samples or a sign test for small samples). Within-treatment tests can also be made without presenting change from baseline summary statistics, but this is a less preferable method of presentation.

• Appropriate statistical tests can be used to compare treatments at each assessment time. Such comparisons could be based either on the recorded values or on changes from baseline.

• If the number of patients is reasonably small, any statistical test should be accompanied by a statement of power.

• If a large number of patients results in "over power" and most comparisons are significant even if the actual magnitude of difference is small, then this fact should be mentioned. This scenario is fairly common with EKG data measured in a large number of patients.

Illustrates a statistical analysis of quantitative electrocardiogram data (group data, single site or study).

TABLE 5.19. Statistical Analysis of Electrocardiogram Variables

Variable	Screen				Treatment				Treatment minus screen		
	N	Mean	SE	Range	N	Mean	SE	Range	N	Mean diff.	p value[a]
Drug A											
Heart rate (beats/min)	72	72.014	14.08	(47–120)	77	83.065	15.88	(55–126)	68	11.500	0.0001[b]
QRS axis (degrees)	72	46.431	33.16	(−64–95)[c]	77	47.065	31.09	(−52–96)[c]	68	−1.324	0.4133
PR interval (sec)	72	0.152	0.02	(0.096–0.200)	77	0.151	0.02	(0.116–0.208)	68	−0.002	0.3676
QRS duration (sec)	72	0.088	0.01	(0.060–0.140)	77	0.092	0.01	(0.072–0.116)	68	0.003	0.0443[b]
QT interval (sec)	72	0.374	0.07	(0.200–0.800)	77	0.357	0.03	(0.300–0.420)	68	−0.022	0.0026[b]
Drug B											
Heart rate (beats/min)	7	67.571	9.38	(55–81)	8	92.500	27.92	(54–146)	7	17.286	0.0703
QRS axis (degrees)	7	49.286	26.68	(−3–84)[c]	8	52.250	24.19	(−2–81)[c]	7	1.286	0.6472
PR interval (sec)	7	0.152	0.02	(0.096–0.200)	8	0.151	0.02	(0.116–0.208)	7	−0.010	0.0920
QRS duration (sec)	7	0.088	0.01	(0.060–0.140)	8	0.092	0.01	(0.072–0.116)	7	0.004	0.3650
QT interval (sec)	7	0.374	0.07	(0.200–0.800)	8	0.357	0.03	(0.300–0.420)	7	−0.019	0.3086

[a]Two-sided tests.
[b]p<0.05.
[c]The second number in the range is a positive number.

• Paired t-test is inappropriate for Drug B group because of small sample size. A sign test would be preferable.
• This table could be expanded to include between-treatment tests.

Illustrates the frequency of abnormal electrocardiogram values (group data, single site or study).

TABLE 5.20. Summary of Electrocardiogram Abnormalities

Treatment	Assessment	Normal EKGs		Abnormal EKGs		Treatment-emergent abnormal EKGs	
		N	%	N	%	N	%
Placebo	Baseline						
	Week 1						
	. . .						
	Week N						
Drug A	Baseline						
	. . .						
	Week N						

• Although all abnormalities are of interest, attention is usually focused on the abnormalities that are not present at baseline or any previous clinic visit.

• Abnormalities that arise during treatment are of sufficient importance that they are almost always listed in an accompanying table.

• Criteria for "identifying" abnormalities should be given to investigators (e.g., heart rate must be above 100 to be classified as sinus tachycardia). Criteria must be consistently followed throughout a study, and the same criteria *must* be used by all investigators in a multicenter study.

• Each week of the study would usually be listed. A summary row for placebo and for drug data could be shown (i.e., total of week 1 to N).

Illustrates identification of patients with electrocardiogram abnormalities during treatment (individual patient data, multiple sites or studies).

TABLE 5.21. Electrocardiographic Changes During Drug Treatment

Study number	Drug dose (mg/kg)	Patient number	Sex	Age	EKG abnormality	Minutes to onset	Duration (min)	Severity	Drug-related	Investigator comments	Treatment required
20-01	0.2[a]	8	M	46	Ventricular bigeminy	2.0	2.0	Mild	No	Related to surgeon cystoscoping and distending the bladder	Hyperventilation
20-01	0.4	14	M	26	Bradycardia	25.0	2.0	Moderate	No	Related to halothane administration	Atropine
20-02	0.2[a]	26	F	34	Bradycardia[b]	25.0	10.0	Mild	No	Related to halothane administration	Atropine
20-02	0.2[a]	28	F	62	Bradycardia	30.0	3.0	Mild	No	Related to halothane administration	Atropine
20-03	0.2[a]	30	M	42	Bradycardia	40.0	5.0	Mild	No	Related to halothane administration	Atropine

[a]Cumulative dose (two 0.10 mg/kg injections received prior to adverse experiences).
[b]Bradycardia accompanied by mild hypotension.

Illustrates treatment-emergent electrocardiogram abnormalities, as opposed to all abnormalities (individual patient data, single site or study).

TABLE 5.22. Specification of Treatment-Emergent Electrocardiogram Abnormalities[a]

Treatment	Assessment	Patient number	Abnormality
Drug A	Week 1	11	Sinus bradycardia
	Week 2	15	Ventricular tachycardia
Drug B	Week 1	31	Second degree block
	Week 2	14	Sinus bradycardia

[a]A definition of a treatment-emergent abnormality must be presented in the table or text.

• In some studies, the investigator rates severity and drug relationship of abnormalities. If available, those data should be included in this presentation.

• If any patient is discontinued due to an EKG abnormality, that fact should be indicated here.

• Patient's age, sex, concurrent drugs, and other relevant characteristics that could affect the EKG are sometimes included.

Illustrates electrocardiogram abnormalities not present at baseline (individual patient data, multiple sites or studies).

TABLE 5.23. Patients with Abnormal Electrocardiograms on Treatment but Not at Baseline

Treatment group	Patient number	Site no.	Abnormality noted[a]	Clinical significance (Y, N)[b]	Related to study drug (Y, N, P, U)[c]	Comment
Placebo	331	3	LVH	Y	N	Not on study drug
Dose A	415	4	LAH	Y	P	Consultant doubted a relationship
Dose B	711	7	RBBB	N	N	Noted in past
Dose B	712	7	LVH	N	N	Artifact due to electrode placement

[a]LAH, left anterior hemiblock; RBBB, right bundle branch block; LVH, left ventricular hypertrophy.
[b]Y, Yes; N, No.
[c]Y, definite; N, not related; P, possible; U, unknown.

• Data from multiple studies may be presented in this format if there are not too many abnormalities.

Illustrates both within- and between-treatment group electrocardiographic data (group data, single site, or study).

TABLE 5.24. Electrocardiogram Within- and Between-Treatment Comparison for Screen Versus Termination

	Number of patients at termination					
	Study drug (N = y)			Placebo (N = x)		
Screen	Normal	Abnormal	NA[a]	Normal	Abnormal	NA[a]
Normal						
Abnormal						
NA						
Total						

[a]NA, not assessed.

Illustrates how electrocardiogram data may be combined across studies (individual data, multiple sites or studies).

TABLE 5.25. Combining Safety Data Across Studies to Develop a Profile of an Adverse Reaction Using the Example of Electrocardiogram Abnormalities

Study	Proportion of patients with EKG abnormalities	Severity of abnormality	Duration of abnormality	Number of reports in study[a]	Countermeasure	Comments
A	0/17	—		0	—	On placebo
B	1/34	Mild	1 hr	2	None	Did not occur on rechallenge
C	1/40	Moderate	1 week	5	Surveillance	
D	1/14	Mild	Persistent	14	None	Occurred at baseline too
E	4/56	Severe	Unknown	14	β-blocker	See Report X
		Mild	Persistent	7	None	None
		Moderate	Unknown	2	Surveillance	None
		Moderate	1 week	5	Surveillance	None
F	2/17	Mild	Unknown	7	None	PVCs possibly associated with drug
		Moderate	Persistent	14	Surveillance	On placebo
Totals:	9/178	Mild = 4 Moderate = 4 Severe = 1	Unknown = 3 Persistent = 3 1 hr = 1 1 week = 2	Range = 2–14 Total of 70 reports in 9 patients	None = 4 Surveillance = 4 β-blocker = 1	One report issued

[a]A maximum of 14 reports for each abnormality were possible per patient in these studies (i.e., each patient's electrocardiogram was evaluated on 14 separate occasions).
• This table would be enhanced by identifying each abnormality or providing a reference to the abnormalities.
• The totals would be enhanced if the totals were given for each of the study treatments.

PHYSICAL EXAMINATIONS

Illustrates specific physical examination abnormalities (individual patient data, multiple sites or studies).

TABLE 5.26. Clinically Significant Abnormalities Noted on Physical Examination During Treatment[a]

Body system	Treatment group	Patient number	Site no.	Specific abnormality	Observed at (weeks)	Severity (M, Mo, S)[b]	Related to study drug (Y, N, P, U)[c]	Action taken
Head and neck	Drug	302	3	Gingival Hyperplasia	4	Mo	N	None
				Gingival Hyperplasia	6	Mo	P	↑ Surveillance
				Skin Rash	8	S	Y	D/C drug
	Placebo	417	4	Lymphadenopathy	6	M	U	↑ Surveillance
Respiratory	Placebo	821	8	Wheezing	10	M	U	None
				Wheezing	14	M	P	↑ Surveillance
				Wheezing	20	Mo	N	D/C other drug

[a]An evaluation should be conducted to determine which abnormalities were present during baseline.
[b]M, mild; Mo, moderate; S, severe.
[c]Y, definite; N, not related; P, possible; U, unknown.

Illustrates a summary of physical examination abnormalities (group data, single site or study).

TABLE 5.27. Physical Examinations—Overall Incidence of Baseline Versus Treatment Abnormalities[a]

	Number of patients					
	Normal baseline			Abnormal baseline		
	Norm. tr.	Abn. tr.	Total	Norm. tr.	Abn. tr.	Total
Study drug (N =)						
Placebo (N =)						
Total						

	Number of reports					
	Norm. bl.	Abn. bl.	Total	Norm. tr.	Abn. tr.	Total
Study drug (N =)						
Placebo (N =)						
Total						

[a]Data from any specialized physical examinations (e.g., neurological) would be presented separately.

Norm., normal; Abn., abnormal; tr., treatment period; bl., baseline period.

Illustrates a presentation displaying how mean values change over time (multiple patients, single or multiple studies).

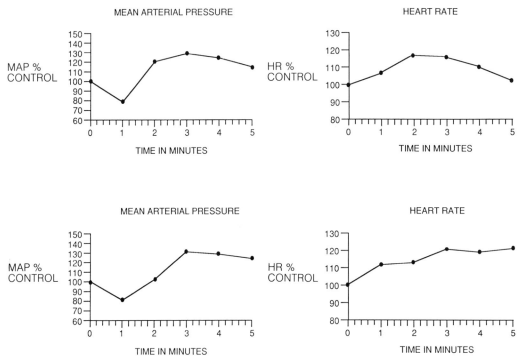

FIG. 5.1. Summary of changes in mean arterial pressure (MAP) and heart rate (HR) during first 5 min after drug administration, for two different drugs.

• Including the standard errors would allow reader to (1) observe overall variability at each assessment time and (2) verify that variability did not change over time.

• The fact that the vertical axis for MAP is 60 to 150 percent whereas the vertical axis for HR is 80 to 130 percent is potentially confusing to readers.

Illustrates superimposing aspects of the study design on mean plots in order to help interpret results (multiple patients, single or multiple sites).

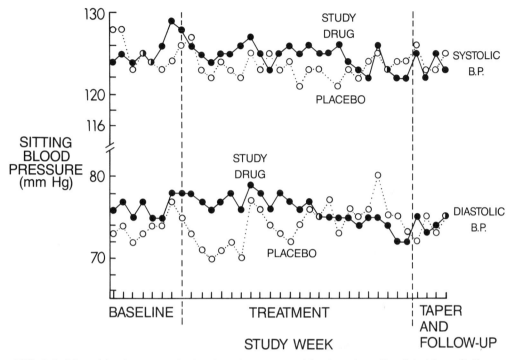

FIG. 5.2. Mean blood pressure by treatment group, combined centers. Reprinted from Spilker (1984) with permission.

• Similar graphs could be prepared to illustrate other vital signs (e.g., pulse rate, temperature).

• Similar graphs could also be prepared to illustrate changes in other parameters (e.g., body weight).

• The break in the y-axis allows both diastolic and systolic blood pressures to be displayed in the same graph.

• With this many data points (i.e., treatment group means) being plotted, the inclusion of standard error indicators would hamper interpretation.

• Units of measurement (although well-known) are specified.

• Individual center summary statistics (which are crucial for efficacy variables) are not often analyzed for safety variables.

• A summary table is often followed by a graph of mean values versus time.

• Both systolic and diastolic blood pressure can be plotted on the same axes.

• Vertical lines, arrows, or symbols "between" baseline and treatment and "between" treatment and posttreatment greatly help understanding of the graph.

**Illustrates how an individual patient's temperature changed over time
(single patient).**

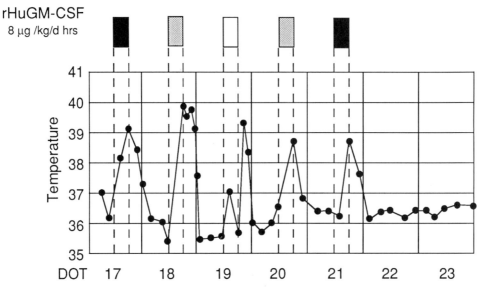

FIG. 5.3. Temperature chart for a patient given rHuGM-CSF. The chart shown is for a patient who did not receive ibuprofen. The original reference also shows a similar chart for another patient who was given ibuprofen. Reprinted from Peters et al. (1988) with permission.

- Information on dosing with rHuGM-CSF is superimposed on display.

- Presenting "side-by-side" plots of two patients (one with and the other without ibuprofen) would allow reader to interpret the effect of ibuprofen on temperature.

- Plots such as this are often used in crossover studies to visually compare a patient's responses to each drug studied.

Illustrates a scatterplot to display relationship between two variables (multiple patients, single or multiple studies).

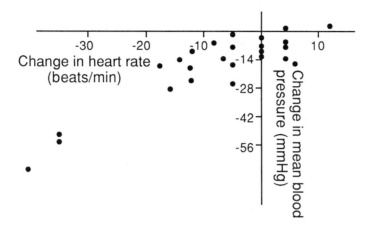

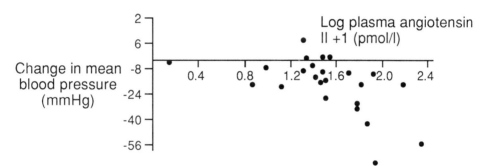

FIG. 5.4. Relation between log plasma angiotensin II value and fall in mean blood pressure and change in heart rate versus change in mean blood pressure. Reprinted from Cleland et al. (1985) with permission.

• A conversion of standard international units (SI) to traditional units of angiotensin II is usually given.

• Spearman's rank correlation may be given.

• The clarity of the ordinate in the upper graph would be enhanced if the label was printed horizontally, as in the lower graph.

Illustrates displaying a series of scatterplots to show effect of drugs on two related variables.

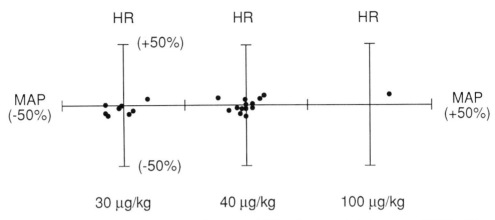

FIG. 5.5. Maximum percent change in heart rate (HR) and mean arterial pressure (MAP) within 5 min of drug administration. Each dot represents the mean of three trials for each patient.

• Individual values may be shown.
• The overall mean value may be shown with a different symbol.
• Results from multiple clinical studies may use this format with one dot per study.
• This format may be used for efficacy variables.

Illustrates physiology data-change in vital signs (individual patient).

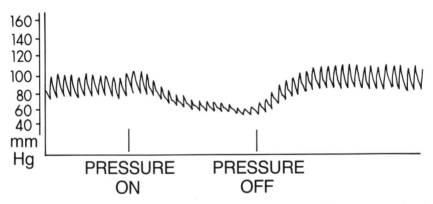

FIG. 5.6. Arterial hypotension following the application of 20 cm H_2O pressure to the airway of a patient under general anesthesia. Reprinted from Dripps et al. (1982) with permission.

• Placing units of measurement (mm Hg) at the bottom of the y-axis is confusing and detracts from the figure's appearance. Units should be placed further to the left or included in the figure legend.
• Indicating a time bar along the x-axis would be helpful.
• Hospital charts of vital sign data measured on the ward, in an intensive care unit, or during a surgical operation may be shown, in separate figures. These would illustrate a graph of multiple measured values over time.

Illustrates physiologic data (individual patient).

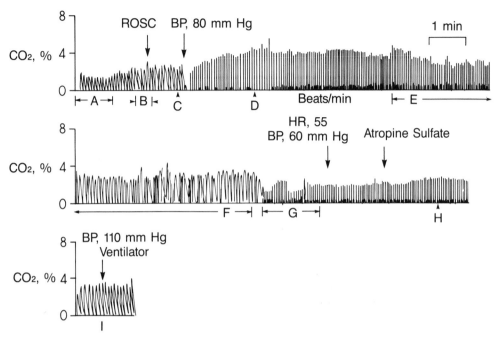

FIG. 5.7. End-tidal carbon dioxide (CO_2) recordings. Reprinted from Garnett et al. (1987) with permission.

• ROSC indicates return of spontaneous circulation; BP, blood pressure; and HR, heart rate (on monitor).

• EKG tracings or other physiologic records could be illustrated in separate figures.

Illustrates a box plot presentation of vital sign data.

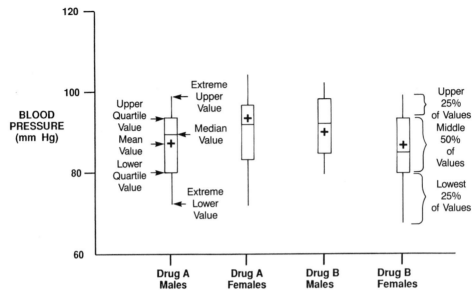

FIG. 5.8. Schematic plot of follow-up diastolic blood pressures to evaluate treatment interactions by gender.

• Another version of the box plot has tails for values within 1.5 times the length of the box. More extreme outlying values are illustrated on the graph with individual marks or symbols.

6

Laboratory Data

Laboratory data, as discussed in this chapter, are results of analytes measured in biological samples (e.g., blood, urine). Other types of laboratory data (e.g., physiological function tests, electroencephalograms, echocardiograms) are not specifically addressed. Those data are presented similarly to data in this chapter or in other chapters in this book (e.g., Chapters 5, 7).

Numerous approaches to developing and presenting summary statistics of overall and abnormal laboratory results are provided in Appendix 2 of *Guide to Clinical Studies and Developing Protocols* (Spilker, 1984). The term abnormality must be carefully defined. It is sometimes used to denote all values outside the normal range, but at other times it refers only to those values that are outside an expanded normal range or are outside the normal range by a prespecified amount.

Two ways of presenting laboratory data are to present means of groups to check for trends, and individual data to evaluate abnormalities and individual changes. Small differences between groups are often statistically significant, but are not clinically important.

SELECTED METHODS OF PRESENTING ABNORMAL LABORATORY DATA IN PUBLICATIONS OR REGULATORY SUBMISSIONS

1. Plot or tabulate the overall number of abnormalities for each parameter in each study and cumulatively for all studies.
2. Conduct subgroup analyses to determine the influence and associations of age, sex, race, and other relevant patient factors.
3. Tabulate (or plot with histograms) the number and severity of abnormalities observed with different drugs or treatments. Compare number and percent of patients on each treatment with different degrees of substantial increases above normal (and those with decreases below normal).
4. Define categories of mildly, moderately, and severely intense abnormalities and plot or tabulate the number of abnormalities in each category.
5. Cross-tabulate data based on whether the baseline laboratory value was normal or abnormally high (or low) with corresponding values obtained during treatment (normal, abnormally high, or abnormally low).
6. If multiple values were obtained, tabulate the number of patients with all values normal, those with no two successive values abnormal, or those with two or more successive abnormalities. If appropriate, further describe data in the latter group.

7. Transform data to standardized scales. If this technique is used it should be followed for all similar and appropriate studies on a drug initiated by a single sponsor.
8. Describe noteworthy abnormalities in the text, presenting sufficient details.
9. List or otherwise present laboratory values that are outside an expanded normal range.
10. List or otherwise present abnormal laboratory values stated to be possibly or probably caused by the drug.
11. Present laboratory abnormalities associated with a specific category or function (e.g., liver function tests). These analytes often do not change independently.

CLINICALLY ORIENTED TRANSFORMATIONS OF LABORATORY DATA

To aid the clinical interpretation of laboratory tests, the data are sometimes subjected to a clinically oriented data transformation. These transformations are not primarily intended to contribute to the statistical analysis of the data.

1. Each study site in a multicenter trial may use different methods to measure a laboratory analyte or have a different reference range that prevents data pooling. It is possible to set the lower point of the reference range at 0 for each analyte and the upper limit of the reference range at 100. All values would be transformed and could then be easily combined across sites (or studies).
2. Similar to the above method, data may be normalized by dividing each value by the upper limit of the normal range for the particular laboratory involved. All analytes would have a reference range up to 1.0 and all transformed values would be positive.
3. Arbitrary categories may be established to grade abnormalities. Three to five distinct groups could express increases, and the same number could express decreases. The cutoffs for each category could be established by medical experts prior to a study. The categories plus 1, plus 2, and plus 3; and minus 1, minus 2, and minus 3 could be created, or names could be associated with the categories (e.g., mildly abnormal elevation, moderately abnormal decrease, severely abnormal elevation). Because the clinical consequences of abnormal elevations and decreases are often unequal, and the range of decreases below normal is often less than possible elevations, the scales associated with each category for a single analyte need not be equal. Data could be expressed in numerous ways using this type of classification (e.g., number or percent of patients in each category, those whose categories changed on treatment).
4. A global score may be created that combines results of multiple laboratory parameters in a clinical study. One such system is presented by Sogliero-Gilbert et al. (1986).
5. Group data of laboratory results may be presented as relative frequencies of different value ranges for one or more clinical states (e.g., diseases, syndromes) or adjusted relative frequencies (Krieg et al., 1988).

The authors are *not* recommending the use of any of these (or other) clinically oriented transformations of laboratory data. Such transformations are not commonly used, primarily because interpretation of the transformed data is often more complicated. Additionally, most physicians are not familiar with these transformations and do not use them.

Each presentation of clinical laboratory data should begin with a list identifying the examinations performed, the units of measurements for each examination, and the associated normal range. An example of such a listing is given in Table 6.1. For small studies, a listing of all measurements similar to the presentation in Table 6.2 may be effective. For larger studies, however, data summarizations are required. Tables 6.3–6.7 provide suggested formats for presenting within-treatment summaries, and Table 6.8 provides a suggested format for presenting between-treatment summarizations. All of the formats for presenting within-treatment summarization could be modified to present between-treatment summarizations. The only real difference in presenting within- and between-treatment summaries is the emphasis of what is being compared. Table 6.9 is a suggested format for presenting both types of summarizations in the same table. The remaining tables in this chapter present formats for summarizing individual patient laboratory abnormalities.

Illustrates a listing of normal ranges and/or expanded normal ranges.

TABLE 6.1. Expanded Reference Range of Clinical Laboratory Values

Examination	Reference range
Blood Chemistry	
Sodium (meq/l)	128–155
Potassium (meq/l)	3.2–5.6
Chloride (meq/l)	94–155
Bicarbonate (meq/l)	16–35
Calcium (mg/dl)	7.9–13.0
Blood glucose (mg/dl)	50–160
Blood urea nitrogen (mg/dl)	2–40
Creatinine (mg/dl)	0.2–2.0
Alkaline phosphatase (m units/ml)	0–230
SGOT (units/l)	0–80
SGPT (units/l)	0–42
CPK (m units/ml)	M: 20–400 F: 17–300
Total bilirubin (mg/dl)	0–2
Total protein (g/dl)	4–11
Albumin (g/dl)	2.5–7.0
Hematology	
Hematocrit (%)	M: 28–64 F: 26–57
WBC (1,000/cu mm)	2.5–20
Hemoglobin (g/dl)	M: 9–21 F: 8–19

• A table similar to this at the start of a series of tables could alleviate the need to include normal ranges in each table.

• The terms reference range and normal range are used interchangeably in this book.

Illustrates a listing of laboratory examination values (individual patient data, single site or study).

TABLE 6.2. Values for Blood Urea Nitrogen[a]

Patient N[b]	Baseline[c]	Week of study							
		1	2	3	4	5	6	7	8
1									
2									
3									
. . .									
N									

[a]Values could be in terms of raw numbers, change from baseline in units of the laboratory analyte, or percent change above ($+$) or below ($-$) baseline.

[b]Instead of individual patients, individual clinical sites could be shown.

[c]Baseline must be carefully defined as values on a specific date, average of two or more values, or with another definition.

Illustrates within-treatment summarization (group data, single site or study).

TABLE 6.3. Within-Treatment Summary Statistics

Treatment	Parameter	Evaluation	N	Mean	Median	SD	SE	Range	p Value[a]
Drug A	Glucose	Screen							
		Week 4							
		Week 8							
	Sodium	Screen							
		Week 4							
		Week 8							

[a]p Value for test of change from screen.

• The within-treatment summary allows one to view any trend across time with each parameter.

• The order of the tests listed should have clinical meaning (e.g., liver function tests are grouped together).

• Normal ranges could be included in this presentation.

• All relevant analytes and all treatment groups would be listed.

Illustrates within-treatment summary and analyses (group data, single site or study).

TABLE 6.4. Summary of Clinical Laboratory Measurements—Screen vs. Posttreatment

		Summary statistics				Paired t-test		
		Screen		Posttreatment				
Examination	Normal range	N	Mean	N	Mean	N	Mean difference	p Value[a]
Blood chemistry								
Sodium (meq/l)	135–145	78	138.90	77	137.90	74	−1.122	0.0012[b]
Potassium (meq/l)	3.5–5.0	78	4.07	77	4.11	74	0.038	0.3267
Chloride (meq/l)	100–106	78	105.40	78	102.19	75	−3.360	0.0001[b]
Bicarbonate (meq/l)	24–30	76	23.51	76	25.91	72	2.389	0.0001[b]
Calcium (mg/100 ml)	8.5–10.5	80	9.08	79	8.82	78	−0.264	0.0001[b]
Magnesium (meq/l)	1.5–2.0	78	1.57	76	1.53	73	−0.042	0.1012
Blood glucose—fasting (mg/100 ml)	70–110	77	99.01	76	105.51	72	5.736	0.0781
BUN (mg/100 ml)	8–25	77	13.30	77	9.99	73	−3.356	0.0001[b]
Creatinine (mg/100 ml)	0.6–1.5	80	0.91	77	0.98	76	0.066	0.0004[b]
Alk phos (iu/l)	13–39	78	22.08	74	24.45	71	2.549	0.4436
SGOT (u/l)	7–27	79	16.46	78	22.59	76	6.961	0.0001[b]
SGPT (u/ml)	1–21	76	14.59	71	13.90	67	−0.373	0.7204
CPK (u/l)	M: 17–148 F: 10–79	77	110.56	77	323.08	73	225.425	0.0001[b]
Total bilirubin (mg/100 mg)	0.0–1.0	80	0.69	79	0.85	78	0.156	0.0001[b]
Total protein (g/100 ml)	6.0–8.4	80	6.27	79	5.99	78	−0.287	0.0004[b]
Albumin (g/100 ml)	3.5–5.0	78	3.81	79	3.62	77	−0.179	0.0003[b]
Globulin (g/100 ml)	2.3–3.5	78	2.47	79	2.37	77	−0.105	0.0157[b]

Hematology			N		N			
Hematocrit (%)	M: 42.0–52.0	F: 37.0–48.0	81	42.61	79	37.96	− 4.613	0.0001[b]
Hemoglobin (g/100 ml)	M: 13.0–18.0	F: 12.0–16.0	81	13.96	79	12.49	− 1.458	0.0001[b]
Total RBC (million/cu. mm)	4.2–5.9		81	4.75	79	4.23	− 0.516	0.0001[b]
MCV (cu. micron)	86–98		81	89.86	79	89.78	− 0.063	0.8266
MCH (micro microgram)	28–33		81	29.47	79	29.57	0.108	0.2705
MCHC (%)	32–36		81	32.76	79	32.93	0.167	0.1943
Total WBC (thousand/cu.mm)	4.3–10.8		81	7.28	79	8.78	1.601	0.0001[b]
Neutrophils (%)	40–75		80	62.82	79	72.29	0.679	0.0001[b]
Bands (%)	01–05		79	0.86	78	0.71	− 0.171	0.7919
Lymphocytes (%)	20–45		80	27.70	79	17.28	− 10.513	0.0001[b]
Monocytes (%)	02–10		80	7.76	78	8.22	0.372	0.4550
Eosinophils (%)	01–06		79	0.68	78	1.12	0.408	0.4101
Basophils (%)	00–01		79	0.18	77	0.32	0.147	0.1463
Urinalysis								
pH			74	6.13	69	6.32	0.177	0.3292
Specific gravity			39[c]	1.02	41	1.01	− 0.006	0.0004[b]

[a]Two-sided tests.
[b]p<0.05.
[c]Text or footnote must explain major discrepancies in numbers between different parameters; e.g., only 39 patients reported values for specific gravity.

• Separate sets of summary statistics could be presented for patients with different diseases.

Illustrates summary statistics of laboratory examinations representing significant changes (group data, multiple sites or studies).

TABLE 6.5. Significant Within-Group Changes from Baseline for Laboratory Values in a Group of Clinical Studies

| Category | Laboratory parameters[b] | Study number | Week 2[a] | | | Week 4 | | | Week 8 | | |
			I or D[c]	Change[d]	p value	I or D	Change	p value	I or D	Change	p value
I. Drug (Dose A)[e]											
II. Drug (Dose B)											
III. Drug (Dose C)											
IV. Placebo											

[a]Each time period of the study may be listed separately.
[b]Depending on the number of abnormalities reported, a separate table could be prepared for each laboratory test where significant changes were observed.
[c]I, increase; D, decrease.
[d]The units of the parameter may be listed as well as some measure of variability.
[e]A dose range may be specified.

• This display is appropriate when combining data from several studies.
• Display needs to include sample size in some form.
• Since only significant changes are included in this table, the p value column for individual time periods could be deleted.
• It would be helpful if the normal ranges for each test were listed.

Illustrates a novel variation of within-treatment summarization (group data, multiple sites or studies).

TABLE 6.6. Summary Statistics of Laboratory Analytes[a]

Study no.	Investigator	Treatment group	No. of patients[d]	Pretreatment			Week X[b]			Change from pretreatment[c]		
				Mean	Median	SD	Mean	Median	SD	Mean	Median	SD
	A	Drug[e]										
		Placebo										
		Difference										
	B	Drug										
		Placebo										
		Difference										
	C	Drug										
		Placebo										
		Difference										
	Etc.											
	Total	Drug										
		Placebo										
		Difference										

[a]Each analyte (e.g., glucose, creatinine, bilirubin) would be listed on a separate sheet and expressed in units measured.
[b]This could be an end of treatment value, average of a few weeks, or defined differently.
[c]Statistically significant differences could be indicated for (1) change from pretreatment within a group, (2) differences between treatment groups at a given time period, or (3) differences among investigators.
[d]If the number of patients is not the same at each time point, then the number of patients at each time point should be presented.
[e]Different doses or dose ranges could be presented separately for analytes which were affected by drug.

Illustrates a within-treatment summary and analysis (group data, single site or study).

TABLE 6.7. Hematology and Urinalysis Measurements—Within-Treatment Group Changes—Combined Centers[a]

| | Study drug | | | | | | | | Within-treatment change scores analysis[d] | |
| | Baseline[b] | | | Termination[c] | | | | | | |
Test	N	Mean ± SE	Range	N	Mean ± SE	Range		N	Mean ± SE	p value[e]
Hematology:										
Hemoglobin (g/dl)										
Hematocrit (%)										
Total WBC count (%/cmm)										
Neutrophils (%)										
Lymphocytes (%)										
Monocytes (%)										
Eosinophils (%)										
Basophils (%)										
Total RBC count (millions/mm²)										
MCV (fl)										
MCH (pg)										
MCHC (g/dl)										
Fibrinogen (mg/dl)										
Reticulocytes (%)										
Prothrombin time (sec)										
Partial thromboplastin time (sec)										
Urinalysis:										
Specific gravity										

Test	Placebo								
	Baseline			Termination			Within-treatment change scores analysis		
	N	Mean ± SE	Range	N	Mean ± SE	Range	N	Mean ± SE	p value
Hematology:									
Hemoglobin (g/dl)									
Hematocrit (%)									
Total WBC count (%/cmm)									
Neutrophils (%)									
Lymphocytes (%)									
Monocytes (%)									
Eosinophils (%)									
Basophils (%)									
Total RBC count (millions/mm²)									
MCV (fl)									
MCH (pg)									
MCHC (g/dl)									
Fibrinogen (mg/dl)									
Reticulocytes (%)									
Prothrombin time (sec)									
Partial thromboplastin time (sec)									
Urinalysis:									
Specific gravity									

[a]Separate tables for each of the individual centers could be constructed.
[b]Baseline, values obtained at week 5 or last baseline visit (other definitions of baseline values may be established, e.g., average of all or specific values).
[c]Termination, values obtained at last visit on study drug (other definitions of termination values may be established).
[d]Change scores, termination minus baseline.
[e]Two-tailed test.

Continued

TABLE 6.7. (Continued)

Test	Baseline			Termination[d]			Within-treatment change scores analysis[b]		
	N	Mean ± SE	Range	N	Mean ± SE	Range	N	Mean ± SE	p value[c]
Calcium (mg/dl)									
Total protein (g/dl)									
Albumin (g/dl)									
Phosphorus (mg/dl)									
Glucose (mg/dl)									
Bilirubin (mg/dl)									
BUN (mg/dl)									
Alk. phosphatase (iu/l)									
Uric Acid (mg/dl)									
LDH (iu/l)									
Cholesterol (mg/dl)									
SGOT (iu/l)									
Sodium (meq/l)									
Potassium (meq/l)									
Chloride (meq/l)									
CO_2 (meq/l)									
Creatinine (mg/dl)									
Serum Iron (µg/dl)									
TIBC (µg/dl)									

Placebo

Test	Baseline			Termination			Within-treatment change scores analysis		
	N	Mean ± SE	Range	N	Mean ± SE	Range	N	Mean ± SE	p value
Calcium (mg/dl)									
Total protein (g/dl)									
Albumin (g/dl)									
Phosphorus (mg/dl)									
Glucose (mg/dl)									
Bilirubin (mg/dl)									
BUN (mg/dl)									
Alk. phosphatase (iu/l)									
Uric acid (mg/dl)									
LDH (iu/l)									
Cholesterol (mg/dl)									
SGOT (iu/l)									
Sodium (meq/l)									
Potassium (meq/l)									
Chloride (meq/l)									
CO_2 (meq/l)									
Creatinine (mg/dl)									
Serum iron (μg/dl)									
TIBC (μg/dl)									

[a]Baseline, values obtained at week 5 or last baseline visit (other definitions of baseline values may be established). mg/dl = mg/100 ml = mg%.

[b]Change scores, termination minus baseline.

[c]Two-tail test.

[d]Termination, values obtained at last visit on study drug (other definitions of termination values may be established). Separate tables for each of the 10 centers could be constructed.

Illustrates between-treatment summary and analysis (group data, single site or study).

TABLE 6.8. Hematology and Urinalysis Measurements—Between-Test Group Changes—Combined Centers[a]

| | Treatment minus baseline[b] | | | | Between-treatment analysis[c] | |
| | Study drug | | Placebo | | | |
Test	N	Mean ± SE	N	Mean ± SE	Mean Diff. ± SE	p value[d]
Hematology:						
Hemoglobin						
Hematocrit						
Total WBC count						
Neutrophils						
Lymphocytes						
Monocytes						
Eosinophils						
Basophils						
Total RBC count						
MCV						
MCH						
MCHC						
Fibrinogen						
Reticulocytes						
Prothrombin time						
Partial thromboplastin time						
Platelet count[e]						
Urinalysis:						
Specific gravity						

[a]Separate tables could be constructed for each of the individual centers.
[b]Alternative approaches to presenting the treatment data are to (1) only list treatment data for study drug and placebo, ignoring the baseline; (2) use baseline minus treatment, especially if this will yield positive numbers; (3) adjust all treatment data for baseline using the least square means technique; (4) use the format in next table.
[c]Between-treatment = (treatment minus baseline for study drug) minus (treatment minus baseline for placebo).
[d]Two-tailed test. Ranges for each laboratory value could be provided.
[e]The terms thrombocytosis and thrombocytopenia are not used in these tables, since they refer to an interpretation of the data, which may be discussed in the text of the report.

• A similar table could be constructed for blood chemistry values.

Illustrates both within- and between-treatment analyses (group data, single site or study).

TABLE 6.9. Hematology and Urinalysis Measurements Within and Between Test Group Changes—Combined Centers[a]

Test	Treatment	Study period	N	Mean	SD	Min. value	Max. value	Normal range	Within-group p value[b]	Between-group p value[c]
Hemoglobin	Study drug	Screen								
		Posttreatment								
	Placebo	Screen								
		Posttreatment								
Other										

[a]Separate tables could be constructed for each of the individual centers.
[b]Two-tailed test comparing the study drug screen and posttreatment values (i.e., within group) with respect to change scores (i.e., posttreatment values minus screen value).
[c]Two-tailed test comparing the study drug and placebo treatment groups (i.e., between groups) with respect to change scores (i.e., study drug posttreatment minus screen value) minus (placebo posttreatment minus screen value).

Illustrates identification of laboratory examination with abnormal posttreatment means (group data, multiple sites or studies).

TABLE 6.10. Laboratory Examinations with Posttreatment Mean Value Outside of Normal Range

Examination	Study number	Normal range	Screen N	Screen Mean	Posttreatment N	Posttreatment Mean
Chloride	05-01	100–106 meq/l	39	104.33	40	99.90[a]
Bicarbonate	07-01	23–28 meq/l	31	27.42	24	29.33[a]
	07-01	23–28 meq/l	26	27.00	22	29.41[a]
Calcium	10-01	8.5–10.5 meq/l	40	9.74	40	11.27
Blood glucose	03-01	70–110 mg/dl	25	218.28	22	115.82[a]
	03-02	65–110 mg/dl	24	100.04	24	110.83
	06-01	70–110 mg/dl	20	229.40	16	136.44[a]
	06-02	65–100 mg/dl	22	116.68	21	116.52
	10-01	65–110 mg/dl	25	99.80	25	118.56
Blood urea nitrogen	02-01	8–25 mg/dl	70	12.21	69	7.84[a]
	03-02	10–20 mg/dl	25	11.08	24	8.63[a]
	07-01	10–20 mg/dl	26	15.19	22	9.05[a]
	10-01	10–20 mg/dl	25	13.96	25	9.60[a]
Total protein	06-01	6.0–8.2 g/dl	20	5.72	16	5.98
SGOT	03-02	9–28 u/l	25	35.40	24	51.17[a]
	06-02	10–30 u/l	21	39.38	21	49.38
	10-01	7.5–40 u/l	25	24.04	25	41.20[a]
SGPT	07-01	3–23 iu/l	29	30.10	26	30.38

[a]Statistically significant change from screen ($p < 0.05$, two-sided paired t-test).

- Presentation of screen is necessary so that one can judge if a "real" change has occurred. A posttreatment mean that is out of range might not be noteworthy if screening mean was also out of range.
- Mean values should be rounded off. There are too many significant figures.
- SD or SE values would be helpful.
- 95% confidence intervals would be helpful.

Illustrates the frequency of clinically important changes (group data, single site or study).

TABLE 6.11. Number of Patients with Clinically Important Changes at Weeks 6 and 12 of Treatment

Analyte	Predefined clinically important change	Week 6 (Days 35–63)	Week 12 (Days 64–98)
BUN	↑ 10 mg%	1/19	1/20
Creatinine	↑ 0.2 mg%	2/19	0/20
Bilirubin	↑ 0.5 mg%	0/19	0/20
SGOT	↑ 20 μ/ml	1/19	0/20
Alkaline phosphatase	↑ 20 units	2/19	0/20
Glucose	↑ 30 mg%	4/19	2/20
	↓ 20 mg%	0/19	0/20
Cholesterol	↑ 50 mg%	0/19	0/20
Uric acid	↑ 2.9 mg%	0/19	0/20
Sodium	↑ 5 meq/l	0/19	1/20
	↓ 5 meq/l	0/19	0/20
Potassium	↑ 0.5 meq/l	0/19	0/20
	↓ 0.5 meq/l	0/19	0/20
Chloride	↑ 5 meq/l	0/19	0/20
	↓ 5 meq/l	1/19	1/20
Hemoglobin	↑ 1.0 gm%	0/19	0/19
	↓ 1.0 gm%	1/19	0/19
Hematocrit	↑ 3.0%	1/19	1/19
	↓ 3.0%	0/19	0/19
White blood cells	↑ 2 ths/cmm	0/19	0/19
	↓ 2 ths/cmm	0/19	0/19
Platelets	↑ 60 ths/cmm	1/19	2/18
	↓ 60 ths/cmm	0/19	0/18

• The range of days should be explained in the text.

Illustrates the frequency of patient values outside of normal range (group data, single site or study).

TABLE 6.12. Abnormalities Observed During Treatment

Number of patients	Albumin	Calcium	Phosphorus	BUN	Creatinine
Above normal					
Below normal					

• "Normal" could be based on (1) real normal range, (2) approximation of normal ranges, or (3) expanded normal range.
   • This table could readily illustrate multiple sites or studies.
   • Interpretation would be enhanced by information on the total number of patients treated.

Illustrates frequency of clinically significant abnormalities (group data, single site or study).

TABLE 6.13. Overall Percent Incidence of Clinically Significant Abnormal Elevations[a] in Hematology and Urinalysis Measurements—Within-Treatment Group Changes—Combined Centers

| | Study drug | | | | | Within-treatment group analysis[e] | | |
| | Baseline[b] | | Treatment[b] | | | | | |
Test	N	% Patients[c]	% Reports[d]	N	% Patients[c]	% Reports[d]	N	p (% Pts.)	p (% Reps.)
Hematology:									
Hemoglobin									
Hematocrit									
Total WBC count									
Neutrophils									
Lymphocytes									
Monocytes									
Eosinophils									
Basophils									
Total RBC count									
MCV									
MCH									
MCHC									
Fibrinogen									
Reticulocytes									
Prothrombin time									
Partial thromboplastin time									
Urinalysis:									
Specific gravity									

Placebo

Test	Baseline			Treatment			Within-treatment group analysis		
	N	% Patients	% Reports	N	% Patients	% Reports	N	p (% Pts.)	p (% Reps.)
Hematology:									
Hemoglobin									
Hematocrit									
Total WBC count									
Neutrophils									
Lymphocytes									
Monocytes									
Eosinophils									
Basophils									
Total RBC count									
MCV									
MCH									
MCHC									
Fibrinogen									
Reticulocytes									
Prothrombin time									
Partial thromboplastin time									
Urinalysis:									
Specific gravity									

[a]The same table for "decreases" in laboratory values would be prepared. Separate tables for each of the separate centers could be constructed.

[b]Baseline, values at week 5 or last baseline visit (other definitions of baseline values may be established). Treatment, any clinically significant value while on study drug is included (other definitions of treatment values may be established).

[c]% Pts., the overall percent of all patients on study drug (or placebo) who experienced a clinically significant abnormal elevation in a specific parameter during baseline or treatment.

[d]% Reps., the overall percent of all reports on study drug (or placebo) in which a clinically significant abnormal elevation was indicated for a specific parameter during baseline or treatment.

[e]Treatment minus baseline.

• The definition of clinically significant must be clarified. It could be a value that moved outside of a pre-specified range (which could be the normal range), it could be a value that required an intervention to treat, or another definition could be used.

• Between-treatment comparisons with respect to proportion of patients experiencing a clinically significant abnormality would be meaningful.

Illustrates identification of patients with clinically significant abnormalities (single patients, multiple sites or studies).

TABLE 6.14. Patients with Clinically Significant Abnormalities in Hematological Parameters[a]

Abnormality	Treatment group (drug, placebo)	Patient number	Site number	Observed at (weeks)	Related to study drug (Y, N, P, U)[b]	Action taken[c]	Outcome
Decreased hematocrit	Drug	204	2	8	N	None	No change
				12	U	↑ Surv.	No change
				16	P	↓ Dose	Improved
	Placebo	215	2	8	Y	↓ Dose	Improved
	Placebo	331	3	12	P	None	No change
				16	P	None	No change
				24	Y	↑ Surv.	No change
Decreased hemoglobin	Drug	111	1	10	N	None	Improved

[a]The same table would be prepared for RBC morphology, blood chemistry, and urinalysis.
[b]Y, definite; N, not related; P, possible; U, unknown.
[c]↑ Surv., increase surveillance; ↓ Dose, decrease dose.

• The definition of clinically significant must be clarified. It could be a value that moved outside of a pre-specified range (which could be the normal range), it could be a value that required an intervention to treat, or another definition could be used.

• Between-treatment comparisons with respect to proportion of patients experiencing a clinically significant abnormality would be meaningful.

Illustrates frequency of clinically significant abnormalities (group data, single site or study).

TABLE 6.15. Overall Percent Incidence of Clinically Significant Abnormal Increases in Blood Chemistry Measurements—Within-Treatment Group Changes—Combined Centers[a]

	Study drug								
	Baseline			Treatment			Within-treatment change scores analysis[d]		
Test	N	% Patients[b]	% Reports	N	% Patients[b]	% Reports[c]	N	p (% Pts.)	p (% Reps.)
Calcium									
Total protein									
Albumin									
Phosphorus									
Glucose									
Bilirubin									
BUN									
Alk. phosphatase									
Uric acid									
LDH									
Cholesterol									
SGOT									
Sodium									
Potassium									
Chloride									
CO_2									
Creatinine									
Serum iron									
TIBC									

continued

TABLE 6.15. Continued

	Baseline			Study drug Treatment			Within-treatment change scores analysis[d]		
Test	N	% Patients	% Reports	N	% Patients	% Reports	N	p (% Pts.)	p (% Reps.)
Calcium									
Total protein									
Albumin									
Phosphorus									
Glucose									
Bilirubin									
BUN									
Alk. phosphatase									
Uric acid									
LDH									
Cholesterol									
Sodium									
Potassium									
Chloride									
CO2									
Creatinine									
Serum iron									
TIBC									

[a]The same table for "decreases" would be prepared. The clinical significance of an abnormal parameter was judged by the investigator. Separate tables for each of the 10 centers could be constructed.

Baseline, values at week 5 or last baseline visit (other definitions of baseline values may be established).

Treatment, any clinically significant value while on study drug is included (other definitions of treatment values may be established).

[b]% Pts., the overall percent of all patients on study drug (or placebo) who experienced a clinically significant abnormal elevation in a specific parameter during baseline or treatment.

[c]% Reps., the overall percent of all reports on study drug (or placebo) in which a clinically significant abnormal elevation was indicated for a specific parameter during baseline or treatment.

[d]Change score, treatment minus baseline.

• The definition of clinically significant must be clarified. It could be a value that moved outside of a pre-specified range (which could be the normal range), it could be a value that required an intervention to treat, or another definition could be used.

• Between-treatment comparisons with respect to proportion of patients experiencing a clinically significant abnormality would be meaningful.

Illustrates frequency of clinically significant abnormalities (group data, single site or study).

TABLE 6.15. Overall Percent Incidence of Clinically Significant Abnormal Increases in Blood Chemistry Measurements—Within-Treatment Group Changes—Combined Centers[a]

| | | | Study drug | | | | Within-treatment change scores analysis[d] | | |
| | Baseline | | | Treatment | | | | | |
Test	N	% Patients[b]	% Reports	N	% Patients[b]	% Reports[c]	N	p (% Pts.)	p (% Reps.)
Calcium									
Total protein									
Albumin									
Phosphorus									
Glucose									
Bilirubin									
BUN									
Alk. phosphatase									
Uric acid									
LDH									
Cholesterol									
SGOT									
Sodium									
Potassium									
Chloride									
CO2									
Creatinine									
Serum iron									
TIBC									

continued

TABLE 6.15. Continued

	Study drug						
	Baseline		Treatment		Within-treatment change scores analysis[d]		
Test	N	% Patients	% Reports	N	% Patients	% Reports	N	p (% Pts.)	p (% Reps.)
Calcium									
Total protein									
Albumin									
Phosphorus									
Glucose									
Bilirubin									
BUN									
Alk. phosphatase									
Uric acid									
LDH									
Cholesterol									
Sodium									
Potassium									
Chloride									
CO_2									
Creatinine									
Serum iron									
TIBC									

[a]The same table for "decreases" would be prepared. The clinical significance of an abnormal parameter was judged by the investigator. Separate tables for each of the 10 centers could be constructed.

Baseline, values at week 5 or last baseline visit (other definitions of baseline values may be established). Treatment, any clinically significant value while on study drug is included (other definitions of treatment values may be established).

[b]% Pts., the overall percent of all patients on study drug (or placebo) who experienced a clinically significant abnormal elevation in a specific parameter during baseline or treatment.

[c]% Reps., the overall percent of all reports on study drug (or placebo) in which a clinically significant abnormal elevation was indicated for a specific parameter during baseline or treatment.

[d]Change score, treatment minus baseline.

• The definition of clinically signficant must be clarified. It could be a value that moved outside of a pre-specified range (which could be the normal range), it could be a value that required an intervention to treat, or another definition could be used.

• Between-treatment comparisons with respect to proportion of patients experiencing a clinically significant abnormality would be meaningful.

Illustrates incidence of clinically significant abnormalities (group data, single site or study).

TABLE 6.16. Overall Incidence of All Reported Abnormalities in RBC Morphology[a]

| Baseline | Anisocytosis | | | | | | | | | | Poikilocytosis | | | | | | | | | |
| | Study drug treatment | | | | | Placebo treatment | | | | | Study drug treatment | | | | | Placebo treatment | | | | |
	Mild	Mod.	Marked	Sev.	N	Mild	Mod.	Marked	Sev.	N	Mild	Mod.	Marked	Sev.	N	Mild	Mod.	Marked	Sev.	N
Anisocytosis																				
Normal																				
Mild																				
Moderate																				
Marked																				
Severe																				
Poikilocytosis																				
Normal																				
Mild																				
Moderate																				
Marked																				
Severe																				

[a]Patients are entered only once in each category, under the maximal intensity observed for anisocytosis and similarly for poikilocytosis. Mod., moderate; Sev., severe; N, number of patients.

• The definition of clinically significant must be clarified. It could be a value that moved outside of a pre-specified range (which could be the normal range), it could be a value that required an intervention to treat, or another definition could be used.

• Between-treatment comparisons with respect to proportion of patients experiencing a clinically significant abnormality would be meaningful.

Illustrates a gross classification of patients based on pretreatment and treatment values (group data, single site or study).

TABLE 6.17. Summary of Patients' Laboratory Values/Changes on Drug[a]

Treatment group	Pretreatment status	Number of patients during treatment at week X[b] (or weeks X to Y) who were			
		Below normal	Normal	Above normal	Total
Drug (Low dose range)	Below normal Normal Above normal Total				
Drug (High dose range)	Below normal Normal Above normal Total				
Placebo	Below normal Normal Above normal Total				

[a]Each analyte (e.g., glucose, creatinine, bilirubin) is listed on a separate sheet. This series of charts could be prepared for each study or for combinations of studies.

[b]This part of the table must cover only one assessment or a single mean or median value, otherwise a single patient could be counted in more than one column.

• This 9-cell display for each group categorizes each patient on the basis of screen value (below, within, above normal range) and posttreatment or treatment value (below, within, above normal range).

• It displays movement out of normal range (or movement into normal range); however, the display "misses" movement which remains within normal range. This could be addressed by plotting screen value versus postvalue.

• Rather than using normal ranges to determine abnormal values, an expanded range might be more realistic.

• A rearrangement of format would allow more than one drug (or more than one patient population) to be presented on the same page.

Illustrates a gross classification of patients based on pretreatment and during treatment values, incorporating dose effects (group data, single site or study).

TABLE 6.18. Normal and Abnormal Laboratory Values (Hematocrit)

| | All doses | | Cumulative dose of drug (mg/kg) | | | | | | | | |
| | | | 0.0–0.135 | | 0.136–0.30 | | 0.31–0.50 | | 0.51–2.00 | |
	N	%	N	%	N	%	N	%	N	%
Normal screening										
Normal posttreatment	156	34	58	48	44	36	38	38	16	14
Abnormal low posttreatment	119	26	30	25	36	29	23	23	30	26
Abnormal high posttreatment	1	0	0	0	0	0	1	1	0	0
Total	276	60	88	72	80	65	62	61	46	40
Abnormal low screening										
Normal posttreatment	31	7	5	4	13	11	7	7	6	5
Abnormal low posttreatment	152	33	29	24	29	24	31	31	63	54
Abnormal high posttreatment	0	0	0	0	0	0	0	0	0	0
Total	183	40	34	28	42	34	38	38	69	59
Abnormal high screening										
Normal posttreatment	3	1	0	0	1	1	1	1	1	1
Abnormal low posttreatment	0	0	0	0	0	0	0	0	0	0
Abnormal high posttreatment	0	0	0	0	0	0	0	0	0	0
Total	3	1	0	0	1	1	1	1	1	1
Grand total	462	101	122	100	123	100	101	100	116	100

Illustrates bar graph presentation of individual patient laboratory values for a single analyte at important study milestones.

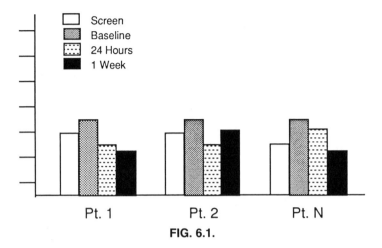

FIG. 6.1.

• The ordinate would usually show the level.

• Many variations on this presentation are possible (e.g., groups of patients, other time points, groups of analytes).

• Error measurements would sometimes be appropriate.

Illustrates using a bar graph to display individual site summary statistics for a single analyte (group data, multiple sites or studies).

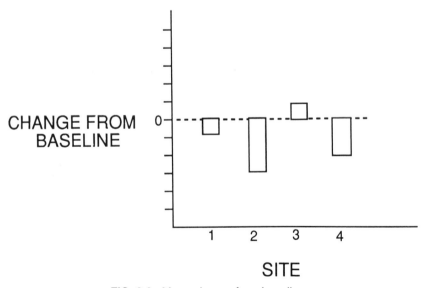

FIG. 6.2. Mean change from baseline.

• Adding standard error bars would allow comprehension of variability.

• Change could be in units or percent.

Illustrates annotating a bar graph in order to provide additional information to assist in extrapolating results.

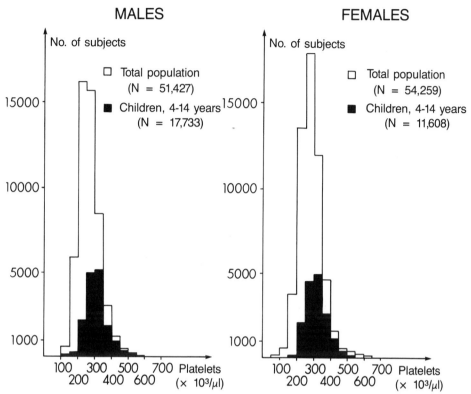

FIG. 6.3. Usual values for platelet count proposed in the literature. Reprinted from Siest et al. (1985) with permission.

Illustrates annotating a histogram with summary statistics of the data being displayed.

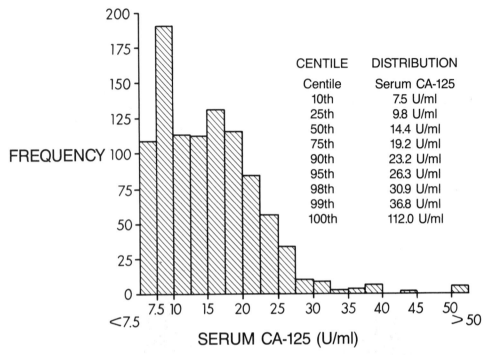

FIG. 6.4. Serum CA-125 results in the study population by 2–5 U/ml groups (N = 1010). Reprinted from Jacobs et al. (1988) with permission.

Illustrates a method for comparing two groups around a common base.

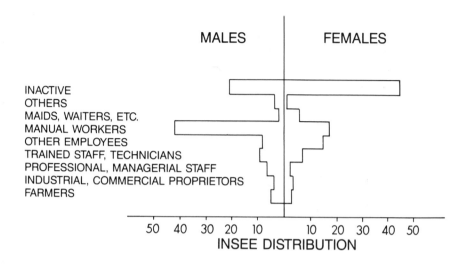

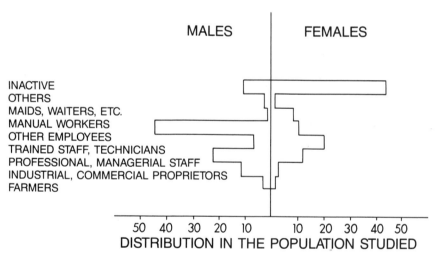

FIG. 6.5. Distribution of subjects as a function of socioprofessional category (adults). Reprinted from Siest et al. (1985) with permission.

• Degree of balance (i.e., symmetry) around vertical reference line is a measure of the "agreement" or similarity between the two groups.

• This presentation describes the population used to establish reference values for laboratory analytes.

• This format may be modified to present results of analytes for two different groups.

Illustrates same approach as preceding figure, but a scale is placed along the common base.

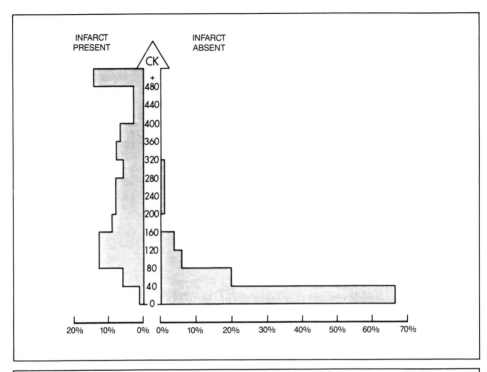

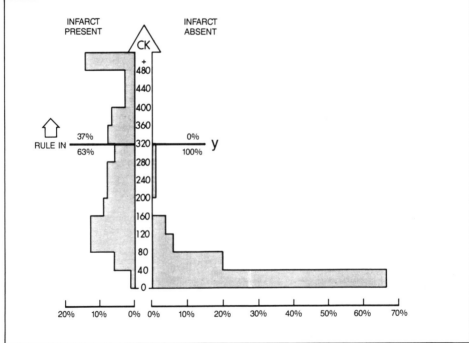

FIG. 6.6. A histogram of maximum creatinine kinase levels when myocardial infarction is present and absent. Reprinted from Sackett, Haynes and Tugwell (1985) with permission.

Illustrates histogram with bars of unequal widths and unequal categories.

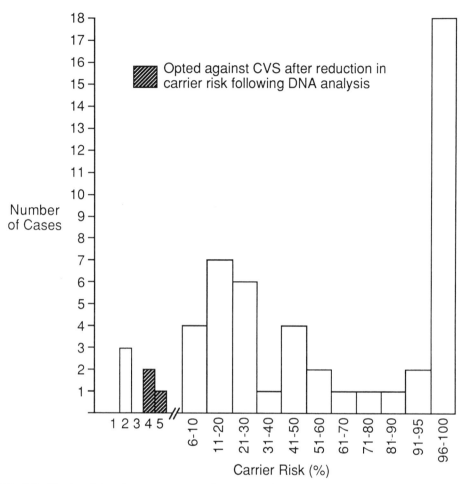

FIG. 6.7. Carrier risks of women requesting prenatal diagnosis. Reprinted from Cole et al. (1988) with permission.

- Note that the identification of some categories is placed 90° to the abscissa.
- Identification of categories at 45° is often used to indicate more categories on the abscissa.
- Clarity would be enhanced if all categories along the abscissa were equal. The hatched bar comments could be placed in the legend or text.
- Note that the first three bars represent a single percent category of carrier risk, and other bars represent categories of five or ten percent carrier risk.

Illustrates how 50%, 75%, 95%, and 100% of a population distribute.

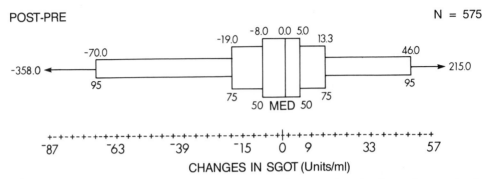

FIG. 6.8. Changes in SGOT (Units/ml) for 575 patients' posttreatment values minus pretreatment values.

- Note the following: (1) The value at "MED" is the median; (2) the middle 95% of the observations fall between the values at the "95" points; (3) the middle 75% of the observations fall between the values at the "75" points; (4) the middle 50% of the observations fall between the values at the "50" points; and (5) the extreme sample values are noted at the ends of the horizontal arrows.
- This is a variation of a box plot (see Fig. 5.8).

Illustrates a three-dimensional histogram.

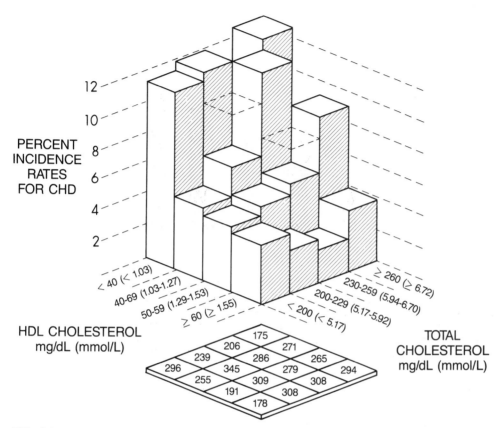

FIG. 6.9. Incidence of coronary heart disease (CHD) in 4 years by high-density lipoprotein cholesterol (HDL) and total plasma cholesterol level for men and women free of cardiovascular disease. Dashed lines indicate two bars that are hidden from view. HDL less than 40 mg/dL (< 1.03 mmol/L), total cholesterol 230 to 259 mg/dL (5.95 to 6.70 mmol/L), rate = 10.7%; HDL 40 to 49 mg/dL (1.03 to 1.27 mmol/L), total cholesterol greater than or equal to 260 mg/dL (6.72 mmol/L), rate = 6.6%. Diagram at bottom shows number of observations from combined sample that fell into each cell and were therefore at risk for CHD. Reprinted from Castelli et al. (1986) with permission.

• Note the helpful reference lines around the back two sides of the cube.

Illustrates superimposing a line representing one variable on top of a histogram displaying a related variable.

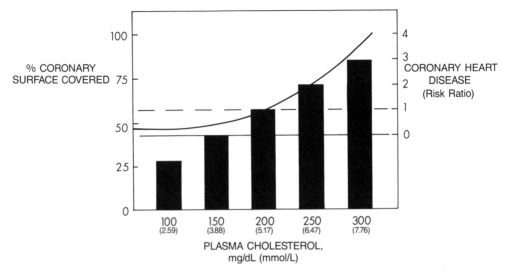

FIG. 6.10. Hypothetical relationships among plasma cholesterol levels, severity of coronary atherosclerosis, and rates of clinical coronary heart disease. This figure suggests that correlation between the plasma cholesterol level and coronary atherosclerosis is linear, but since a critical amount of atherosclerosis is required for clinical coronary heart disease, the relationship between the latter and the plasma cholesterol level is curvilinear. Reprinted from Grundy (1986) with permission.

• Could present dose-response data similarly.

Illustrates fitting a curvilinear relationship to related variables, each of which was measured in two studies.

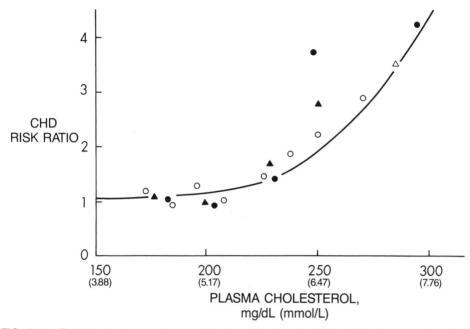

FIG. 6.11. Relation between plasma cholesterol level and relative risk of coronary heart disease (CHD) in three prospective studies: Framingham Heart Study (solid circles), Pooling Project (triangles), and Israeli prospective study (open circles). Reprinted from Grundy (1986) with permission.

Illustrates presenting comparison graphs, each comparing one variable to a related second variable.

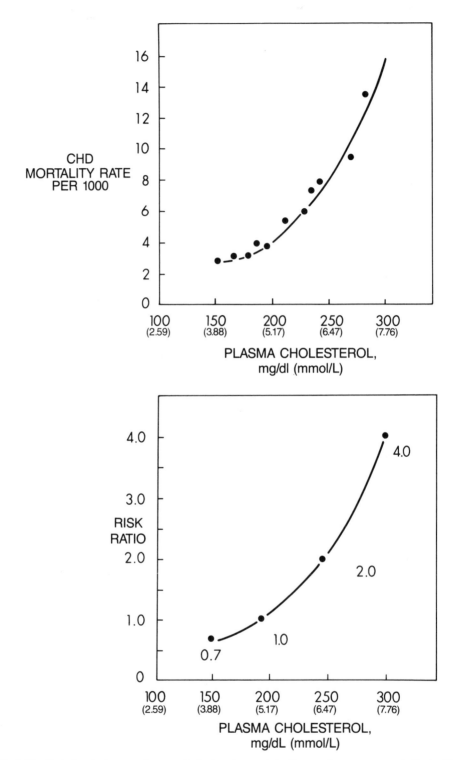

FIG. 6.12. Relation between plasma cholesterol concentration and coronary mortality in Multiple Risk Factor Intervention Trial participants. **Top**, coronary mortality for all individuals who were normotensive at screening expressed as yearly rates per 1,000. **Bottom**, coronary mortality expressed by risk ratios. Reprinted from Grundy (1986) with permission.

Illustrates plotting both percent reduction and relative reduction on same set of axes.

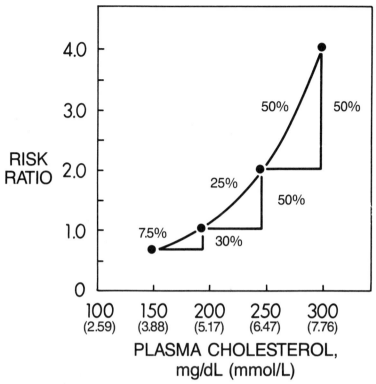

FIG. 6.13. Hypothetical effects of reduction of cholesterol levels on coronary heart disease mortality among Multiple Risk Factor Intervention Trial participants. On left is shown percentage reduction of coronary risk resulting from 50 mg/dL (1.29 mmol/L) decrease in plasma cholesterol level. On right is shown relative reduction in coronary risk resulting from 50 mg/dL (1.29 mmol/L) decrease in plasma cholesterol level as function of cholesterol level at time of identification. From the latter it can be seen that the higher the initial level of plasma cholesterol, the greater will be the absolute reduction in risk with treatment. Reprinted from Grundy (1986) with permission.

• This graph could also be considered as an efficacy presentation.

Illustrates indicating study design information on a graph of laboratory data for patients on drug or placebo.

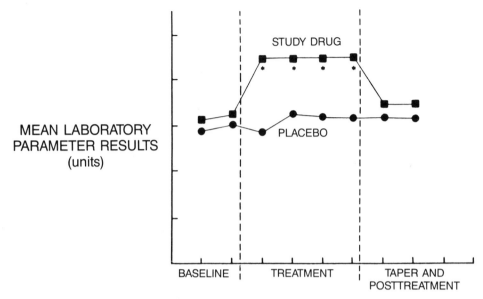

FIG. 6.14. Prototype of mean laboratory parameter results versus time by treatment group, combined centers. *$p < 0.05$, change from baseline.

- Using different symbols for drug and placebo lines is helpful.
- Asterisks indicate time where observed differences are statistically significant.

Illustrates plotting data from two studies on the same set of axes.

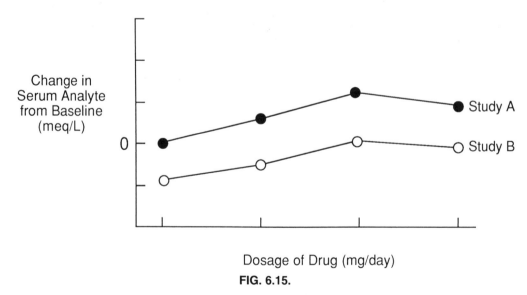

Dosage of Drug (mg/day)

FIG. 6.15.

- Different patients, formulations, routes of administration, or other factors could be similarly graphed. The percent change from baseline could be illustrated.

Illustrates plotting data from eight subgroups on the same set of axes, and providing the key to the plot within the "frame" of the plot.

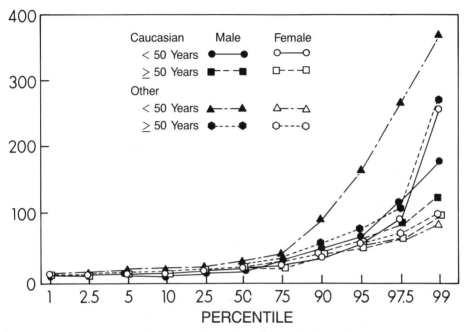

FIG. 6.16. Serum activities of gamma-glutamyltransferase for the reference sample of 5,560 patients. Reprinted from Thompson et al. (1987) with permission.

Illustrates another presentation of multiple subgroups.

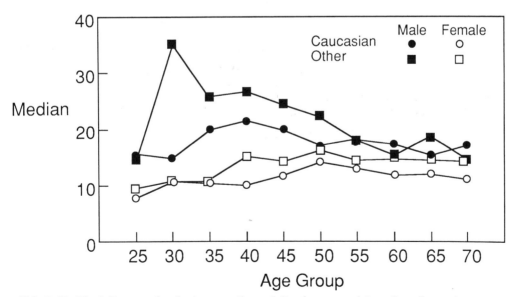

FIG. 6.17. The influence of patient age on the activity of gamma-glutamyltransferase in serum is shown for four groups of patients classified by gender and racial origin. Each point represents the median value of serum for one patient group. Reprinted from Thompson et al. (1987) with permission.

**Illustrates a vertical stack of line graphs each displaying data from a different
laboratory examination, and shading in the normal range associated with each
examination.**

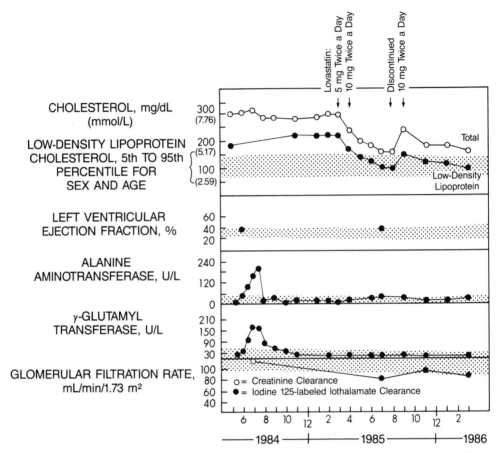

FIG. 6.18. Clinical indices since combined heart and liver transplantation in February 1984.
In July 1984, patient had episode of probable mild hepatic rejection. Lovastatin therapy was
begun in March 1985, discontinued in August 1985, and restarted in September 1986. (Stippled areas represent normal range). Reprinted from East et al. (1986) with permission.

• Note inclusion of dosing information at top of "frame."

Illustrates a method of displaying percent error of estimation techniques, also illustrates the inclusion of a horizontal reference line.

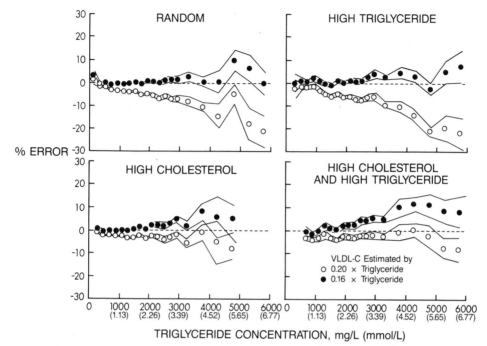

FIG. 6.19. Mean percent error of estimated low-density lipoprotein cholesterol relative to measured low-density lipoprotein cholesterol for two triglyceride coefficients (0.20 and 0.16). Data are given for random and for three hyperlipidemic recall groups. VLDL-C indicates very low-density lipoprotein cholesterol. Reprinted from DeLong et al. (1986) with permission.

Illustrates plotting normalized data, and using a vertical reference line to indicate time of dosing.

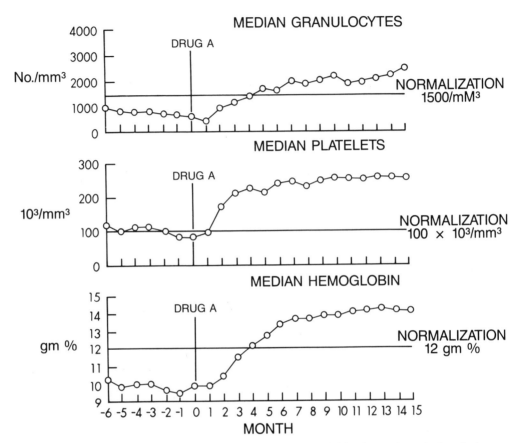

FIG. 6.20. Median values for the three hematologic variables for patients in the study.

Illustrates graphing percent of patients who have exhibited at least one abnormal laboratory value as a function of time.

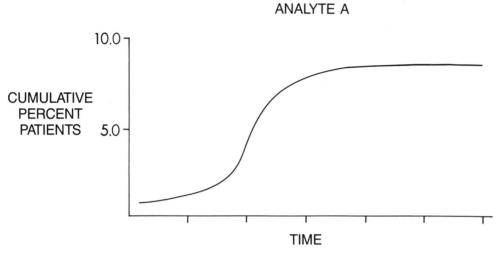

FIG. 6.21. Incidence of abnormal values for analyte A.

Illustrates plot of mean values (with variability indicators) of a laboratory examination over time.

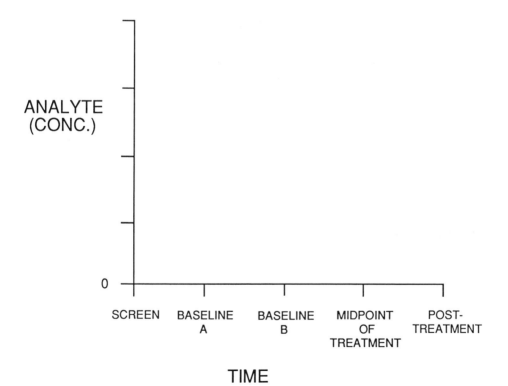

FIG. 6.22. Plot of mean concentration of analyte A versus time in study for individual patients and/or groups.

Illustrates transforming laboratory examination values to a percent change from baseline and then plotting the mean value of transformed data versus time.

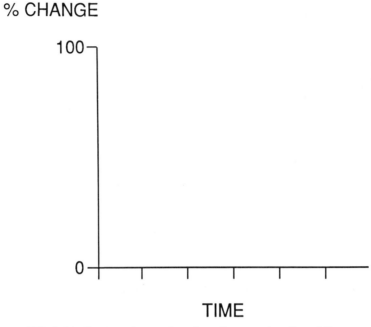

FIG. 6.23. Percent change from baseline as a function of time.

- An alternative transformation would be to use percent of baseline.
- Presenting only positive values in the ordinate implies that only increases are possible, or that absolute values are graphed.

Illustrates plotting levels of an analyte versus time.

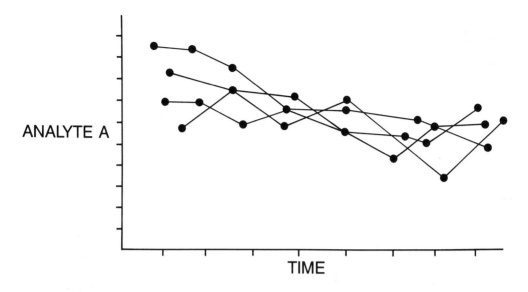

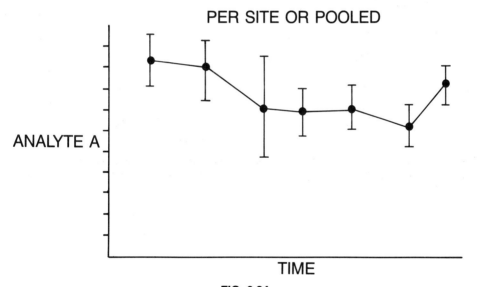

FIG. 6.24.

• Different patients' or groups' laboratory data plotted in a straightforward manner.

• Ordinate would usually be expressed in units.

Illustrates plotting three variables, each with a different y-axis scale, against a common variable.

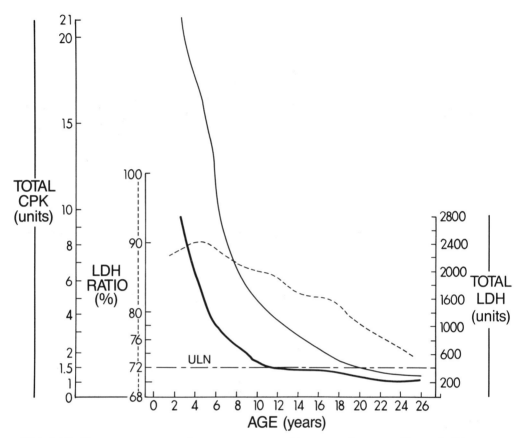

FIG. 6.25. The average curve of serum enzyme and isozyme changes with age in 76 cases of Duchenne Dystrophy (ULN, upper limit of normal). Reprinted from Hooshmand (1975) with permission.

Illustrates enhancing a scatterplot of data collected at one time period by drawing a straight line from each patient's value at that time to his/her value at a subsequent assessment.

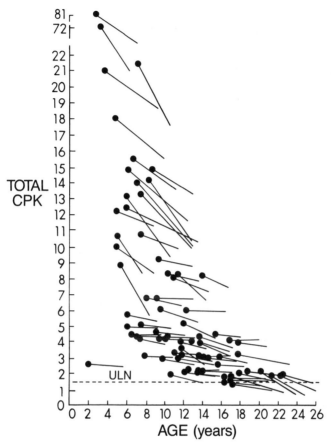

FIG. 6.26. Serial total serum CPK (Tanzer Unit). Changes in 76 cases of Duchenne Dystrophy (ULN, upper limit of normal). Reprinted from Hooshmand (1975) with permission.

Illustrates presentation of laboratory data as percent of control.

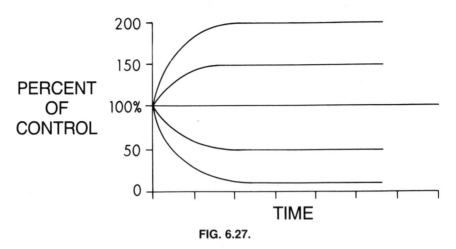

FIG. 6.27.

• Both increases and decreases may be shown.
• Each curve may be a different group of patients, a single patient for showing multiple analytes, or a single group of patients showing multiple analytes.

Illustrates false and true positives and negatives for screening level of a blood analyte.

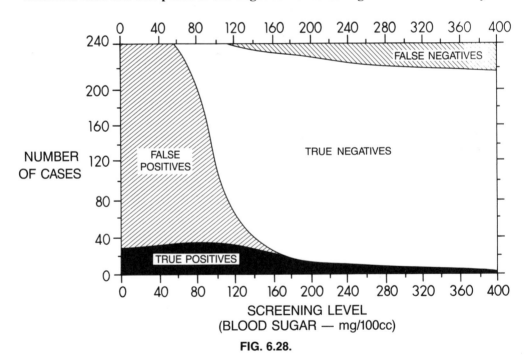

FIG. 6.28.

Illustrates use of shading to demonstrate a range of values of particular interest.

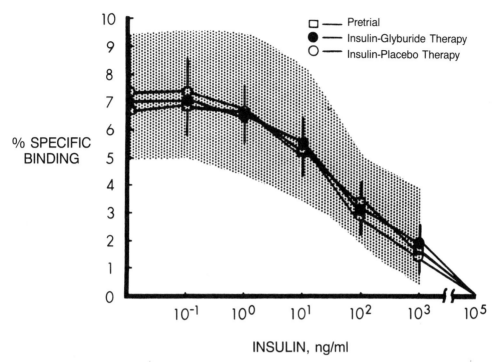

INSULIN, ng/ml

FIG. 6.29. Displacement of labeled insulin from erythrocytes in patients before initiation of study (pretrial) during 4 months of insulin-glyburide therapy, and during 4 months of insulin-placebo therapy. Shaded area is normal range (mean $\pm$ 2 SDs). Logarithmic abscissa provides concentration of unlabeled insulin added to incubation medium to displace iodine[125]-labeled insulin. One nanogram per ml is equivalent to approximately 25 μU/ml of insulin. Data are shown as mean $\pm$ SD. Reprinted from Schade et al. (1987) with permission.

Illustrates a simple scattergram of analyte results for patients receiving drug or placebo.

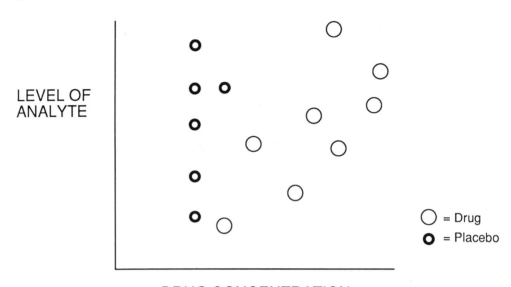

DRUG CONCENTRATION

FIG. 6.30.

• Each mark represents a separate patient.

• The level of analyte may be at the end of treatment, greatest change from control, or any other defined point.

Illustrates connecting pretreatment and posttreatment assessments on each patient in order to show the change in analytes.

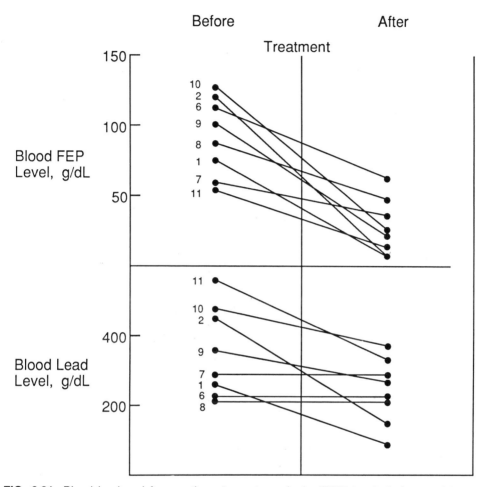

FIG. 6.31. Blood lead and free erythrocyte protoporphyrin (FEP) levels before and 3 to 5 weeks after treatment. Numbers indicate patient numbers. Reprinted from Hershko et al. (1984) with permission.

Illustrates a laboratory relationship in individual patients from two different groups.

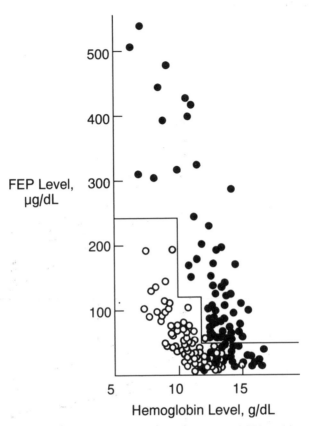

FIG. 6.32. Relation between free erythrocyte protoporphyrins (FEP) and hemoglobin levels in subjects with blood lead levels above 30 μg/dL (closed circles) and in subjects with iron deficiency defined as coexistence of serum ferritin levels less than 12 ng/mL and transferrin saturation less than 15% (open circles). The solid line shows that all but one of 41 patients with normal hemoglobin (i.e., above 12 g/dL) and an FEP above 50 μg/dL had increased lead burdens. All patients with mild anemia (hemoglobin 10 to 12 g/dL) and moderate anemia (hemoglobin less than 10 g/dL) with FEP levels above 120 and 240 μg/dL, respectively, had lead poisoning. Reprinted from Hershko et al. (1984) with permission.

• The solid line emphasizes the conclusion drawn from the data.

Illustrates adding linear regression line to a scatterplot.

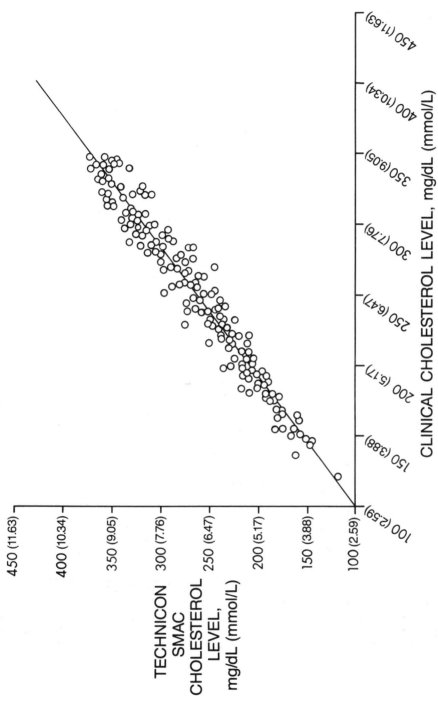

FIG. 6.33. Linear regression of cholesterol results on Technicon SMAC and Lipid Research Clinics-standardized cholesterol method. N = 377, slope = 1.0798, intercept = −5.9866, STD error regression = 8.0129, and R^2 = 0.9510. Reprinted from Blank et al. (1986) with permission.

Illustrates a series of data transformations.

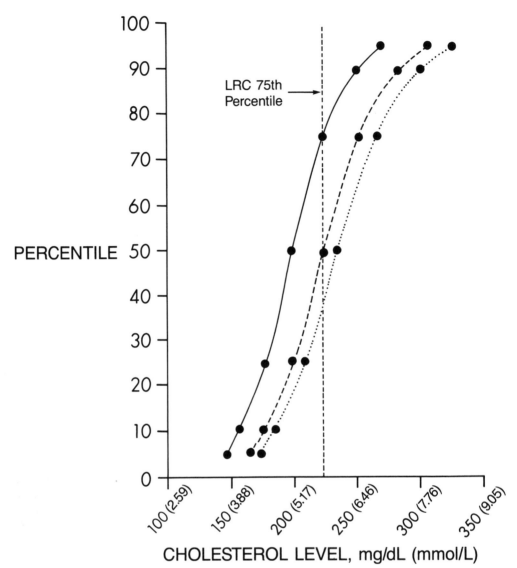

FIG. 6.34. Lipid Research Clinics (LRC) cumulative data for cholesterol values of white men 35 to 39 years old. **Solid curve** is LRC method results; **dash curve**, transformation of LRC to Technicon SMAC; and **dotted curve**, transformation of LRC to Du Pont *aca*. **Vertical dashed line** delineates 75th percentile as defined by original LRC curve. Reprinted from Blank et al. (1986) with permission.

Illustrates "cross-hatching" a scatterplot with the normal ranges.

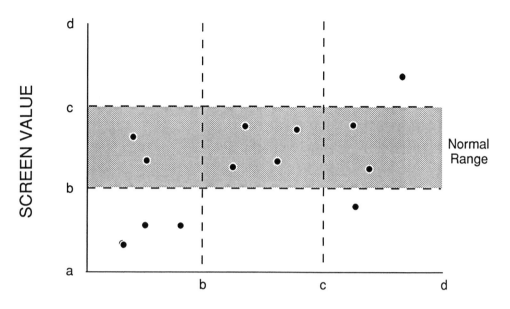

POSTTREATMENT VALUES

FIG. 6.35. Cross classification of baseline and posttreatment values.

- A separate graph is needed for each laboratory analyte.
- Values may be transformed prior to graphing.

Illustrates a 45° reference line (i.e., the line of equivalence).

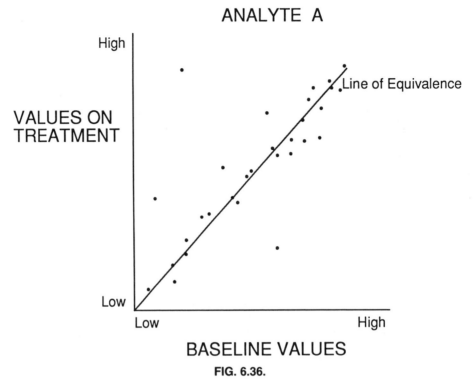

FIG. 6.36.

• The number of values above and below the line of equivalence may be compared, as well as their distance from the line.

Illustrates whether patients' laboratory results were within the normal range on baseline and on treatment.

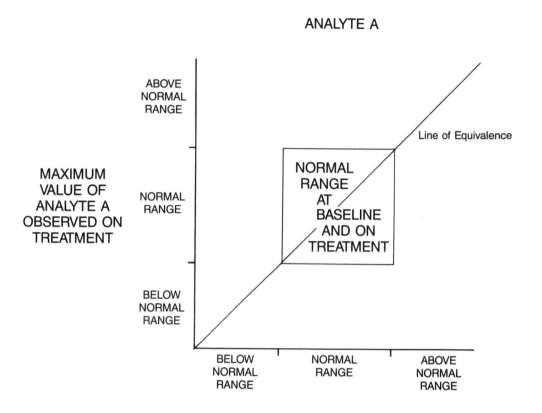

FIG. 6.37. Comparison of individual patient data at baseline and on treatment. Each patient may be represented by one mark on this graph (e.g., the drug group are indicated with an X and the placebo group by a circle).

• The value on treatment could be the final value, the mean of the last W clinic visits, the mean of all clinic visits, or others.

• This figure could be divided into nine quadrants to illustrate possible changes between the 3 × 3 comparisons (i.e., below normal, normal, and above normal).

Illustrates a two-dimensional scatterplot for various subgroups of patients with range of normal values shown.

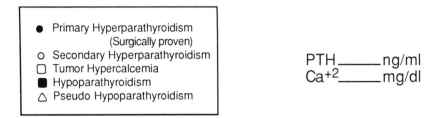

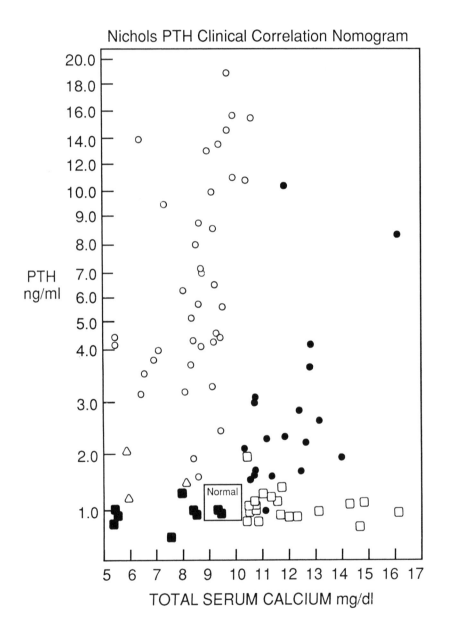

Illustrates picture of isozyme patterns.

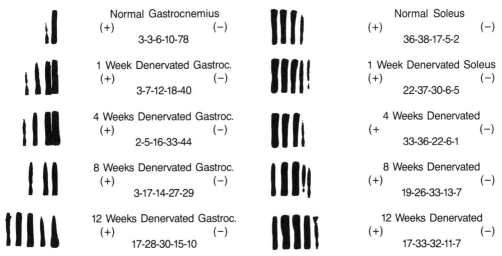

Normal Gastrocnemius
(+)   (−)
3-3-6-10-78

Normal Soleus
(+)   (−)
36-38-17-5-2

1 Week Denervated Gastroc.
(+)   (−)
3-7-12-18-40

1 Week Denervated Soleus
(+)   (−)
22-37-30-6-5

4 Weeks Denervated Gastroc.
(+)   (−)
2-5-16-33-44

4 Weeks Denervated
(+   (−)
33-36-22-6-1

8 Weeks Denervated Gastroc.
(+)   (−)
3-17-14-27-29

8 Weeks Denervated
(+)   (−)
19-26-33-13-7

12 Weeks Denervated Gastroc.
(+)   (−)
17-28-30-15-10

12 Weeks Denervated
(+)   (−)
17-33-32-11-7

FIG. 6.39. Note similarity between isozyme patterns of gastrocnemius and soleus 12 weeks after denervation. Reprinted from Hooshmand (1975) with permission.

FIG. 6.38. Reprinted with permission of the Radioassay-Endocrine Laboratory of North Carolina Memorial Hospital, using data generated from the Nichols Institute Reference Laboratory.

Illustrates a novel presentation of an analyte's profile.

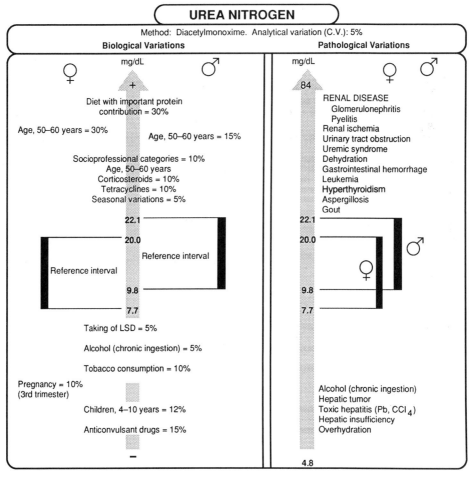

FIG. 6.40. Biological and pathological variations in plasma urea nitrogen concentration. Reprinted from Siest et al. (1985) with permission.

Illustrates transport pathways.

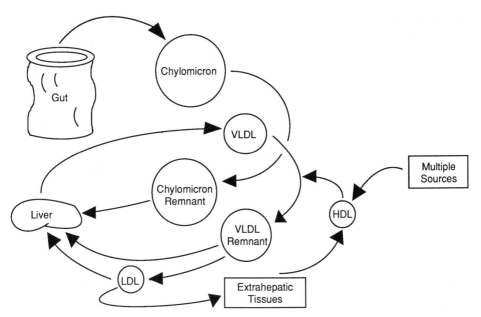

FIG. 6.41. Lipoprotein transport. See text for description of pathways. VLDL indicates very low-density lipoprotein; HDL, high-density lipoprotein; and LDL, low-density lipoprotein. Reprinted from Grundy (1986) with permission.

• A similar figure could be used to display absorption, distribution, metabolism, or elimination pathways.

Illustrates a nomogram.

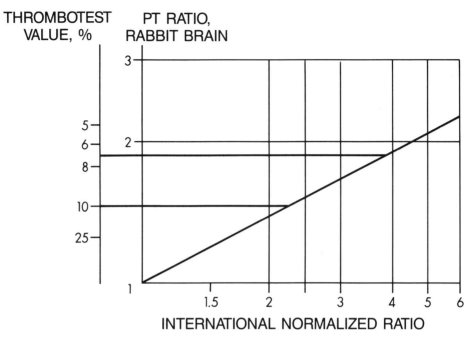

FIG. 6.42. Conversion of prothrombin time (PT) using one of commercial rabbit brain thromboplastins shown in Table 1 to international normalized ratio. Horizontal lines intersecting with thrombotest value of 7 percent to 10 percent corresponds to international normalized ratio of 2.8 to 3.6, and PT ratio using less responsive thromboplastin of 1.5 to 1.7. Reprinted from Hirsh and Levine (1987) with permission.

Illustrates a series of printouts from a laboratory instrument.

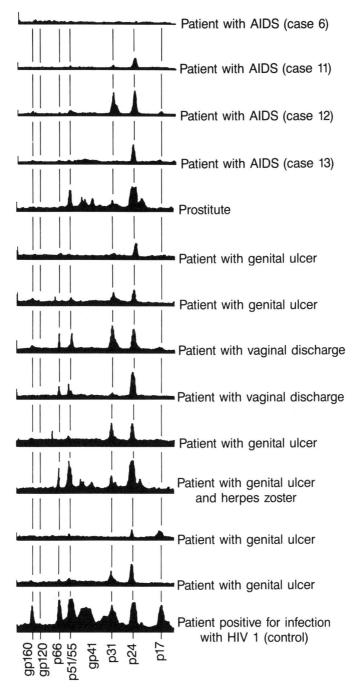

FIG. 6.43. Western blots against HIV 1 of 13 serum samples from patients positive for antibody to HIV 2 by competitive ELISA. Reprinted from Mabey et al. (1988) with permission.

**Illustrates a flow diagram used to interpret laboratory data and help plan
further studies.**

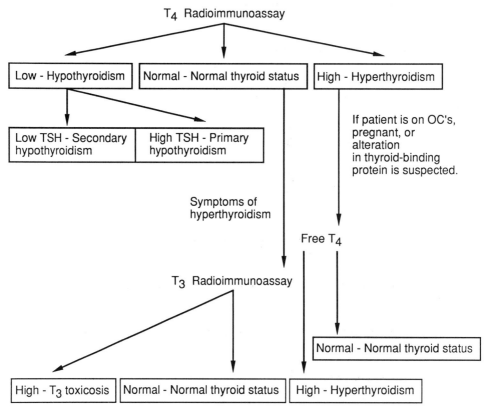

FIG. 6.44. Laboratory diagnostic approach for evaluation of thyroid function.

Illustrates a frequency distribution of two groups for laboratory values measured.

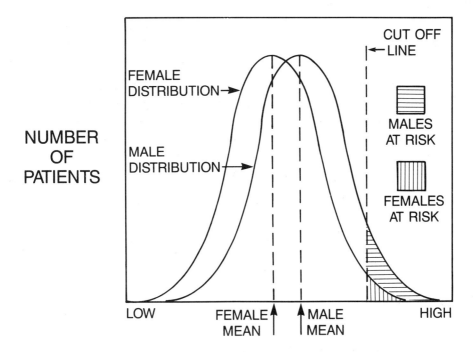

VALUE OF LABORATORY ANALYTE

FIG. 6.45. Hypothetical distribution of an analyte's values for males and females, where values above a given number plotted on the abscissa place patients at risk.

• This type of plot could be constructed for any two (or more) groups and for almost all laboratory analytes that are measured on a continuous scale.
• Ranges for different laboratories could be shown similarly.

Illustrates a means of showing how different groups of patients may (or may not) be differentiated on the basis of a laboratory result.

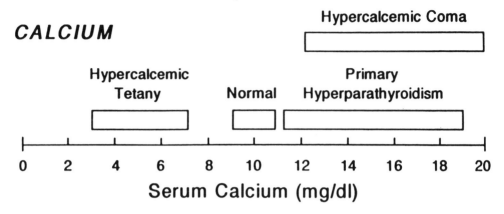

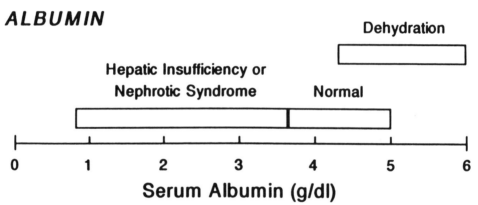

FIG. 6.46. Selected examples of ranges of serum values for calcium and albumin for various diseases. This illustrates a number of patterns that may be obtained. Reprinted from Spilker (1986) with permission.

• Differences for males and females could be shown for any category where differences were observed. Symbols for males and females could be shown on the graph to identify groups.

7

Adverse Reactions

This chapter describes the presentation of specific adverse reactions not covered in earlier chapters on vital signs (Chapter 5), physiological tests (Chapter 5), or laboratory changes (Chapter 6). The term adverse reactions should not be implied to indicate any causality. Other terms used include adverse events and adverse experiences. Adverse reactions are primarily symptoms reported by patients voluntarily or in response to either general or specifically worded questions. Many clinical signs of which a patient is unaware (e.g., heart murmur, altered deep tendon reflexes, mild nystagmus) are also included in this category.

In many presentations, the presenter desires to group reported adverse reactions into common categories. When this is done, the presentation should include a dictionary that explains the categorization. Table 7.1 is an example of one such dictionary. Tables 7.2 and 7.3 provide prototype tables where adverse reactions are listed, and Tables 7.4 to 7.12 provide sample displays of adverse reaction summarizations. Often, one singles out a specific set of adverse reactions (e.g., those which caused a patient to withdraw from a study) and studies additional information associated with them. Tables 7.13 to 7.17 are useful in those instances. Tables 7.18 to 7.26 provide additional examples of adverse reaction summaries. Although tables are more frequently used than graphs when presenting adverse reaction data, Figs. 7.1 to 7.10 provide examples of common graphic displays. Numerous formats in other chapters may also be used to present adverse reaction data (e.g., Figs. 1.20 to 1.24 and 1.58; Table 1.3).

NUMBER AND FREQUENCY OF ADVERSE DRUG REACTIONS (ADRs)

The number of ADRs (i.e., numerator of the incidence ratio) may be expressed in many ways (e.g., 1–8 below). Examples 9–13 show comparisons.

1. X cases of a specific ADR were observed.
2. X cases of liver-related ADRs were observed.
3. X cases of any ADR were observed.
4. X cases of severe (or mild) ADRs were observed.
5. X cases of irreversible ADRs were observed.
6. X cases of clinically important ADRs were observed.
7. X cases of ADRs of longer than 2 weeks duration were observed.
8. X cases of ADRs were observed that were judged to be definitely (probably, definitely not) related to drug.

9. X cases of ADR "M" were observed in patients on drug and Y cases of ADR "M" were observed in patients on placebo.
10. X cases of ADR "M" were observed in patients at dose P and Y cases of ADR "M" were observed in patients at dose Q.
11. X cases of ADR "M" were observed during dose ascension and Y cases were observed during maintenance therapy (or dose taper, or dose withdrawal).
12. X cases of ADR "M" were observed in patients under 16 years of age, Y cases in patients from 16 to 65, and Z cases in patients over 65.
13. X cases of ADR "M" were observed in patients receiving formulation R and Y cases in patients receiving formulation S.

None of the above are adequately informative on their own to reach a judgment because they do not provide information on the rate of occurrence. An almost unlimited number of combinations and variations of the examples above may be listed. Many completions are possible for the first example (i.e., X cases of ADR "M" were observed). These include: by a physician; at a study site; in a study; in treatment group 1, 2, or 3; in all treatment groups; on active drug; on placebo; across all studies using a specific protocol; and across all studies of a specific type.

Each of these numerators should have a denominator (e.g., per 1,000 patients treated, per million prescriptions, per million units sold) to provide incidence or prevalence information. Prevalence refers to the number of cases of a disease, problem, or event (e.g., Z patients per 100,000 people currently have the disease). For short-term and acute diseases (e.g., common cold), incidence is greater than prevalence. For chronic diseases, prevalence is greater than incidence. Incidence refers to the number of new cases of a disease, problem, or event per unit of time (e.g., number of patients per number of population per period of time). More specifically, one could discuss Z new cases of adverse reaction Q per 100,000 people using the drug per year. Other examples are:

$$1. \quad \frac{\text{Number of patients with the specific adverse reaction who received drug for at least X days (or weeks)}}{\text{Total number of patients who received drug for at least X days (or weeks)}}$$

$$2. \quad \frac{\text{Number of episodes (events) of a specific adverse reaction reported in a study}}{\text{Total number of possible episodes (events) of the specific adverse reaction which could have been reported}}$$

The total number of possible episodes equals the number of patients multiplied by the number of clinic visits, or multiplied by the number of occasions when adverse reactions are collected.

$$3. \quad \frac{\text{Number of patients with a specific adverse reaction that is severe}}{\text{Total number of patients treated with the drug for at least X weeks (or other time)}}$$

4. $$\frac{\text{Number of patients with severe adverse reactions of any specific type (e.g., cardiovascular, dizziness, palpitations)}}{\text{Total number of patients with mild, moderate, or severe adverse reactions of the same specific type}}$$

5. $$\frac{\text{Number of patients in the study with a specific adverse reaction that is severe}}{\text{Total number of patients in the study treated with the drug}}$$

6. $$\frac{\text{Number of patients treated in the clinical practice who had the adverse reaction}}{\text{Total number of patients treated in the clinical practice with the drug}}$$

7. $$\frac{\text{Number of patients with the specific adverse reaction}}{\text{Total number of patient years of treatment with the drug}}$$

The number of patients treated is important to mention if this ratio is presented. The number of patients treated allows some perspective on whether many patients are treated for short periods or few patients are treated for long periods.

8. $$\frac{\text{Number of episodes of the adverse reaction lasting over X hours}}{\text{Total number of episodes of the adverse reaction possible}}$$

9. $$\frac{\text{Number of patients with the specific adverse reaction}}{\text{Number of units of the drug sold}}$$

10. $$\frac{\text{Number of patients with the specific adverse reaction}}{\text{Number of people exposed}}$$

11. Number of patients with the specific adverse reaction per million prescriptions.

12. These ratios may also be based on the patient's age, sex, race, type of disease, dose of drug given, or any other treatment, demographic, or prognostic variable.

CATEGORIZING MORTALITY

Presentations of data from the following categories could be made in tables or graphs for deaths or number of live patients in a treatment group, study, or group of studies.

1. Number or percent of patients alive (dead) in each treatment group.
2. Number of patients alive (dead) versus number expected to be alive (dead).
3. Ratio of number alive (dead) to number expected to be alive (dead).

These presentations also could be used for specific subgroup analyses, for example:

    a. Patients who received the full dose of drug.
    b. Patients who were compliant and those who were noncompliant.
    c. Patients treated at specific treatment centers.
    d. Patients in a specific demographic group (e.g., males versus females, old versus young, blacks versus whites).
    e. Patients with the best (worst) prognostic characteristics.

Other displays of these data could present:

1. Only data obtained at clinically recommended doses. This would be particularly relevant for observational studies where patients were taking a wide variety of doses, some of which were above or below clinically recommended doses.
2. Case studies.
3. Data from patients who survived at least the first X days on treatment. This would have the advantage of removing moribund patients who were near death and only received one or a limited number of doses of a drug, and could not be expected to respond.

Illustrates the association of terms referring to adverse reactions in a coding system.

TABLE 7.1. Use of Standardized Terms in an Adverse Reaction Dictionary

Standardized term	Reported term	
Term 1	ADV_1 ADV_2 . . . ADV_n	List of reported adverse reaction terms which are referred (i.e., mapped) to the first standardized term
Term 2	ADV_1 . . . ADV_n	Terms which are referred to by the second standardized term

- To summarize adverse reactions, reported terms are often grouped into more general terms based on a standardized dictionary (e.g., dizzy, dizziness, and lightheaded could all be referred to by a standardized term such as dizziness).
- COSTART and WHO are standard dictionaries of adverse reaction terms. If neither of these nor other standard dictionaries suffice, a company may develop its own dictionary for a single drug or for all of its drugs.
- Many dictionaries group standardized terms by body system to form more general categories.
- When a dictionary is used, care must be taken to insure consistent, across-study referrals. The term used for referrals or associations is *mappings*. This is usually done with a computer and a single person is responsible for reviewing all associations.
- Care must be used when interpreting summarizations based on standardized terms. Some of the mappings are counterintuitive—e.g., in COSTART "tired" maps to "asthenia" but "feels sedated" maps to "somnolence."
- Some mappings result in strange connotations due to "everyday" usage of various words, e.g., in COSTART "lack of appetite" maps to "anorexia."

Illustrates listing of adverse reactions reported during study (individual patient data, single site or study).

TABLE 7.2. Adverse Reactions Observed During the Double-Blind Treatment Period[a]

Patient number	Age	Sex	Adverse reaction	Onset (day)	Duration (days)
Drug					
441	39	M	Otitis externa	16	9
			Otitis externa	37	18
			Cystitis	40	1
			Vestibular disorder (labyrinthitis)	36	12
442	47	F	Edema	60	1
450	58	M	Arrhythmia (paroxysmal atrial fibrillation)	83	1
452	54	M	Cervical vein distention	1	1
Placebo					
455	35	M	Diarrhea	17	15
			Diarrhea	80	11
			Diarrhea	91	51

[a]Listings such as this generally should include severity, relationship to drug, and possibly other information (e.g., action taken); see Table 7.3 for example.

- Onset could be confusing. Presumably time is measured since the beginning of the double-blind treatment period.
- A listing like this is appropriate and most useful if the total number of reported adverse reactions is small so that the complete table can fit on one or two pages.

Illustrates more extensive listing of adverse reactions (i.e., includes more descriptions) reported during study (individual patient data, single site or study).

TABLE 7.3. Adverse Reactions for Patients Receiving Drugs A or B

Dose (mg/kg)	Patient no.	Reactions	Minutes to onset after dose	Duration (min)	Severity	Relationship to drug
Drug A						
0.25	81	Flush	1.00	4.00	Mild	Possible
	82	Flush	1.00	7.00	Mild	Possible
	84	Flush	1.00	4.00	Mild	Possible
	85[a]	Flush	1.00	5.00	Mild	Possible
	86	Flush	0.00	3.00	Mild	Possible
	87	Flush	1.50	2.50	Mild	Possible
	89[a]	Flush	1.00	8.00	Mild	Possible
	93	Flush	1.50	5.50	Mild	Possible
	94	Flush	1.00	9.00	Mild	Possible
	94	Bronchospasm	3.00	6.00	Mild	None
	95	Flush	1.00	3.00	Mild	Possible
	97[a]	Flush	1.00	5.00	Mild	Possible
	97	Hypothermia	205.00[b]	120.00	Mild	Possible
	98	Flush	1.50	5.00	Mild	Possible
0.27	131	Flush	1.00	4.00	Mild	Possible
	132	Flush	1.00	4.00	Mild	Possible
	133	Slow resp. rate	172.00[b]	10.00	Moderate	None
	133	Slow resp. rate	237.00[b]	45.00	Moderate	None
	135	Flush	1.00	5.00	Mild	Possible
	137	Flush	1.17	4.00	Mild	Possible
	138	Flush	2.00	4.00	Mild	Possible
	139	Flush	1.00	4.00	Mild	Possible
0.30	123	Flush	1.00	7.00	Mild	Possible
	124	Wheezing sound, bilateral	10.00	183.00	Severe	Yes
	125	Flush	1.00	5.00	Mild	Possible
	126	Flush	1.00	5.00	Mild	Possible
	129	Flush	1.00	8.00	Mild	Possible
Drug B						
0.52	64	Flush	1.50	5.50	Mild	Possible
	68	Flush	1.00	4.00	Mild	Possible
0.60	51	Flush	1.00	4.00	Mild	Possible
	52	Erythema—veins, inj. site	15.00	44.00	Mild	Yes
	54	Flush	2.00	4.00	Mild	Possible
	57	Flush	0.50	5.00	Mild	Possible
	58	Erythema—veins, inj. site	12.00	40.00	Mild	Yes

[a]Patient also experienced greater than a 20% decrease in mean arterial blood pressure.
[b]In recovery room.

Illustrates basic summary of the number of patients reporting at least one adverse reaction (group data, multiple sites or studies).

TABLE 7.4. Overall Incidence of Total Adverse Reactions (A.R.) by Treatment Group and Phase for Each Center

| | Study drug | | | | | | Placebo | | | | | |
| | Baseline | | Treatment period | | | | Baseline | | Treatment period | | | |
Center	No. pts. with A.R.	Total no. pts.	No. pts. with A.R.	Total no. pts.	No. rep. of A.R.	Total no. of ass.	No. pts. with A.R.	Total no. pts.	No. pts. with A.R.	Total no. pts.	No. rep. of A.R.	Total no. ass.
01												
02												
03												
04												
05												
06												
07												
08												
09												
10												
Total patients	X	X	X	X			X	X	X	X		
Total reports or assessments					X	X					X	X

Ass., assessments (number of times that an A.R. was potentially able to be observed); Rep., reports (actual number of occurrences of an A.R.).

• This basic summary is on a per patient basis. Each patient either has at least one adverse reaction or has none.

• Treatment groups can then be compared with respect to proportion having an adverse reaction. Fisher's Exact Test is a good test to use for this comparison.

• Summary can also be expanded to include a posttreatment phase.

• This table has entries for each center of the multiple center study. Usually adverse reaction data are only summarized across all centers combined.

• If study involves more than one dose or dosing regimen or study drug, they are all grouped together in this summary. A follow-up summary table would then be dose- and dosing regimen-specific.

• Presence of an adverse reaction is related to the number of assessments—the more assessments, the more likely the occurrence.

• This summary is independent of severity and causality. It is a general presentation.

Illustrates a summarization of number of reports, gives indication of adverse reaction prevalence (group data, single site or study).

TABLE 7.5. Frequency of Patients with a Given Number of Reports of Adverse Reactions

No. of reports	Study drug (N = a)		Placebo (N = b)	
	No. of patients	Percent of patients	No. of patients	Percent of patients
0				
1				
3				
4				
5				
6–8				
9–12				
13–15				
16–18				
19–21				
More than 21				

- Separate tables for each individual center of a multicenter study could be prepared.
- A similar table that is a composite of multiple studies could be prepared.

Illustrates frequency distribution of individual adverse reactions (group data, single site or study).

TABLE 7.6. Frequency Distribution of Adverse Reactions in Two Groups of 400 Patients[a]

	Group 1[b]	Group 2
Headache	9	11
Dizziness	0	84
Vomiting	92	9
Headache and dizziness	85	4
Headache and vomiting	21	102
No adverse reactions	193	190
Total	400	400

[a]Percents could be added in parentheses. The rows and columns could be switched.
[b]Groups 1 and 2 could refer to two doses, two different drug treatments, or another aspect. Data from additional groups could be shown.

• Note inclusion of row for "no adverse reactions." This allows reader to compute how many patients reported at least one adverse reaction. Alternatively, a row for "at least one adverse reaction" could be added.

Illustrates frequency distribution of adverse reactions grouped by body system (group data, single site or study).

TABLE 7.7. Clinical Adverse Reactions by Body System (%)

	Drug (N = 167)	Placebo (N = 169)
Body as a whole	1 (0.6)	3 (1.8)
Cardiovascular	1 (0.6)	1 (0.6)
Central nervous system	1 (0.6)	1 (0.6)
Digestive	9 (5.4)	7 (4.1)
Integumentary	2 (1.2)	3 (1.8)
Metabolic/nutritional/immune	2 (1.2)	0 (0.0)
Musculoskeletal	1 (0.6)	2 (1.2)
Nervous and psychiatric	5 (3.0)	9 (5.3)
Respiratory	5 (2.4)	4 (2.4)
Tegumentary	2 (1.2)	2 (1.2)
Special senses	1 (0.6)	0 (0.0)
Urogenital	3 (1.8)	2 (1.2)
At least one adverse reaction	22 (13.2)	22 (13.0)

Illustrates frequency distribution of adverse reactions and reports of adverse reactions (grouped by body system) by study phase (group data, multiple sites or studies).

TABLE 7.8. Overall Incidence of Specific Adverse Reactions by Treatment (Study Drug vs. Placebo), Combined Centers[a]

	Study drug				Placebo			
	Baseline % of patients (N = X)	Treatment period			Baseline % of patients (N = C)	Treatment period		
		Percent of patients (N = Y)	No. of reports	Percent of reports[b]		Percent of patients (N = D)	No. of reports	Percent of reports[b]
Adverse reaction								
Behavioral								
Neurological								
Autonomic								

Cardiovascular

Other

Total no. of reports

Total no. of assessments

[a]Separate tables could be constructed for each of the individual centers in a multicenter study.
[b]This column is the total number of reports obtained for each adverse reaction in the treatment period of the placebo (or study drug) group divided by the total number of assessments for that symptom in the group studied (i.e., placebo or study drug) during that treatment period ($\times$ 100).

• Could be expanded to include a posttreatment phase.

• Differs from previous table (Table 7.7) in that this is a summary of each specific adverse reaction.

• Note grouping by body system.

• Within each body system, adverse reactions could be listed in alphabetical order. It might be better, however, to order them in terms of decreasing incidence.

• Data are most meaningful if they are entirely based on COSTART (or another dictionary) terms.

• Presentation is independent of relationship to study drug. A follow-up table might be based only on those adverse reactions which the investigator regarded as possibly or probably related to study drug, or to those which the investigator judged to be clinically important.

• Table might be restricted to treatment emergent reactions. A treatment emergent adverse reaction would be one that either first appeared during the treatment period or that increased in severity during the treatment period.

Illustrates frequency distribution of adverse reactions (grouped by body system) by study phase and duration of exposure to study drug (group data, multiple sites or studies).

TABLE 7.9. Incidence of Adverse Reactions by Assessment Period, Combined Centers[a]

Adverse reaction	Percent of patients											
	2 (Baseline) (N = a)	4 (Baseline) (N = b)	Study drug treatment: Study week									
			6 (N = c)	8 (N = d)	10 (N = e)	12 (N = f)	15 (N = g)	18 (N = h)	21 (N = i)	24 (N = k)	27 (Posttreatment) (N = m)	
Behavioral												
Neurological												
Autonomic												

	A	B	C	D	E	F	G	H	J	K	M
Cardiovascular											
Other											
Total no. of patients reporting at least one symptom											

[a]This table would have a second page for "Placebo treatment." All of these data could be plotted with a different adverse reaction on each graph.

• Separate tables for each of the individual centers in a multicenter study could be constructed.

• The actual incidences presented would be affected by how data were collected—spontaneous reports, generally worded probes, or specific probes.

• A good follow-up table would be to restrict attention to adverse reactions which the investigator judged to be possibly or probably related to the study drug, or to those judged clinically important.

Illustrates frequency distribution of adverse reactions and reports of adverse reactions (grouped by body system) by study phase and severity of report (group data, multiple sites or studies).

TABLE 7.10. Overall Intensity of Adverse Reactions, Combined Centers[a]

	Study drug							Placebo						
	Baseline period % of patients (N = a)			Treatment period					Baseline period % of patients (N = c)			Treatment period				
				% of patients (N = b)			% of reports						% of patients (N = d)			% of reports		
Adverse reaction	Mild	Mod.	Sev.	Mild	Mod.	Sev.	Mild	Mod.	Sev.	N[b]	Mild	Mod.	Sev.	Mild	Mod.	Sev.	Mild	Mod.	Sev.	N[b]
Behavioral																				
Neurological																				

Autonomic

_____

_____

Cardiovascular

_____

_____

Other

_____

_____

Total (% reports)
Total (% patients)

[a]Separate tables for each of the individual centers in a multicenter study could be constructed.
[b]N, number of assessments.
Mod., moderate; Sev., severe.

- Since patients could easily report any particular adverse reaction at more than one severity, this summarization should be based on each patient's maximum recorded severity for each adverse reaction.
- By adding severity, this table provides a more sensitive comparison than mere incidence rates.
- Separate tables could be prepared for each dose of drug.

Illustrates frequency distribution of adverse reactions and reports of adverse reactions (grouped by body system) by relationship to drug (group data, multiple sites or studies).

TABLE 7.11. Relationship Between Adverse Reactions and Treatment, Combined Centers[a]

	Study drug (N = A)										Placebo (N = B)									
	% of patients					% of reports					% of patients					% of reports				
Adverse reaction	Yes	Poss.	Unk.	No	N	Yes	Poss.	Unk.	No	N	Yes	Poss.	Unk.	No	N	Yes	Poss.	Unk.	No	N
Behavioral																				
Neurological																				

Autonomic

_____

Cardiovascular

_____

Other

_____

Total (%)

[a]Treatment period only. Only the most definite relationship will be considered (i.e., "yes" before "possible," "possible" before "unknown," "unknown" before "not related").

Poss., possible; Unk., unknown; No, not related; Yes, definite; N, number of patients or reports.

• Different dosages or dosing regimens could be presented.
• Separate tables for each of the centers could be prepared.
• The identity of the individual who assigned the relationship (e.g., investigator, sponsor) should be stated in a footnote or in the text.

Illustrates frequency distribution of adverse reactions and reports of adverse reactions (grouped by body system) by action taken to treat adverse reaction (group data, multiple sites or studies).

TABLE 7.12. Action Taken as a Result of Adverse Reactions for Patients Receiving Study Drug (N = A), Combined Centers[a]

Adverse reaction	None		Increase surveillance		Contra-active Rx		Change dose		D/C study drug	
	No. pts.	No. reps.	No. pts.	No. reps.	No. pts.	No. reps.	No. pts.	No. reps.	No. pts.	No. reps.
Behavioral										
Neurological										

Autonomic

Cardiovascular

Other

aSame table would be prepared for placebo. Separate tables could be prepared for each center in a multicenter study. Additional actions include (1) nondrug treatment, (2) hospitalization, and (3) temporary suspension of study drug. If only a few patients require treatment as a result of adverse reactions, then a more detailed listing of individual patients would be preferable to this table.
Pts., patients; reps., reports.

Illustrates listing of relevant data associated with adverse reactions that required treatment (individual patient data, multiple sites or studies).

TABLE 7.13. Adverse Reactions that Required Treatment

Study number	Patient number	Drug dose[a] (mg/kg)	Route of admin.	Patient's age	Patient's sex	Adverse reaction	Time of onset (min, hr)	Approx. duration	Severity	Action taken	Results	Comments

[a] If more than a single drug is referred to in this table, a separate column for drug name is essential.
• A column for concomitant drugs would be helpful.

Illustrates listing of relevant data associated with adverse reactions that were severe (individual patient data, multiple sites or studies).

TABLE 7.14. Patients with Severe Adverse Reactions Whose Treatment Was Not Discontinued

Treatment group	Patient no.	Age	Sex	Site no.	Drug week	Dose (mg/day)	Adverse reaction	Intensity (M, Mo, S)[a]	Related to drug study (Y, N, P, U)[b]	Action taken
Drug	440									
	681									
Placebo	112									
	145									
	268									
	294									
	412									
	654									

[a]M, mild; Mo, moderate; S, severe. The text should indicate the definitions of these terms.
[b]Y, definite; N, not related; P, possible; U, unknown.

Illustrates list of relevant data associated with all adverse reactions that necessitated a patient's being withdrawn from study (individual patient data, multiple sites or studies).

TABLE 7.15. Patients Whose Treatment Was Discontinued Because of an Adverse Reaction

Treatment group	Patient no.	Age	Sex	Site no.	Drug week	Dose (mg/day)	Adverse reaction	Intensity (M, Mo, S)[a]	Related to drug study (Y, N, P, U)[b]	Patient outcome
Drug	420			4						
	682			6						
	943			9						
Placebo	174			1						
	560			5						
	592			5						

[a]M, mild; Mo, moderate; S, severe.
[b]Y, definite; N, not related; P, possible; U, unknown.

Illustrates summary of incidence of adverse reactions and of adverse reactions causing patient withdrawal (group data, multiple sites or studies).

TABLE 7.16. Adverse Reactions and Reasons for Withdrawal from Treatment Among 1884 Patients[a]

Category	Adverse reaction[b]		Withdrawal due to reaction[c]	
	Placebo (N)	Drug (N)	Placebo (N)	Drug (N)
Cardiac failure, nonfatal	63	73	20	27
Pulmonary edema, nonfatal	7	16	2	8
Heart rate <40 beats/min	3	47[d]	2	37[d]
Hypotension	15	29[e]	11	26[e]
Atrioventricular block, 2nd or 3rd degree	5	4	3	3
Sinoatrial block	7	8	7	6
Claudication	27	31	5	13
Cold hands and feet	6	73[d]	0	4
Raynaud's phenomenon	1	6	0	0
Bronchial obstruction	7	18[e]	4	10
Cerebrovascular disease	20	27	6	10
Thrombotic or embolic disease (excluding central nervous system)	9	16	3	2
Appearance of hyperglycemia	18	30	0	0
Hypoglycemia	2	0	1	0
Nausea or digestive disorders	57	71	5	11
Urogenital disorders	17	26	0	2
Nervous system disorders	23	24	2	3
Psychiatric disorders	35	28	1	6
Asthenia or fatigue	11	45[d]	1	4
Dizziness	34	53	0	11[f]
Syncope	13	10	0	0
Skin disorders	25	25	4	2
Musculoskeletal disorders	38	35	1	1
Pneumonia or bronchitis	27	45[e]	0	0
Other infections	34	41	0	1
Trauma	12	11	0	2
Malignant processes	11	8	3	2
Miscellaneous	59	73	1	5
Arrhythmia requiring treatment >21 days	38	13[d]	38	13[d]
Condition requiring beta-adrenergic blockade	68	32[d]	68	32[d]
Unconsciousness after heart arrest	—	—	6	4
Nonmedical withdrawal reasons	—	—	25	30

[a]Transient occurrences complicating recurrent infarctions are included only if they caused withdrawal.

[b]When an adverse reaction recurred in a patient, it is listed only once.

[c]Only principal reason for withdrawal in each patient is listed.

[d]$p < 0.001$.

[e]$p < 0.05$.

[f]$p < 0.01$.

Illustrates listing of relevant data from patients who died during study (individual patient data, multiple sites or studies).

TABLE 7.17. Deaths in Patients Treated with Drug X[a]

Country	Study no.	Pt. no.	Age	Sex	Immediate cause	Concomitant drugs	Concurrent condition	Drug dose	Route of administration

[a]Other parameters that could be included: indication for which drug was given, duration of treatment, time since last dose when episode occurred (or at time of death), blood level, and comments.

• "Death" is not an adverse reaction, but it is an outcome of an adverse reaction.

Illustrates comparison of treatments with respect to increases in incidence between the baseline and treatment phases (group data, single site or study).

TABLE 7.18. Percent Incidence of Adverse Reactions for Study Drug vs. Placebo[a]

A. Percent of patients

Adverse reaction	Study drug (S) $(t-b)^b$	Placebo (P) $(t-b)^b$	Study drug − Placebo $S(t-b)$ − $P(t-b)$ (Percentage units difference)
Effect M	+7	+17	+10
Effect N			
Effect O			
Other			
[c] -------			
Effect P	+4	−11	−15
Effect Q			
Effect R			
Other			

B. Percent of reports

Effect N			
Effect O			
Effect J			
Effect Q			
Other			
[c] -------			
Effect V			
Effect X			
Effect Y			
Other			

[a]For all adverse reactions where $S(t-b)$ − $P(t-b)$ is 10 percent or more units different. This factor of 10 can be raised (or lowered) as deemed appropriate.

[b]t, treatment; b, baseline.

[c]This dashed line divides those adverse reactions for which patients (reports) were more prevalent in the study drug group (above the lines) from those for which the percent of patients (reports) was greater in the placebo group (below the lines).

• Instead of including only adverse reactions where the incidence difference was 10% (or some other fixed percentage), one could include all adverse reactions or only those that have an incidence greater than any prespecified percent.

• Summary is based on treatment period occurrences. Baseline and posttreatment occurrences are not included.

Illustrates using various statistical techniques to investigate the incidence of selected adverse reactions (group data, single site or study).

TABLE 7.19. Percentage of Patients Based on Three Analyses of Complaint Reporting

Complaint	Survival analysis (%)		Cumulative (%)		Cross-sectional (1 yr) (%)	
	Drug	Placebo	Drug	Placebo	Drug	Placebo
Blacking out or losing consciousness	9.9	11.6	9.1	10.4	1.7	1.8
Unusual tiredness or fatigue during ordinary activities	68.7	65.7	66.9	62.3	22.6	21.3
Frequent depression that interfered with work, recreation, or sleep	42.8	42.3	40.7	39.8	11.1	10.4
Recurrent bronchospasm (wheezing in the chest)	34.0	29.2	31.2	27.1	10.5	8.9

• Note use of both survival analysis (incorporating duration of exposure prior to occurrence of adverse reactions) and chi-square analysis (based only on incidence).

• Survival analysis is relatively "sophisticated" and probably should be applied only to the most frequent and/or most serious adverse reactions.

Illustrates relative frequency of all adverse reactions on drug within clinical trials and in clinical practice (group data, multiple studies).

TABLE 7.20. Percentage Distribution of Adverse Reactions to Metoprolol for Different System-Organ Classes, Reported in Clinical Studies and in Clinical Practice (1975–1981)

| | Percentage of adverse drug reaction reports | |
System-organ class	Clinical studies	Clinical practice[a] 1975–1981
Skin and appendage system	2.4	25.3
Musculoskeletal system	0	2.1
Collagenous system	0	1.4
Central and peripheral nervous system	22.0	8.9
Autonomic nervous system	19.0	11.8
Vision	2.4	11.2
Hearing and vestibular system	0	1.2
Special senses, other	0	0.4
Psychiatric	10.4	15.3
Gastrointestinal system	19.6	3.7
Liver and biliary system	0	2.3
Metabolic and nutritional system	0	1.7
Cardiovascular system	0.1	1.1
Myo-endo-pericardial and valve	0.1	0.4
Heart rate and rhythm	0	0.4
Vascular (extracardiac)	0.6	2.1
Respiratory system	7.0	6.0
Platelet, bleeding and clotting	0	0
Urinary system	0	0
Reproductive system	0	0.2
General disorders	16.4	4.3

[a]The total number of reported adverse reactions to metoprolol was 658, and the use of the drug was 4 million patient years during this period.

Reprinted from Johnsson et al. (1984) with permission.

Illustrates incidence of different adverse reactions according to route of drug administration (group data, multiple studies).

TABLE 7.21. Incidence of Patients with Adverse Drug Reactions

| Adverse drug reaction | Route of administration | | | | | | Total N |
| | Intravenous | | Intraarterial | | Oral | | |
	N	%	N	%	N	%	
Central nervous system							
a. _____							
b. _____							
c. _____							
d. _____							
Cardiovascular							
a. _____							
b. _____							
c. _____							
d. _____							
Respiratory							
a. _____							
b. _____							
c. _____							
d. _____							
Gastrointestinal							
a. _____							
b. _____							
c. _____							
d. _____							

Illustrates a simple table focusing on dosing regimen (group data, multiple sites or studies).

TABLE 7.22. Summary of Adverse Reactions by Dosing Regimen[a,b]

| Adverse reaction | Dosing Regimen | | | | Total no. of patients reporting an adverse reaction |
	qd	bid	tid	qid	
Amblyopia	0 (0)	0 (0)	1 (100)	0 (0)	1
Anorexia	0 (0)	0 (0)	2 (100)	0 (0)	2
Anxiety	0 (0)	0 (0)	1 (100)	0 (0)	1
Arthritis	0 (0)	0 (0)	1 (100)	0 (0)	1
Asthenia	0 (0)	1 (25)	2 (50)	1 (25)	4
Bronchospasm	0 (0)	0 (0)	1 (33)	2 (67)	3
Chills	0 (0)	0 (0)	0 (0)	1 (100)	1
CNS stimulation	0 (0)	0 (0)	4 (100)	0 (0)	4
Conjunctivitis	0 (0)	0 (0)	1 (100)	0 (0)	1
Constipation	0 (0)	0 (0)	2 (100)	0 (0)	2
Cough	0 (0)	0 (0)	1 (50)	1 (50)	2
Diarrhea	0 (0)	0 (0)	1 (100)	0 (0)	1
Dizziness	0 (0)	0 (0)	5 (100)	0 (0)	5
Dry mouth	0 (0)	0 (0)	22 (85)	4 (15)	26

[a]Numbers in parentheses are row percentages within each treatment group.
[b]The numbers of patients on each regimen would be listed in a separate table.

• Many variations of expanded dosing regimen data could be presented using other formats in this chapter.

• Adverse reactions starting with letters E through Z would also be included in this table.

Illustrates a means of identifying patterns in the onset and duration of a specific adverse reaction (individual patient data, single site or study).

TABLE 7.23. Time of Occurrence and Duration of Specific Adverse Reactions in a Study

Patient number	Adverse reaction = Dry mouth			Week 4 (on-site)	Treatment drug X		Patient status
	Day 1 (on-site)	Day 1–week 2	Week 2–week 4		Week 4–week 8	Week 8–week 16	
104					X	X	Continuing in study as of wk 16
115		X	X				Continuing in study as of wk 16
119		X	X				Discontinued study
228		X	X				Continuing in study as of wk 16
309					X		Continuing in study as of wk 16
312		X					Continuing in study as of wk 16
606		X					Continuing in study as of wk 16
607		X					Continuing in study as of wk 16
610		X				X	Continuing in study as of wk 16
612		X	X		X		Entered open-label study
613		X					Continuing in study as of wk 16
615			X			X	Continuing in study as of wk 16
703		X		*****	*****	*****	Discontinued study
805						X	Continuing in study as of wk 16
816		X	X				Continuing in study as of wk 16
906		X		*****	*****	*****	Entered open-label study
907		X	X	*****	*****	*****	Entered open-label study
908		X	X	*****	*****	*****	Entered open-label study
926					X		Continuing in study as of wk 16
928		X					Discontinued study
1006		X					Continuing in study as of wk 16
1023		X					Continuing in study as of wk 16
1106		X	X	X			Continuing in study as of wk 16
1107				X			Continuing in study as of wk 16
1113					X		Continuing in study as of wk 16
1117						X	Continuing in study as of wk 16

*****, Adverse reaction data are not available.

X, Adverse reaction occurred during the indicated interval.

Illustrates the relative risk of two treatments based on incidence of adverse reactions (group data).

TABLE 7.24. Determining the Relative Risk of Treatment X over Treatment Y

Adverse reaction (AR)	Treatment X (incidence)[a]	Treatment Y[b] (incidence)	Relative risk (X ÷ Y)	95% Confidence interval	Range
AR$_1$ (e.g., MI)[c]					
AR$_2$ (e.g., stroke)					
. . .					
AR$_N$					
Total (AR$_1$ to N)[d]					

[a]Incidence should only consider associations that are possibly, probably, or definitely drug related. Associations that are unknown should be considered as possibly drug related in most situations.

[b]Treatment Y could be placebo, a different drug, no treatment, different treatment, or a different dose of the same drug as treatment X.

[c]Adverse reactions could be limited to moderate and severe intensity only or could include all reports.

[d]This row usually may be eliminated since the overall addition of different types and severities of adverse reactions makes little inherent clinical sense in most situations.

Illustrates the pattern of time to onset of an adverse reaction in a population and also illustrates its duration (group data, single site or study).

TABLE 7.25. Percent of Patients with Adverse Reactions Over Time

Adverse reaction	Week (or month) of therapy				
	1	2	3	4	5
	% (N = 88)	% (N = 86)	% (N = 86)	% (N = 85)	% (N = 80)
A	0	0	1	0	0
B	0	1	2	17	19
C	2	7	6	4	1
D	2	40	45	36	22
E	10	12	11	9	9

Illustrates selected ratios for evaluating risk (group data).

TABLE 7.26. Examples to Determine the Increased or Decreased Risk of Treatment X

1. Expected number of a specific event (e.g., MI) without treatment X

   Observed number of a specific event (e.g., MI) with treatment X

2. Expected number of all events of one type (e.g., CV) without treatment X

   Observed number of all events of one type (e.g., CV) with treatment X

3. Expected number of all events of all types without treatment X

   Observed number of all events of all types with treatment X

MI, myocardial infarction; CV, cardiovascular.

• The parameters of treatment X must be established (e.g., dose range, dosage form, duration of treatment) and specified.

Illustrates using a horizontal bar chart to present percent incidence of adverse reactions (group data, single site or study).

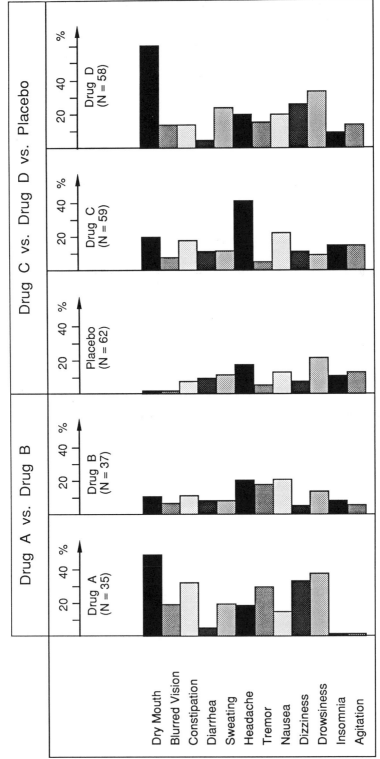

FIG. 7.1. Incidence of selected adverse reactions.

• Data are displayed from two studies. If at least one treatment occurs in both studies, the reader can compare incidence between, as well as within, studies.

• An indication of severity and other characteristics should be provided in other graphs, figures, tables, or in the text.

Illustrates how numbers of patients in multiple studies with a specific condition may be shown (group data, multiple sites or studies).

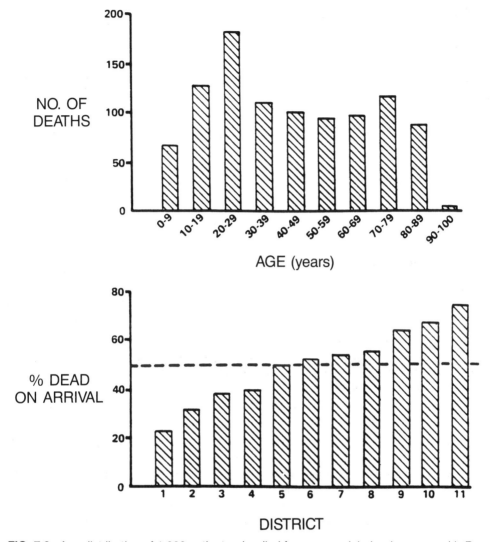

FIG. 7.2. Age distribution of 1,000 patients who died from severe injuries (upper graph). Percentage of patients who were dead on arrival at hospital in the 11 districts studied (lower graph). Reprinted from Anderson et al. (1988) with permission.

• Listing the groups or categories under the x-axis at a 45° angle (upper graph) enables these identifiers to be read more easily than if they are placed at 90°.

• Note how the reference line in the bottom display greatly enhances the histogram.

Illustrates using a line graph to display incidence of adverse reactions during therapy (group data, single or multiple studies).

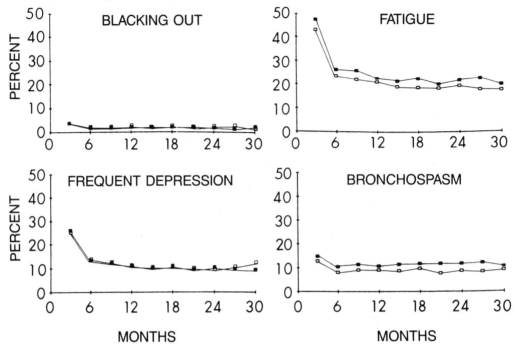

FIG. 7.3. The percentage of patients reporting complaints during any 3-month interval in the BHAT (**filled squares** = propranolol group; **open squares** = placebo group). Reprinted from Davis et al. (1987) with permission.

  • Using different symbols for the different treatment groups facilitates interpretation.

  • Even though lines are very close, some indication of variability (e.g., standard error) would help.

  • Given the relatively long duration of the study (2.5 years), presumably dropouts occur and imply that the sample size is not constant across time; hence, presentation is potentially misleading without that information.

  • The term percent on the ordinate could be displayed horizontally.

Illustrates using a life table approach to evaluate cumulative proportions (group data, single or multiple studies).

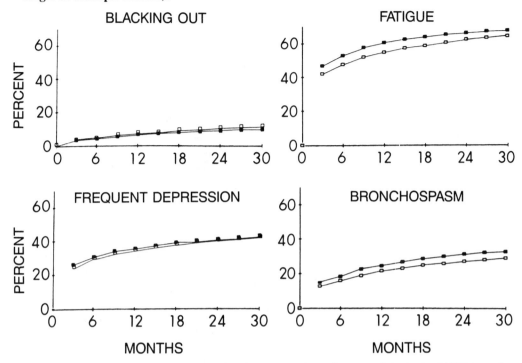

FIG. 7.4. The cumulative percentage of patients reporting a first complaint in the BHAT based on the survival analysis approach (**filled squares** = propranolol group; **open squares** = placebo group). Reprinted from Davis et al. (1987) with permission.

Illustrates superimposing study design indicators (timing of "Dear Doctor" letters), a line graph of drug usage, and two histograms of adverse reaction incidence (group data, multiple sites or studies).

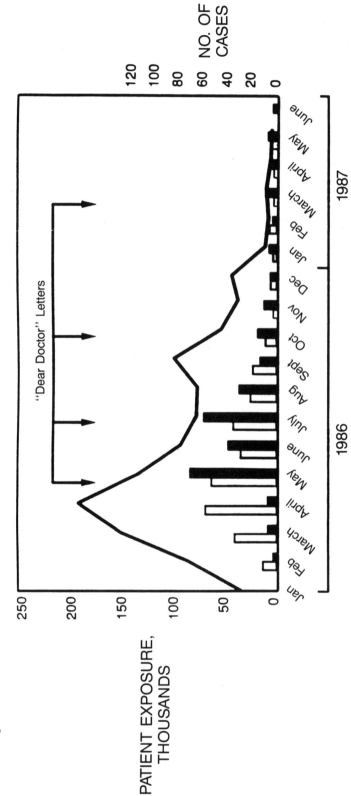

FIG. 7.5. Suprofen use and reports of associated flank pain syndrome. **Solid line** represents suprofen use; **open bars** represent adverse drug reactions by month of onset; and **filled bars** represent adverse drug reactions by month of report. Reprinted from Rossi et al. (1988) with permission.

- Note the use of a line graph to provide information on a third variable.
- This is an effective graph that combines histogram and line graph elements.
- Note the use of both a left and right y-axis.

Illustrates how a line graph may express a relationship between an adverse reaction and another factor for two (or more) groups (group data, single or multiple sites or studies).

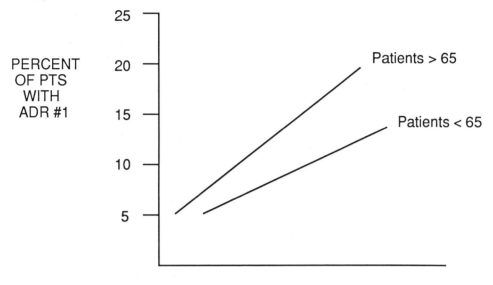

FIG. 7.6. Relationship of adverse reaction incidence and blood drug levels.

• Various subgroups may be shown.

Illustrates the increasing risk of experiencing any specific adverse reaction as dosage increases (group data, single or multiple sites or studies).

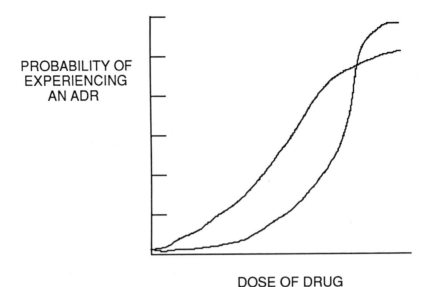

FIG. 7.7. Risk of experiencing an adverse reaction as a function of dose.

• Presumably either the same patients were studied at increasing dosage levels, or different groups at each level were studied. In either event, the number of patients studied at each dose should be indicated.

• Vertical axis for "Percent of patients experiencing adverse reaction" would be equally informative.

• Groups of adverse reactions (e.g., central nervous system, renal) may be illustrated similarly.

Illustrates a comparison of adverse reaction rate at specific times on treatment.

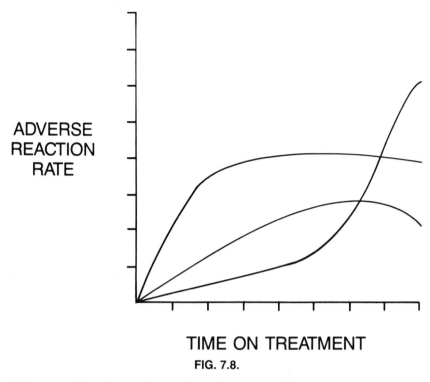

ADVERSE
REACTION
RATE

TIME ON TREATMENT

FIG. 7.8.

- This type of graph may be used to plot:

    1. individual adverse reactions;
    2. crude rates, adjusted rates, cumulative rates, or others;
    3. rates of one adverse reaction in different studies;
    4. rates of one adverse reaction using different doses; and
    5. rates of one adverse reaction for patients using different concomitant drugs.

304

Illustrates using a scatterplot to relate the number of adverse reactions to therapy duration (individual data, single or multiple studies).

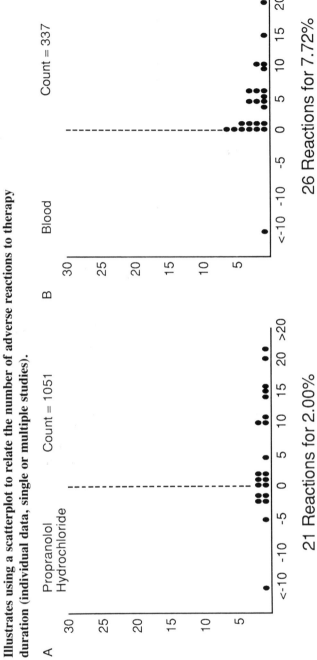

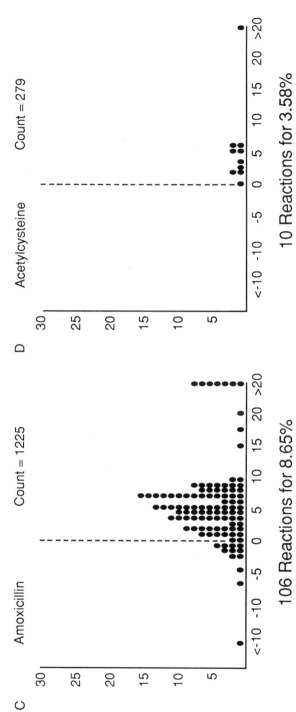

FIG. 7.9. Scattergrams relate number of cutaneous reactions (each mark, vertical axis) to number of days before or after onset of therapy with indicated drug (horizontal axis). Drugs not associated with rashes (example A) have low reaction rates and have reactions randomly distributed before and after onset of therapy. Drugs associated with rashes (examples B through D) have reactions cluster within 7 days after onset of therapy and have a reaction rate more than twice the mean rate. Mean reaction rates in first stage (examples A, B, and C) and second stage (example D) were 2.3% and 0.8%. Count indicates number of persons exposed. Reprinted from Bigby et al. (1986) with permission.

• Both duration and incidence are shown.
• Horizontal and vertical axes should be labeled to provide greater clarity.

Illustrates presence of adverse reactions by hatched squares (individual patient data, single site or study).

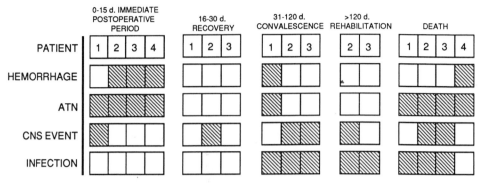

FIG. 7.10. Complications occurring in Patients 1 through 4 (B.C., W.S., M.H., and J.B., respectively) during each postoperative time period. **ATN**, acute tubular necrosis; **CNS**, central nervous system; **hatched boxes**, complication seen; and **open boxes**, complication not seen. Reprinted from DeVries (1988) with permission.

Illustrates a series of scales to compare drugs used for a single disease and to relate adverse reactions to efficacy.

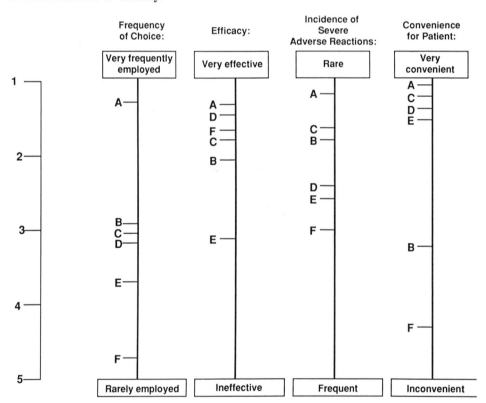

FIG. 7.11. Characterization of various drugs along an arbitrary scale. Each letter stands for a different drug.

• Data used to support the placements should be provided in a table or references should be given.

8
Efficacy

Of the categories of data described in this book, efficacy data vary most from study to study. Nonetheless, most efficacy data presented in clinical reports appear to use a small number of generally similar formats. These formats have a great deal in common with the presentations of safety data.

Patients are usually evaluated at discrete time points to measure both safety and efficacy parameters. For *outpatient studies,* these evaluations generally occur during clinic visits that are scheduled at baseline and at specified times in terms of days, weeks, months, or years after the initiation of treatment. For *inpatient studies,* most evaluations also occur at prescheduled times. It is also possible to wait for a pre-specified change in function, behavior, or clinical endpoint to occur and to evaluate the patient at that time. Measurements of efficacy variables, as well as safety variables and possibly pharmacokinetic or quality of life parameters, are made at these times. Values obtained may then be compared with those obtained both at baseline (active or historical) and during treatment to get a rough (or precise) indication of how well the patient is responding to treatment (e.g., test drug, active drug used as control, placebo).

Data are usually presented to closely mimic a clinician's way of thinking about a patient or group of patients. This is usually in terms of the patient's (1) present state versus previous state before treatment, (2) present state versus previous state on treatment, (3) degree of improvement or change observed versus degree of improvement desired as a goal, or (4) degree of improvement observed versus that observed in other patients in the study. Additionally, data may be evaluated in terms of a trend of major parameter(s), or in other ways. The clinical questions being addressed in a study can be directly translated into creation of appropriate tables and figures for data presentation.

Because there are a limited number of basic questions that one may ask about changes of efficacy parameters in a study, there are a limited number of ways of presenting the data obtained with any one parameter. As was the case for safety data, presentations may logically and systematically proceed from consideration of a single patient, to a single group of patients according to treatment or by a subgroup analysis, to a single study site, to a single multicenter study, and to combining or comparing multiple studies. Unlike safety presentations where all data obtained must be included in a presentation, efficacy analyses often exclude patients who were discontinued or dropped out of a study. Presentations may focus on comparisons of effective doses, ratios of benefit to risk, comparison of dose response curves, or many other procedures.

The tables included in this chapter have been grouped into three basic categories: presentations of individual patient data (Tables 8.1 to 8.5), presentations of grouped data from a single or multiple studies (Tables 8.6 to 8.21), and presentations of data from observational studies (Tables 8.22 to 8.28). Because of the "interchangeability" of visual displays among those three categories, no similar distinction is used to classify the figures. The relatively large number of figures illustrates numerous variations. Most figures in Chapter 1, as well as the figures in other chapters, could be used to illustrate efficacy data.

ILLUSTRATING SUBJECTIVE DATA

Subjective data may relate to efficacy measures (e.g., global impressions) or to safety data (e.g., adverse reactions). Both types may be presented similarly.

Some common approaches to illustrating subjective data are the following:

1. Convert subjective data to quantitative responses (e.g., 0 to 4 for different types of responses). Example: 0, none at all; 1, a few times per year; 2, about once a week; 3, several times a day; 4, almost continuously.
2. Have patients complete visual analogue scales and illustrate responses as described in that section (see Chapter 1).
3. List responses verbatim, by type and by category.
   • List responses for all patients.
   • List responses separately for different categories of patients.
   • Graph responses (e.g., line graph, histogram).

PRESENTATIONS OF GROUP DATA

Examples of Efficacy Data that May Be Combined Across Studies

1. Specific values or scores obtained in standardized tests or any tests that are used in a standard way. These tests measure physical performance, laboratory measures, or other objective parameters. Data combined across studies may be chosen as either one or more values for each test. If one value per patient per test is used, it may be the first value obtained, last value obtained, mean value, median value, or modal value of all applications of the test. Other choices may be made but should be defined in advance. If multiple values from a single patient's test are combined across studies, consultation with a statistician is strongly advised to insure that appropriate methods and approaches are followed.
2. Data from patient diaries (e.g., number of events, maximum or mean intensity of events, maximum or mean duration of events, scores of events using an arbitrary scale, number of entries).
3. Data from efficacy scales obtained and measured by written tests or verbal interviews (patient and/or investigator completed).
4. Clinical global impression scores (patient and/or investigator completed).
5. Scores of disease severity.
6. Percentages of patients improved or cured at different time points.

7. Drug formulations, dosing regimens, and combinations of drugs used by patients where maximum efficacy was observed.
8. Dosages found to elicit a maximum therapeutic effect.

Raw data should be combined whenever possible, before converting it to percent response or using another data transformation where the nature of the effects measured becomes less clear. Normalization of data is one method of transforming data that usually causes little distortion of raw data. Patient populations should be similar for defined characteristics in the studies being combined. If different scales were used in different studies to measure efficacy, then broad categories (e.g., improved, unchanged, deteriorated) are a possible (though often undesirable) means of transforming data so that dissimilar data may be combined.

Observational Studies and Subjective Data

Most efficacy data come from well-controlled clinical studies. In such studies the study drug (and often a control drug—either placebo or a known active drug) is administered to patients under controlled situations. A protocol is followed and clinical evaluations are made at scheduled intervals. In other studies, only the study drug is administered, and physicians "prescribe" the drug as they would use it in clinical practice. Clinical evaluations are still made at scheduled intervals.

Observational studies are another kind of efficacy study. Although these studies are not confirmatory in practice, they generate data which can be scrutinized in an exploratory hypothesis-generating manner. Relationships discovered can then be tested in subsequent controlled studies. In observational studies, data are often generated retrospectively. That is, records (e.g., hospital records, census records, school records) are searched retrospectively and data are gathered to describe the existing situation.

Formats and displays used to present such data often differ from displays of data from controlled efficacy studies. Tables 8.22 to 8.28 and various figures depict typical displays for observational data.

Illustrates data from a crossover study for individual patients using three scales, plus components of one of those scales (individual patient data, single site or study).

TABLE 8.1. Means of Physicians' Ratings for Chlordiazepoxide (C) and Placebo (P) for Each Patient[a]

Patient numbers:	2		3		4		6		7		8	
Treatments:	C (df = 12)	P	C (df = 9)	P	C (df = 12)	P	C (df = 11)	P	C (df = 12)	P	C (df = 12)	P
Global physician rating	3.0	4.0	3.8	6.0 (p<.001)	3.9	5.1 (p<.05)	4.3	4.2	3.9	3.8	3.9	4.0
Hamilton Anxiety Rating Scale	5.8	14.0 (p<.05)	17.8	32.8 (p<.001)	14.0	25.1 (p<.001)	4.6	5.0	12.0	9.6	12.6	12.4
Brief Psychiatric Rating Scale	2.0	2.7	2.5	3.8	3.8	4.6	1.1	1.2	3.6	3.5	2.6	2.9
Somatic anxiety	1.4	2.0	3.5	6.8 (p<.001)	3.3	5.1 (p<.005)	1.4	1.3	3.3	3.3	3.9	3.7
Emotional withdrawal	1.0	1.0	1.8	2.5	1.0	1.3	4.0	3.5	2.0	1.8	3.3	3.3
Conceptual disorganization	0.5	0.6	1.0	1.8 (p<.05)	1.4	2.0	1.7	1.7	1.0	1.0	1.1	1.0
Guilt feelings	0.4	0.4	1.5	5.3 (p<.001)	3.3	3.7	1.3	1.0	1.0	1.0	2.3	3.0
Tension	1.4	2.3 (p<.05)	3.2	6.8 (p<.001)	3.3	4.4 (p<.05)	3.0	3.7	2.9	2.5	3.8	3.4
Mannerism & posturing	0.5	0.6	1.2	2.5 (p<.01)	1.5	1.1	3.9	4.0	1.0	1.1	3.5	3.4
Grandiosity	0.4	0.4	1.0	1.0	1.3	1.0	1.0	1.0	1.0	1.0	1.0	1.0
Depressive mood	2.0	2.3	3.2	4.5	3.9	4.0	2.3	1.8	3.0	1.6 (p<.05)	3.4	3.6

Hostility	0.4	0.4	1.0	3.3 (p<.005)	2.9	3.9	1.9	1.7	1.0	1.1	1.5	1.6
Suspiciousness	0.5	0.9	1.0	3.7 (p<.001)	2.9	3.9	1.1	1.0	2.0	2.4	1.1	1.0
Hallucinatory behavior	0.4	1.3 (p<.05)	1.0	2.3	1.0	2.6 (p<.05)	1.0	1.2	1.0	1.0	1.0	1.0
Motor retardation	2.0	2.4 (p<.05)	1.8	1.3	1.4	1.1	3.1	2.8	2.7	2.1 (p<.05)	3.3	2.9
Uncooperativeness	0.4	0.4	1.0	1.0	1.4	1.3	1.3	1.0	1.0	1.3	1.0	1.0
Unusual thought content	0.8	0.7	1.3	3.0 (p<.001)	2.0	3.1 (p<.05)	2.1	2.0	2.0	1.5	1.0	1.1
Blunted affect	2.1	2.1	2.8	2.7	1.0	1.0	3.6	3.5	2.8	2.4	3.8	3.4
Excitement	0.5	0.4	2.3	6.2 (p<.001)	2.4	3.4 (p<.05)	1.4	2.0	1.0	1.0	2.3	2.7
Disorientation	0.4	0.4	1.0	1.0	1.0	1.0 (p<.05)	1.3	1.0	1.0	1.0	1.0	1.0

[a]Reprinted from Kellner et al. (1975) with permission.

- Includes statistical comparisons.
- Using an asterisk(s) to indicate statistical significance is an alternative means of presenting this information.

Illustrates both individual and combined data (individual patient data, single site or study).

TABLE 8.2. Results of a Clinical Study

Drug A Patient number	Number of weeks					
	0	1	2	3	4	5
2	4	4	3	3	2	2
5	5	4	3	3	2	0
7	3	2	1	—[b]	—[b]	—[b]
10	4	4	3	4	2	1
11	4	4	—[a]	—[a]	—[a]	—[a]
14	4	3	2	2	1	—[a]
15	5	5	3	2	2	1
17	4	3	2	1	—[b]	—[b]
18	5	5	4	2	3	3
20	4	3	3	2	1	0
Mean	4.2	3.8	2.7	2.2	1.8	1.0
(N)	(10)	(9)	(9)	(9)	(8)	(7)
Drug B						
1	5	5	—[b]	—[b]	—[b]	—[b]
3	4	3	3	3	2	1
4	4	3	2	2	2	1
6	5	5	4	3	3	3
8	3	2	1	0	0	0
9	5	5	3	2	3	2
12	4	3	3	2	—[b]	0
13	5	5	—[a]	—[a]	—[a]	—[a]
16	4	4	3	—[a]	—[a]	—[a]
19	5	3	3	3	2	2
Mean	4.4	3.8	2.8	2.5	2.1	1.3
(N)	(10)	(10)	(8)	(8)	(8)	(7)

[a]Patient dropped out of study.
[b]Missing observation.

• Values of means could also be given for individual patients across a selected period (e.g., plateau treatment dose).

• Values for specific parameters at one or more times could be presented in lieu of data for a single parameter.

• One or more horizontal lines could be deleted.

Illustrates data from a single patient study (single patient, single study).

TABLE 8.3. Evidence of Primary Process[a]

Session number	Medication	Raw scores		Trend-adjusted scores	
		Session score	Sequence average	Session score	Sequence average
0	None	5	5.0	—	—
1	Placebo	4	4.0	2.2	2.2
2	Chlordiazepoxide	2		0.6	
3	Chlordiazepoxide	1	1.7	0.0	0.7
4	Chlordiazepoxide	2		1.4	
5	Placebo	5		4.8	
6	Placebo	2	2.3	2.2	2.5
7	Placebo	0		0.6	
8	Chlordiazepoxide	0		0.9	
9	Chlordiazepoxide	0	0.0	1.3	1.3
10	Chlordiazepoxide	0		1.7	
Placebo session means		2.75		2.45	
Chlordiazepoxide session means		0.83		0.98	

[a]Reprinted from Bellak and Chassan (1964) with permission.

- Both raw and adjusted data are given, as well as means on each of two treatments.
- Error measurements and p values could be added to the means and their comparison.

Illustrates single patient data for eight characteristics evaluated under two treatment conditions (single patient, single study).

TABLE 8.4. Effects: Raw and Trend-Adjusted Scores[a]

	Average raw scores		Average trend-adjusted scores	
	Chlordiazepoxide	Placebo	Chlordiazepoxide	Placebo
Primary process	0.83	2.75	0.98	2.45
Anxiety	0.75	1.75	1.40	2.15
Confusion	0.67	2.00	1.37	2.40
Hostility	0.83	1.50	1.63	2.05
"Sexual flooding"	0.83	1.75	0.98	1.45
Depersonalization	0.67	2.75	1.45	3.32
Ability to communicate	0.50[b]	1.75[b]	0.35[b]	1.37[b]
Depression	1.00	1.25	—[c]	—[c]

[a]Reprinted from Bellak and Chassan (1964) with permission.
[b]The lower the numerical score, the better the ability to communicate.
[c]Depression is the only item for which a decreasing trend was not evident from the data.

Illustrates clinical characteristics in 30 individual cases (individual patient data, single study).

TABLE 8.5. Clinical Manifestations in 30 Cases of Primary Varicella Pneumonia[a]

Case no.	Patient	Date of admission	Age in years	Sex	Day of onset of cough	Cough	Dyspnea	Cyanosis	Hemoptysis	Rales	Pulmonary consolidation on X-ray study	White cell count	Complications
1	C.B.	6-18-56	26	F	2	+++	+++	+++	+++	++	+++	12,800	Pulmonary edema; death
2	J.R.	3-3-58	51	M	3	+++	+++	+++	+++	+++	+++	8,000	Pulmonary abscesses; gastric ulcers; death
3	E.W.	4-5-57	44	M	4	+++	+++	+++	++	++	—	—	Hepatitis; death
4	E.Wo.	11-26-59	33	F	1	+++	+++	+++	++	++	+++	7,700	Hodgkin's disease; pulmonary abscesses; death
5	F.R.	5-14-58	6	M	3	+++	+++	++	0	+++	++	12,000	Leukemia; death
6	O.R.	1-28-56	27	M	5	+++	+++	+++	+++	+++	+++	10,700	Subcutaneous emphysema; pleural effusion
7	J.F.	1-25-59	82	M	2	+++	+++	++	+	+++	+++	4,950	None
8	C.L.	6-13-56	24	M	3	+++	+++	+++	++	++	+++	12,600	None
9	E.R.	4-4-59	32	F	3	+++	++	0	++	+	++	16,200	Hepatitis; pleural effusion

			Age	Sex								WBC	Complications
10	M.Ve.	6-1-58	38	M	2	+++	++	+	++	++	+++	7,700	None
11	Ro.M.	3-28-56	29	M	5	+++	+++	+	+	++	+++	15,500	Hepatitis
12	R.R.	3-25-58	27	M	3	++	+	0	+	++	+++	—	None
13	S.S.	5-14-58	4	F	2	+++	+++	0	0	+++	+++	5,000	None (leukemia)
14	J.W.	5-26-58	24	M	2	+++	+++	0	0	+	+++	—	None
15	E.M.	1-29-56	38	M	2	+++	+++	0	0	+++	+++	9,600	None
16	M.V.	6-20-56	34	F	2	+++	+++	0	0	++	+++	7,800	None
17	E.M.	3-26-60	26	F	1	++	+	0	0	+	+++	6,200	None
18	A.G.	4-23-56	56	M	2	++	+	0	0	+	+++	8,900	Pleural effusion
19	A.B.	3-30-60	24	M	1	+	0	0	0	+	0	5,100	None
20	A.O.	1-6-60	35	M	1	+	0	0	0	++	+	4,000	Hepatitis
21	M.M.	3-21-56	42	M	2	++	+	0	0	+	++	5,400	None
22	R.M.	2-21-56	29	M	3	++	+	+	0	0	+	8,600	None
23	G.T.	3-26-56	36	M	2	+	0	0	0	+	+	—	None
24	M.P.	6-5-58	20	M	2	+	+	0	0	+	+	4,500	None
25	R.D.	2-12-59	28	M	3	+	+	0	0	+	+	5,150	None
26	D.L.	1-21-57	47	M	2	+	+	0	0	+	+	10,000	None
27	J.M.	1-15-60	30	M	1	+	+	0	0	+	+	8,950	None
28	M.R.	5-5-60	30	M	2	++	+	0	+	+	+	8,250	None
29	J.C.	6-17-60	36	F	2	+	+	0	0	+	+	5,100	None
30	J.Ro.	6-19-60	70	F	1	+	0	0	0	0	+	10,200	None

aReprinted from Krugman and Ward (1973) with permission.

+++, severe; ++, moderate; +, mild; 0, none

• Note that the headings combine demographics, medical history, laboratory values, clinical signs, and an indication of complications.

Illustrates group values and basic statistical information for variations of a single parameter at various times under two conditions (drug 1 and drug 2) (group data, single site or study).

TABLE 8.6. Summary Statistics for Primary Efficacy Variable

Treatment	Time of assessment	N	Mean	Median	SD	SE	Range
Drug 1	0						
	1						
	2						
	3						
Drug 2	0						
	1						
	2						
	3						

• If "N" is the same for all assessments it need not be printed in each row.

• The order of the first two columns could be interchanged, depending on what the presenter wishes to emphasize.

• Space permitting, it is helpful to give both mean and median. However, only standard deviation (SD) or standard error (SE) is necessary.

• Range is usually exceptionally helpful.

• If the study has more than one efficacy variable, the primary efficacy variable should be summarized in a table by itself. Other (i.e., secondary) efficacy variables may be summarized either in one big table or in a separate table for each variable.

• If the first assessment is a baseline assessment, then a similar summarization of change from baseline may be warranted. If so, a column for the p value of change from baseline may be appropriate.

• This table is often associated with a graph where, for each treatment, the mean (or median) value at each assessment is plotted on the y-axis, and the assessment time is on the x-axis. If the mean is plotted, error bars are sometimes added.

Illustrates cumulative responses over time for four treatment groups (group data, single or multiple studies).

TABLE 8.7. Cumulative Number (%) of Patients with Healed Ulcers

Weeks (days) on treatment	Drug dose group (mg)			
	40 hs N = 88	20 bid N = 83	40 bid N = 92	Placebo N = 98
Week 1 (days 2–8)[a]	0 (0)	0 (0)	0 (0)	0 (0)
Week 2 (days 9–15)	21 (24)	25 (30)	20 (22)	8 (8)
Week 3 (days 16–22)	31 (35)	35 (42)	32 (34)	16 (16)
Week 4 (days 23–29)	47 (53)	49 (58)	50 (54)	24 (25)
Week 5 (days 30–36)	62 (70)	57 (68)	70 (75)	30 (31)
Week 6 (days 37–43)	62 (70)	59 (70)	70 (75)	30 (31)
Week 7 (days 44–50)	63 (71)	59 (70)	70 (75)	30 (31)
Week 8 (days 51–57)	70 (79)	62 (74)	72 (77)	39 (40)

[a]Day 1 was the day of the baseline evaluation. Patients started taking drug at bedtime on day 1. All weekly day ranges start with day 2.

Illustrates simple means of presenting subgroup analyses to identify factors that are important to the outcome (group data, single or multiple studies).

TABLE 8.8. Frequency and Percent of Patients with a Healed Ulcer
Stratified by Selected Factors

Factor	Level	Treatment			
		40 mg hs	20 mg bid	40 mg bid	Placebo
Ulcer size (cm)	0.5–0.9	45/50 (90%)	37/43 (86%)	37/48 (77%)	29/54 (54%)
	1.0–1.4	22/28 (79%)	18/26 (69%)	26/30 (87%)	13/31 (42%)
	1.5—2.5	8/11 (73%)	14/15 (93%)	14/15 (93%)	2/12 (17%)
Ulcer history	None	26/29 (90%)	34/40 (85%)	27/31 (87%)	14/25 (56%)
	Single	18/22 (82%)	16/19 (84%)	19/23 (83%)	15/29 (52%)
	Multiple	31/38 (82%)	19/25 (76%)	31/39 (80%)	15/43 (35%)
Esophagus	Normal	56/67 (84%)	47/57 (83%)	62/76 (82%)	25/66 (38%)
condition	Abnormal	19/22 (86%)	22/27 (82%)	15/17 (88%)	19/31 (61%)
Drinking history	No	59/71 (83%)	58/72 (81%)	66/79 (84%)	34/84 (41%)
	Yes	16/18 (89%)	11/12 (92%)	11/14 (79%)	10/13 (77%)
Smoking history	No	30/34 (88%)	29/33 (88%)	31/37 (84%)	19/38 (50%)
	Yes	45/55 (82%)	40/51 (78%)	46/56 (82%)	25/59 (42%)
No. of ulcers	1	64/74 (87%)	56/69 (81%)	67/82 (82%)	40/84 (48%)
	2 to 4	11/15 (73%)	13/15 (87%)	10/11 (91%)	4/13 (31%)

Illustrates use of recurrence values as an efficacy variable to evaluate different treatments (group data, single or multiple studies).

TABLE 8.9. Duodenal Ulcer Relapse Rates by Treatment Groups

Time		Treatment group		
		40 mg hs	20 mg hs	Placebo
Period 1	No. relapsed	0 (0%)	1 (2%)	8 (13%)
(days 1–42)				
	No. dropped out[a]	8	5	11
	Total number	49	49	62
	Cumulative relapse rate	0%[b]	2%[c]	13%
Period 2	No. relapsed	7 (17%)[b]	8 (19%)[c]	20 (47%)
(days 43–105)				
	No. dropped out[a]	15	8	6
	Total number	41	43	43
	Cumulative relapse rate	17%[b]	20%[b]	53%
Period 3	No. relapsed	3 (16%)	2 (7%)[b]	6 (35%)
(days 106 or later)				
	No. dropped out[a]	16	25	11
	Total number	19	27	17
	Cumulative relapse rate	30%[b]	26%[b]	70%

[a]A large number of these patients had been in the maintenance phase for less than the required length of time and are still continuing in the study.
[b,c]Significantly different from placebo, p < 0.01, p < 0.05, respectively.

Illustrates means of segmenting groups of investigators and combining results (group data, multiple sites or studies).

TABLE 8.10. Healing Reported by Investigators with at Least 15 Patients—Number (%) Healed

Invest.[a]	40 mg hs				20 mg bid				40 mg bid			
	N	Wk 2	Wk 4	Wk 8	N	Wk 2	Wk 4	Wk 8	N	Wk 2	Wk 4	Wk 8
1	6	0 (0)	1 (17)	6 (100)	4	2 (50)	3 (75)	3 (75)	5	2 (40)	4 (80)	5 (100)
2	7	2 (29)	5 (71)	5 (71)	7	2 (29)	3 (43)	5 (71)	6	3 (50)	5 (83)	5 (83)
3	10	3 (30)	5 (50)	5 (50)	8	4 (50)	5 (63)	6 (75)	9	0 (0)	8 (89)	9 (100)
4	8	4 (50)	8 (100)	8 (100)	9	3 (33)	5 (56)	5 (56)	6	1 (17)	3 (50)	3 (50)
5	7	4 (57)	6 (86)	7 (100)	8	3 (38)	7 (88)	8 (100)	7	5 (71)	7 (100)	7 (100)
Subtotal	38	13 (34)	25 (66)	31 (82)	36	14 (39)	23 (64)	27 (75)	33	11 (33)	27 (82)	29 (88)
Pool[b]	51	15 (24)	37 (73)	43 (84)	48	18 (38)	33 (69)	42 (88)	60	20 (33)	42 (70)	46 (77)
Total	89	28 (32)	62 (70)	74 (83)	84	32 (38)	56 (67)	69 (82)	93	31 (33)	69 (74)	75 (81)

[a] Invest., investigator.
[b] All other investigators combined.

illustrates two methods of presenting antibiotic data, based on clinical response to different organisms or sites of infections (group data, single site or study).

TABLE 8.11. Summary of Six Controlled, Randomized, Non-Blind Studies Comparing the Efficacy of Antibiotic A vs. Antibiotic B in Serious Systemic Infections

Infection	Antibiotic A Clinical response			Antibiotic B Clinical response		
	Resolved N (%)	Improved N (%)	Failed N (%)	Resolved N (%)	Improved N (%)	Failed N (%)
Lower respiratory	19 (59.3)	10 (31.2)	3 (9.3)	15 (55)	9 (31)	4 (14)
Intraabdominal	5 (33.3)	8 (53.3)	2 (13.3)	2 (15)	5 (39)	6 (46)
Hepato-biliary	2 (67)		1 (33)	2 (33)	3 (50)	1 (17)
Urinary tract	15 (88)		2 (12)	9 (82)		2 (18)
Gynecologic	3 (43)	3 (43)	1 (14)	2 (25)	4 (50)	2 (25)
Skin & skin structures	24 (48)	23 (44)	4 (8)	18 (42)	15 (35)	10 (23)
Septicemia	8 (67)	1 (8)	3 (25)	10 (77)		3 (23)
Bone & joint	1 (33)	2 (67)		1 (20)	2 (40)	2 (40)

Infection/organism	Antibiotic A Bacteriologic response			Antibiotic B Bacteriologic response		
	Eliminated N (%)	Moderately reduced N (%)	Persisted N (%)	Eliminated N (%)	Moderately reduced N (%)	Persisted (i.e., not eradicated) N (%)
Lower respiratory						
S. pneumoniae	11 (100)			6 (100)		
H. influenzae	9 (100)			2 (100)		
K. pneumoniae/sp.	4 (66.7)	1 (16.6)	1 (16.6)	1 (25)	2 (50)	1 (25)
P. mirabilis	4 (100)			5 (83)	1 (17)	
Pseudom. aerug/sp.			1 (100)	1 (100)		
E. coli	2 (66.7)		1 (33)	4 (80)		1 (20)
Bacteroides sp.	3 (100)					
Intraabdominal						
E. coli	7 (70)	1 (10)	2 (20)	4 (40)	2 (20)	4 (40)
P. mirabilis	1 (50)	1 (50)			1 (50)	1 (50)
Klebsiella sp.	3 (75)	1 (25)			2 (67)	1 (33)
Pseudomonas sp.	1 (50)	1 (50)		1 (100)		
Strep. faecalis	1 (100)					
Bacteroides sp.	2 (100)					
Peptococcus sp.	1 (100)					
Peptostrep sp.	1 (100)					

• This is a poor display of percentages. Decimal points should line up (e.g., for 50 and 100) and fractions of a decimal should be rounded off.

Illustrates how cumulative mortality may be summarized (group data, single site or study).

TABLE 8.12. Summary of Life Tables, Endpoint: All Deaths—Total Mortality (Intention-to-treat Approach)

	Cumulative mortality probability (%)													
	High risk group			Reinfarction group			Low risk group			Risk groups combined				
Follow-up time at month	P^a	T^a	Reduction in T	P	T	Reduction in T	P	T	Reduction in T	P	T	Reduction in T	p value
6	8.8	5.8	33.9	10.3	7.9	23.9	2.3	1.8	18.7	7.6	5.3	30.0	0.05
12	11.8	7.5	36.6	16.1	12.4	23.2	6.3	4.1	34.9	11.3	7.6	32.5	0.008
24	16.2	9.4	42.2	23.4	19.3	17.7	9.2	4.1	55.3	15.9	10.1	36.5	0.0005
34	23.0	12.3	46.6	27.2	24.6	9.5	15.2	5.5	63.7	21.9	13.3	39.4	0.0003

[a]P, placebo; T, treatment.

Illustrates a 2 × 2 table (group data, single site or study).

TABLE 8.13. Numbers of Patients with Pressor or Depressor Responses Based on Their Peripheral Renin Values

	Drug response		
	Depressor	Neutral or pressor	Total
Peripheral renin ≥ 13 and renal vein renins positive	42 (93.3%)	3 (6.7%)	45
Peripheral renin ≤ 13 and renal vein renins negative or inconclusive	27 (14.1%)	165 (85.9%)	192

- Data in 2 × 2 tables are often compared by chi-squared analyses or by a Fisher's Exact Test.
- In many such tables all patients fit one of the four cells and no overlap may occur.

Illustrates benefit to patients in terms of time added to life expectancy (group data, single site or study).

TABLE 8.14. Effect of Treatment on Patient Survival

	To end of trial		To April 1, 1987[c]	
	Total[a]	Time lost (%)[b]	Total	Time lost (%)[b]
AIDS treatment group	18.55	0	47.55	4.5
AIDS placebo group	19.36	5.1	48.36	19.9
ARC treatment group	19.60	0	48.60	1.0
ARC placebo group	19.90	3.3	48.90	10.7

[a]Average potential time on study had all patients continued to end of trial (September 19, 1986).
[b]Time lost due to death as a percent of total time in study.
[c]April 1, 1987 is the last date for which data are available.

Illustrates that measuring time to a prespecified endpoint (e.g., recovery) may be divided into any number of categories (group data, multiple studies).

TABLE 8.15. Effect of Inhalation Agents on Duration of Neuromuscular Blockade Caused by Drug X

Study (by inhalation agent)	Dose (mg/kg)	Duration to beginning recovery (min)			Duration to 25% recovery (min)			Duration to 95% recovery (min)		
		Inhal.	Bal.	Inhal./Bal.	Inhal.	Bal.	Inhal./Bal.	Inhal.	Bal.	Inhal./Bal
Halothane vs. balanced										
02-01, 05-01	0.36–0.40	29.2	30.8	0.95	44.9	35.9	1.25	65.2	64.8	1.01
03, 06	0.36–0.40	28.7	20.5	1.40	43.3	45.3	.96	66.7	56.0	1.19
Enflurane vs. balanced										
08-01	0.36–0.40	31.6	23.1	1.37	53.4	37.6	1.42	74.1	59.2	1.25
09-01	0.36–0.40	25.4	20.1	1.26	40.9	31.6	1.29	61.9	50.5	1.23
Isoflurane vs. balanced										
07-01	0.21–0.25	26.4	25.9	1.02	34.7	35.8	0.97	56.4	50.8	1.11
10-01	0.26–0.30	27.4	19.0	1.44	39.8	32.3	1.23	67.2	42.2	1.59

Illustrates that measuring time to a prespecified endpoint (e.g., recovery) may be based on doses studied as well as conditions of the study (group data, multiple studies).

TABLE 8.16. Time to Beginning of Recovery from Neuromuscular Blockade[a,b]

	Initial dose (mg/kg)														
	0.21–0.25			0.26–0.30			0.36–0.40			0.50			0.60		
Study (by inhalation agent)	N	Mean	(SE)	N	Mean	(SE)	N	Mean	(SE)	N	Mean	(SE)	N	Mean	(SE)
Mechanical twitch response															
A. Balanced anesthesia															
02-01				10	18.2	(1.70)	10	30.8	(2.38)	10	34.9	(3.75)	10	42.2	(2.90)
07-01	5	25.9	(4.06)							5	37.2	(4.49)			
08-01							18	23.1	(1.56)	10	26.4	(2.14)			
09-01	5	11.5	(1.15)				5	20.1	(2.40)	5	25.5	(3.51)			
10-01				5	19.0	(2.84)	5	25.0	(4.04)						
B. Halothane anesthesia															
05-01							10	29.2	(1.89)						
C. Enflurane anesthesia															
08-01							10	31.6	(3.22)						
09-01							9	25.4	(2.25)						
D. Isoflurane anesthesia															
07-01	5	26.4	(3.72)												
10-01				10	27.4	(2.32)									

[a] Time to 25%, 50%, or another percent recovery could be shown.
[b] Time to onset of response, time to peak response, or another related parameter could be shown.

Illustrates multiple parameters that changed by more than specified percents in three separate studies (group data, multiple studies).

TABLE 8.17. Increases in Hemodynamic Values

Parameter[a]	Change	Total		Study A				Study B				Study C			
				0.2 mg/kg		0.4 mg/kg		0.2 mg/kg		0.4 mg/kg		0.2 mg/kg		0.4 mg/kg	
		N	%	N	%	N	%	N	%	N	%	N	%	N	%
SYS	≥20%	3/39	(7.7)	1/4	(25)	2/4	(50)	0/7	(0)	0/8	(0)	0/8	(0)	0/8	(0)
	≥30%	2/39	(5.1)	1/4	(25)	1/4	(25)	0/7	(0)	0/8	(0)	0/8	(0)	0/8	(0)
	≥40%	2/39	(5.1)	1/4	(25)	1/4	(25)	0.7	(0)	0/8	(0)	0/8	(0)	0/8	(0)
DIA	≥20%	5/39	(12.8)	2/4	(50)	1/4	(25)	0/7	(0)	0/8	(0)	2/8	(25.0)	0/8	(0)
	≥30%	2/39	(5.1)	1/4	(25)	1/4	(0)	0/7	(0)	0/8	(0)	0/8	(0)	0/8	(0)
	≥40%	1/39	(2.6)	1/4	(25)	0/4	(0)	0/7	(0)	0/8	(0)	0/8	(0)	0/8	(0)
MAP	≥20%	3/39	(7.7)	2/4	(50)	1/4	(25)	0/7	(0)	0/8	(0)	0/8	(0)	0/8	(0)
	≥30%	3/39	(7.7)	2/4	(50)	1/4	(25)	0/7	(0)	0/8	(0)	0/8	(0)	0/8	(0)
	≥40%	3/39	(7.7)	2/4	(50)	1/4	(25)	0/7	(0)	0/8	(0)	0/8	(0)	0/8	(0)
HR	≥20%	2/39	(5.1)	0/4	(0)	1/4	(25)	0/7	(0)	0/8	(0)	1/8	(12.5)	0/8	(0)
	≥30%	2/39	(5.1)	0/4	(0)	1/4	(25)	0/7	(0)	0/8	(0)	1/8	(12.5)	0/8	(0)
	≥40%	2/39	(5.1)	0/4	(0)	1/4	(25)	0/7	(0)	0/8	(0)	1/8	(12.5)	0/8	(0)
CVP	≥20%	12/39	(30.8)	2/4	(50)	2/4	(50)	0/7	(0)	2/8	(25)	3/8	(37.5)	3/8	(37.5)
	≥30%	9/39	(23.1)	2/4	(50)	2/4	(50)	0/7	(0)	0/8	(0)	2/8	(25.0)	3/8	(37.5)
	≥40%	8/39	(20.5)	2/4	(50)	2/4	(50)	0/7	(0)	0/8	(0)	2/8	(25.0)	2/8	(25.0)

CO	≥20%	2/39	(5.1)	1/4	(25)	0/4	(0)	0/7	(0)	0/8	(0)	1/8	(12.5)	0/8	(0)
	≥30%	0/39	(0)	0/4	(0)	0/4	(0)	0/7	(0)	0/8	(0)	0/8	(0)	0/8	(0)
	≥40%	0/39	(0)	0/4	(0)	0/4	(0)	0/7	(0)	0/8	(0)	0/8	(0)	0/8	(0)
CI	≥20%	2/39	(5.1)	1/4	(25)	0/4	(0)	0/7	(0)	0/8	(0)	1/8	(12.5)	0/8	(0)
	≥30%	0/39	(0)	0/4	(0)	0/4	(0)	0/7	(0)	0/8	(0)	0/8	(0)	0/8	(0)
	≥40%	0/39	(0)	0/4	(0)	0/4	(0)	0/7	(0)	0/8	(0)	0/8	(0)	0/8	(0)
SV	≥20%	4/39	(10.3)	1/4	(25)	0/4	(0)	1/7	(14.3)	0/8	(0)	1/8	(12.5)	1/8	(12.5)
	≥30%	0/39	(0)	0/4	(0)	0/4	(0)	0/7	(0)	0/8	(0)	0/8	(0)	0/8	(0)
	≥40%	0/39	(0)	0/4	(0)	0/4	(0)	0/7	(0)	0/8	(0)	0/8	(0)	0/8	(0)
SVR	≥20%	7/39	(17.9)	3/4	(75)	1/4	(25)	0/7	(0)	0/8	(0)	2/8	(25.0)	1/8	(12.5)
	≥30%	4/39	(10.3)	2/4	(50)	1/4	(25)	0/7	(0)	0/8	(0)	0/8	(0)	1/8	(12.5)
	≥40%	3/39	(7.7)	2/4	(50)	1/4	(25)	0/7	(0)	0/8	(0)	0/8	(0)	0/8	(0)
MPAP	≥20%	2/16	(12.5)	—	—	—	—	—	—	—	—	1/8	(12.5)	1/8	(12.5)
	≥30%	2/16	(12.5)	—	—	—	—	—	—	—	—	1/8	(12.5)	1/8	(12.5)
	≥40%	1/16	(6.3)	—	—	—	—	—	—	—	—	0/8	(0)	1/8	(12.5)
PCWP	≥20%	1/16	(6.3)	—	—	—	—	—	—	—	—	0/8	(0)	1/8	(12.5)
	≥30%	1/16	(6.3)	—	—	—	—	—	—	—	—	0/8	(0)	1/8	(12.5)
	≥40%	1/16	(6.3)	—	—	—	—	—	—	—	—	0/8	(0)	1/8	(12.5)

[a]SYS, systolic blood pressure; DIA, diastolic blood pressure; MAP, mean arterial pressure; HR, heart rate; CVP, central venous pressure; CO, cardiac output; CI, cardiac index; SV, stroke volume; SVR, stroke volume resistance; MPAP, mean pulmonary arterial pressure; PCWP, pulmonary capillary wedge pressure.

• Values for different types of treatment groups could be presented.

Illustrates overall hemodynamic values in various treatment groups (group data, single site or study)

TABLE 8.18. Hemodynamic Values in 12 Postoperative Patients[a]

	Isoproterenol (μg/kg per min)			Dopamine (μg/kg per min)		
	Control	0.0125	0.0250	Control	2.5	5.0
Pressures (mm Hg)						
Right arterial mean	8 ± 2.4	7 ± 2.5	7 ± 1.8	7 ± 2.5	7 ± 2.6	7 ± 2.0
Pulmonary arterial mean	24 ± 7.6	23 ± 7.5 (−4%)	23 ± 6.0 (−4%)	22 ± 5.7	19 ± 4.4 (−14%)	22 ± 6.6
Left atrial mean	12 ± 5.9	10 ± 5.5[b] (−17%)	10 ± 5.1[b] (−17%)	11 ± 6.0	8 ± 3.4[b] (−27%)	9 ± 5.1[b] (−18%)
Arterial mean	98 ± 11.5	92 ± 10.1[b] (−6%)	93 ± 6.7[b] (−5%)	95 ± 7.7	87 ± 11.8[b] (−9%)	92 ± 13.8 (−3%)
Cardiac output (liters/min)	5.2 ± 0.9	6.4 ± 1.1[b] (+23%)	7.1 ± 1.6[b] (+37%)	4.7 ± 0.9	5.6 ± 1.1[b] (+23%)	6.6 ± 1.6[b] (+43%)
Cardiac index (liters/min per m²)	2.9 ± 0.5	3.6 ± 0.7	3.9 ± 0.8	2.7 ± 0.5	3.3 ± 0.6	3.9 ± 0.8
Heart rate (beats/min)	108 ± 15.0	126 ± 12.0[b] (+18%)	135 ± 11.8[b] (+28%)	110 ± 18.5	111 ± 17.5	116 ± 18.3 (+5%)
Stroke volume (ml)	49 ± 11.7	51 ± 10.1 (+5%)	53 ± 14.0 (+8%)	43 ± 6.6	51 ± 9.0[b] (+23%)	57 ± 11.3[b] (+35%)
Pulmonary vascular resistance (dynes sec cm^{-1})	189 ± 84.2	172 ± 74.4 (−9%)	150 ± 52.4[b] (−21%)	194 ± 61.3	170 ± 64.5 (−12%)	155 ± 58.9[b] (−20%)
Systemic vascular resistance (dynes sec cm^{-1})	1430 ± 363	1110 ± 324[b] (−22%)	1020 ± 287[b] (−29%)	1560 ± 319	1200 ± 284[b] (−23%)	1060 ± 208[b] (−32%)

[a]Values expressed as mean ± SD, with percent change from control shown in parentheses.

[b]$p < 0.05$.

• Comparable tables could illustrate pulmonary, gastrointestinal, or other categories of data.

• This table probably has too much data. It is particularly difficult to comprehend the percentages, since they are on different rows.

Illustrates a presentation of all data of one type from multiple studies (group data, multiple studies).

TABLE 8.19. Specialized Type of Study (e.g., Cardiovascular)[a]

Variable[b]	Study number	Baseline value (control)	N	Results Time after drug (dose = L)[c]			p value (ANOVA)
				X min or hr (N)	Y min or hr (N)	Z min or hr (N)	
A (units)	1						
	2						
	3						
	4						
B (units)	1						
	2						
	3						
	4						
C (units)	1						
	2						
	3						
	4						
D (units)	1						
	2						
	3						
	4						

[a]Data from each study could be presented separately.
[b]Many variables could be listed.
[c]Dose of drug could be a range or fixed dose.

Illustrates a presentation of dose-response data obtained under various experimental conditions (group data, multiple studies).

TABLE 8.20. Summary of Dose-Response Analyses Across Several Studies

Study	N	ED_{50} (mg/kg)	ED_{95} (mg/kg)
Mechanical twitch response			
A. Balanced anesthesia			
02	50	0.12	0.17
07	20	0.09	0.11
08	53	0.17	0.26
09	15	0.15	0.23
10	15	0.12	0.27
B. Halothane anesthesia			
05	30	0.10	0.17
C. Enflurane anesthesia			
08	24	0.11	0.19
09	31	0.10	0.18
D. Isoflurane anesthesia			
07	20	0.06	0.10
10	30	0.07	0.13
EMG twitch response			
A. Balanced anesthesia			
03	30	0.15	0.23
B. Halothane anesthesia			
06	30	0.11	0.20

• A graphic approach is usually desirable for one or a few dose-response curves, but a table can more simply present results of many curves that are similar.

Illustrates how relative risks may be presented for many patient groups (group data, multiple sites or studies).

TABLE 8.21. Risks Associated with Stability and Change of Body Mass Index from Age 55 Years to Age 65 Years[a]

Body mass index	Relative risk (95% confidence interval)
Duration of overweight[b]	
Men	
70th percentile, ages 55 and 65 years	2.0 (2.3, 3.2)
70th percentile, age 65 years only	1.0 (0.5, 1.9)
Women	
70th percentile, ages 55 and 65	2.1 (1.4, 3.0)
70th percentile, age 65 only	1.4 (0.8, 2.5)
Change in body mass index from age 55 to age 65	
Men	
% Change from body mass index at age 55[c]	
Loss of $\geq$10%	1.9 (1.1, 3.2)
Loss of 0%–9%	1.4 (1.0, 1.9)
Gain of 0%–9%	1.0 (Referent)
Gain of $\geq$10%	1.5 (0.9, 2.4)
Body mass index percentile at age 65[d]	
70th	1.8 (1.2, 2.7)
30th–69th	1.4 (0.9, 2.0)
10th–29th	1.0 (Referent)
0–9th	1.6 (0.9, 2.7)

TABLE 8.21. Continued

Body mass index	Relative risk (95% confidence interval)
Change in body mass index from age 55 to age 65	
Women	
% Change from body mass index at age 55[c]	
Loss of ≥10%	1.8 (1.2, 2.6)
Loss of 0%–9%	1.1 (0.8, 1.4)
Gain of 0%–9%	1.0 (Referent)
Gain of ≥10%	1.6 (0.8, 1.7)
Body mass index percentile at age 65[d]	
70th	2.1 (1.5, 2.9)
50th–69th	1.5 (1.0, 2.2)
30th–49th	1.0 (Referent)
0–29th	1.4 (1.0, 2.0)

[a]Reprinted from Harris et al. (1988) with permission.
[b]Comparison to body mass index of 23.0 to 25.2 kg/m² in men and 24.1 to 26.1 kg/m² in women and controlling for other levels of body mass index.
[c]Controlling for weight percentiles at age 65 years.
[d]Controlling for percentage of change.

Illustrates changes in numbers or rates over time (group data, observational studies).

TABLE 8.22. Annual US Mortality of Persons Younger than 15 Years of Age, Selected Cancers, 1950 and 1977–1980, per Million[a]

Year	Leukemia		Non-Hodgkin's lymphoma		Hodgkin's disease		Bone[b]		Kidney		Other	
	Rate	N	Rate	N	Rate	N	Rate	N	Rate	N	Rate	N
1950	38.6	1,584	4.5	186	1.5	61	3.3	140	6.2	254	29.1	1,919
1977	19.8	1,055	3.1	181	0.3	24	1.7	105	1.4	64	21.4	1,057
1978	18.5	961	2.9	157	0.3	19	1.4	92	1.8	83	19.1	918
1979	17.6	905	2.8	154	0.3	19	1.6	99	1.8	89	19.6	965
1980	16.8	874	2.5	137	0.3	22	1.7	102	1.5	73	20.0	965

[a]Rates are age adjusted. Reprinted from Miller and McKay (1984) with permission.
[b]Reference year for bone cancer only was 1951.

- This is good presentation displaying how the status quo changed between 1950 and 1977–1980.
- Comparisons should be made on the rate, not the raw numbers.
- Improvement would be to add footnote identifying what cancers comprise the "other" category.
- Improvement would be to add a column describing death rates from all kinds of cancer—the presented table breaks down that unpresented column.

Illustrates rates and risks of a problem according to demographic characteristics (group data, observational studies).

TABLE 8.23. Rates of Hospitalizations for Pelvic Inflammatory Disease (PID)[a]

Characteristics	N	Rate[b]	Risk[c]
Age (years)			
15–19	42,000	4.0 (±0.2)	1.1
20–24	72,100	7.0 (±0.2)	2.0
25–29	62,700	6.7 (±0.2)	1.9
30–34	43,200	5.3 (±0.2)	1.5
35–39	26,700	4.0 (±0.2)	1.1
40–44	20,500	3.6 (±0.2)	1.0
Race			
White	187,900	4.3 (±0.1)	1.0
All others	79,300	10.6 (±0.4)	2.5
Marital status			
Single	82,200	4.8 (±0.2)	1.0
Married	129,000	4.9 (±0.1)	1.0
Divorced	28,900	8.4 (±0.4)	1.8
Separated	15,700	7.6 (±0.4)	1.6
Geographic region			
Northeast	44,000	4.0 (±0.2)	1.0
North Central	76,400	5.7 (±0.2)	1.4
South	104,600	6.3 (±0.2)	1.6
West	42,200	4.4 (±0.2)	1.1
Total PID	267,200	5.3 (±0.1)	—

[a]Among women aged 15 to 44 years, by age, race, marital status, and geographic region, United States, 1975 to 1981. Reprinted from Washington et al. (1984) with permission.
[b]Hospitalized PID for each 1,000 women. SE in parentheses.
[c]Relative risk of hospitalized PID compared with index group with lowest rate.

- Footnote "c" would be confusing to any reader not familiar with the term "index group with lowest rate."
- Inclusion of SE with rates is informative.

Illustrates how ordering causes from most prevalent to least prevalent highlights one aspect of the data and assists in the interpretation (group data, observational studies).

TABLE 8.24. Electric Products that Contributed to Bathtub-Related Electrocutions, United States, 1979 to 1982[a]

Product	Bathtub-related electrocutions	
	N	%
Hair dryer	57	60.0
Television	10	10.5
Electric wire and wiring system	10	10.5
Lamp	7	7.4
Electric heater	3	3.1
Water heater	1	1.1
Fan	1	1.1
Not classified	6	6.3
Total	95	100.0

[a]Reprinted from Budnick (1984) with permission.

- Similar to displays from controlled studies.
- Designed to display status during the years 1979–1982—study does *not* evaluate any drug or nondrug intervention.
- Alternative ordering of data, e.g., alphabetical order, would not be nearly as informative.

Illustrates a straightforward means of presenting survey data (group data, single study).

TABLE 8.25. Presenting Data from Surveys and Questionnaires

Question asked	Number obtained to each possible response					Total number of responses	Percent of each possible response				
	1	2	3	4	5		1	2	3	4	5
A											
B											
C											
. . .											
N											
Total Number											

- Possible responses may include: not home, declined comment, none of the above.
- Responses may be assigned a point score and the totals per question averaged and analyzed statistically and a measure of variability expressed (e.g., SD, SE, range, 95% confidence limits).

Illustrates population data showing mortality rates (group data, observational data).

TABLE 8.26. Estimated Years of Potential Life Lost Before 65 and Cause-specific Mortality, by Cause of Death—United States, 1984

Cause of mortality (Ninth revision ICD)	Years of potential life lost by persons dying in 1984[a]	Cause-specific mortality[b] (rate/100,000)
All causes (total)	11,761,000	866.7
Unintentional injuries [c] (E800-E949)	2,308,000	40.1
Malignant neoplasms (140-208)	1,803,000	191.6
Diseases of the heart (390-398, 402, 404-429)	1,563,000	324.4
Suicide, homicide (E950-E978)	1,247,000	20.6
Congenital anomalies (750-759)	684,000	5.6
Prematurity[d] (765, 769)	470,000	3.5
Sudden infant death syndrome (798)	314,000	2.4
Cerebrovascular disease (430-438)	266,000	65.6
Chronic liver diseases and cirrhosis (571)	233,000	11.3
Pneumonia and influenza (480-487)	163,000	25.0
Chronic obstructive pulmonary diseases (490-496)	123,000	29.8
Diabetes mellitus (250)	119,000	15.6

[a]For details of calculation, see footnotes for Table V, MMWR 1986;35:27. Reprinted from Leads from the MMWR (1986) with permission.
[b]Cause-specific mortality rates as reported in the MVSR are compiled from a 10% sample of deaths.
[c]Equivalent to accidents and adverse effects.
[d]Category derived from disorders relating to short gestation and respiratory distress syndrome.

Illustrates population data ranking mortality rates and changes (group data, observational data).

TABLE 8.27. Ranking of Leading Causes of Years of Potential Life Lost (YPLL) Before Age 65 and Percentage of Change in Rates—United States, 1979 and 1986[a]

Cause of mortality	Ranking 1979	Ranking 1986	YPLL rate change 1979–1986 (%)
All causes	—	—	(− 13.3)
Unintentional injuries	1	1	(− 21.3)
Malignant neoplasms	2	2	(− 6.7)
Diseases of the heart	3	3	(− 16.1)
Suicide-homicide	4	4	(− 5.7)
Congenital anomalies	6	5	(− 17.1)
Prematurity	5	6	(− 45.5)
Sudden infant death syndrome	7	7	(− 17.2)
Acquired immunodeficiency syndrome	—[b]	8	—[c]
Cerebrovascular disease	8	9	(− 25.9)
Chronic liver diseases and cirrhosis	9	10	(− 28.1)
Pneumonia and influenza	10	11	(− 21.6)
Chronic obstructive pulmonary diseases	12	12	(+ 8.3)
Diabetes mellitus	11	13	(+ 6.2)

[a]Reprinted from Leads from the MMWR (1988a) with permission.
[b]Unranked.
[c]Not calculable.

Illustrates population data showing mortality rates and ratios by type of neoplasm and by sex (group data, observational data).

TABLE 8.28. Years of Potential Life Lost Before 65 Years (YPLL), YPLL Rates per 100,000 Population Under 65 Years, and YPLL Rate Ratios, By Nine Specific Groups of Malignant Neoplasms and By Sex—United States, 1983[a]

Malignant neoplasm group	Total YPLL	YPLL rate	YPLL rate ratio[b]
Lip, oral cavity, and pharynx			
Male	28,847	28.1	
Female	11,332	10.9	2.6
Digestive organs and peritoneum			
Male	186,769	182.7	
Female	127,710	122.9	1.5
Respiratory and intrathoracic organs			
Male	287,446	279.8	
Female	144,095	138.7	2.0
Breast			
Male	810	0.8	
Female	214,104	206.1	0.004
Genital organs			
Male	31,324	30.5	
Female	110,168	106.1	0.3
Urinary organs			
Male	33,168	32.3	
Female	17,347	16.7	1.9
Leukemia			
Male	83,694	81.5	
Female	59,820	57.6	1.4
Lymphoma and multiple myeloma			
Male	76,300	74.3	
Female	47,157	45.4	1.6
Other and unspecified sites			
Male	203,370	198.0	
Females	146,073	140.6	1.4

[a]Reprinted from Leads from the MMWR (1986) with permission.
[b]For males compared with females within each site-specific category.

Illustrates a novel way of presenting relative risks.

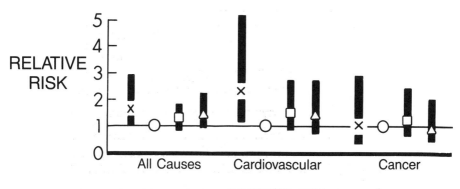

FIG. 8.1. Body mass index and mortality in men at age 65 years by relative risks and 95% confidence intervals (closed bars). Study design controlled for systolic blood pressure, blood glucose level, serum cholesterol level at age 65 years, tobacco use at examination 1, and cardiovascular disease before age 65 years in Cox models. **X**'s indicate below 10th percentile; **open circles**, 10th to 29th percentiles; **open squares**, 30th to 69th percentiles; and **open triangles**, 70th percentile and above. Reprinted from Harris et al. (1988) with permission.

Illustrates building a histogram with blocks which identify and describe a characteristic of individual patients.

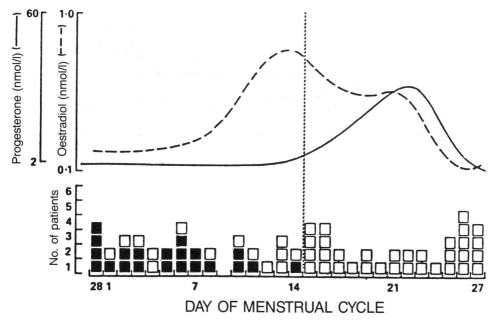

FIG. 8.2. Distribution of 68 assessable samples that are positive **(filled-in squares)** and negative **(open squares)** for estrogen receptor obtained by fine needle aspiration from premenopausal women with normal breasts on different days of menstrual cycle. Changes in serum concentrations of estrogen and progesterone using typical 28-day cycle are shown for comparison. Reprinted from Markopoulos et al. (1988) with permission.

Illustrates an example of data shown with a Gantt chart.

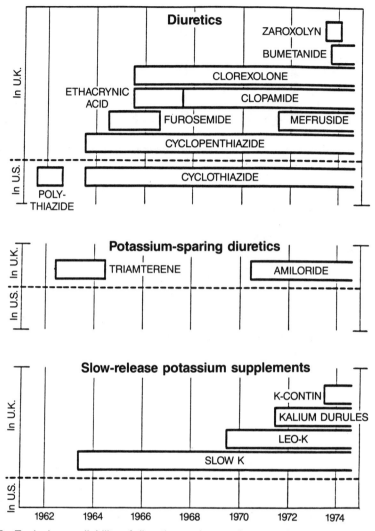

FIG. 8.3. Exclusive availability of diuretics and potassium supplements in two countries.

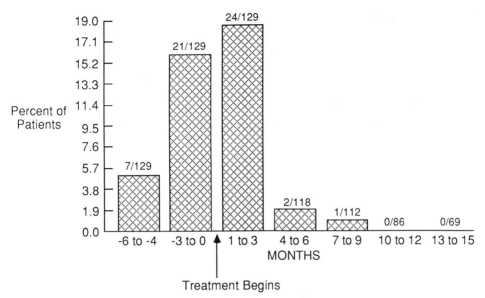

FIG. 8.4. Percent of patients who fit any defined category.

Illustrates annotating histograms and displaying healing in four groups over time.

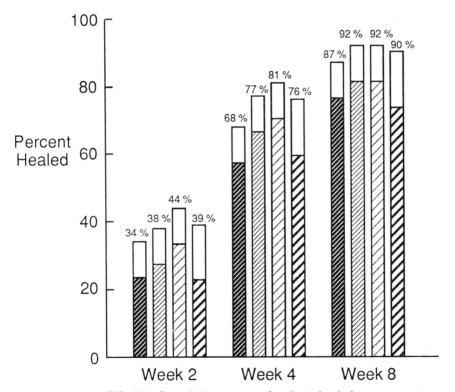

FIG. 8.5. Cumulative percent of patients healed.

• A legend should explain the shading within bars.

Illustrates one means of comparing false positive results of different tests alone and in combination.

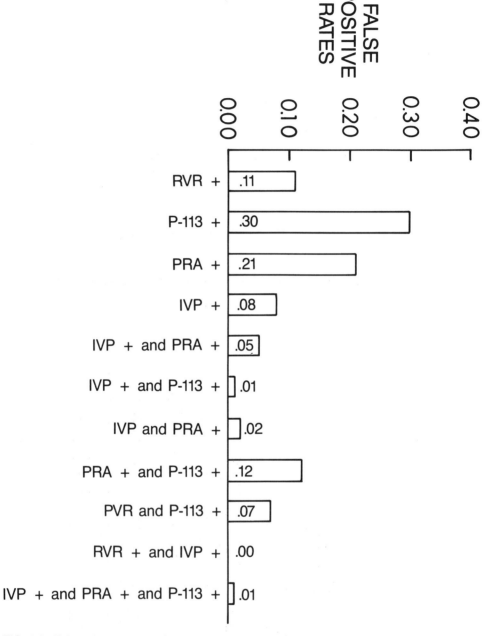

FIG. 8.6. False positive rates of tests P-113, PRA, IVP, and RVR (plasma renin activity, intravenous pyelogram, renal vein renin); alone and in combination.

• Numbers and axis labels should be oriented in the same direction.

Illustrates how two histograms sharing a common base provide an overall perspective of a population's age distribution and allows readers to compare populations.

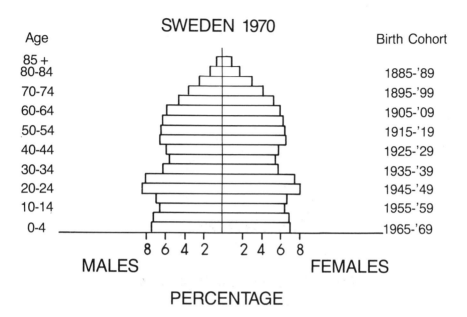

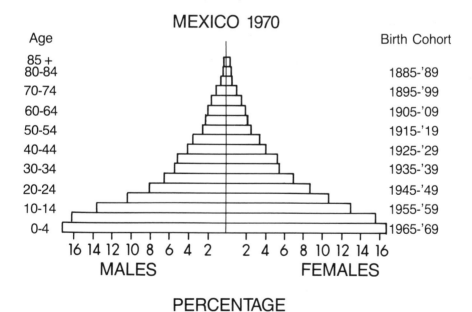

FIG. 8.7. The distribution of the populations of Sweden and Mexico by age and sex, 1970. Reprinted from Ewbank (1986) with permission.

- This graph is also known as a pyramid chart.
- Note that alternate bars are labeled.

Illustrates an easy means of comparing numbers of people in different age cohorts by viewing vertically, or comparing two aspects (gender in this case) of the same cohort by viewing horizontally.

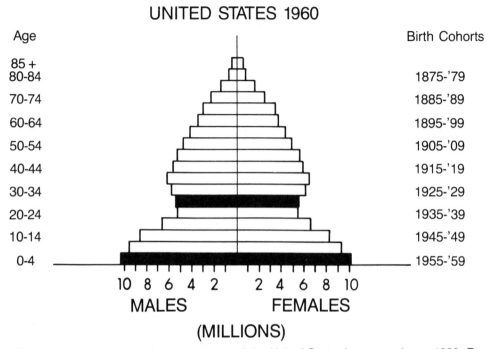

FIG. 8.8. The distribution of the population of the United States by age and sex, 1960. Reprinted from Ewbank (1986) with permission.

• Although this graph presents demographic results it may be readily used to illustrate efficacy data.

Illustrates table and graph combined.

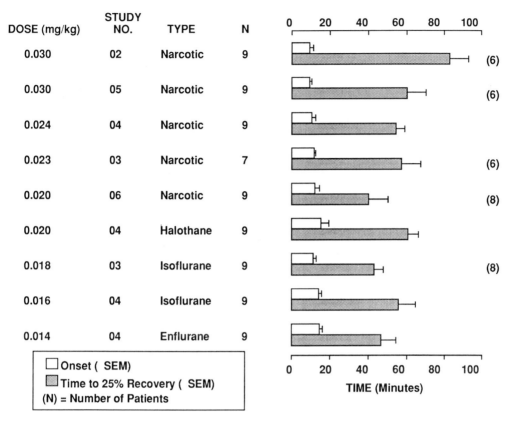

DOSE (mg/kg)	STUDY NO.	TYPE	N
0.030	02	Narcotic	9
0.030	05	Narcotic	9
0.024	04	Narcotic	9
0.023	03	Narcotic	7
0.020	06	Narcotic	9
0.020	04	Halothane	9
0.018	03	Isoflurane	9
0.016	04	Isoflurane	9
0.014	04	Enflurane	9

☐ Onset (SEM)
▨ Time to 25% Recovery (SEM)
(N) = Number of Patients

TIME (Minutes)

FIG. 8.9. Onset and duration of clinically effective neuromuscular block.

• Almost any type of graph may be combined with a table.

Illustrates use of a histogram to vividly display different results for patients found to be responders or nonresponders to treatment.

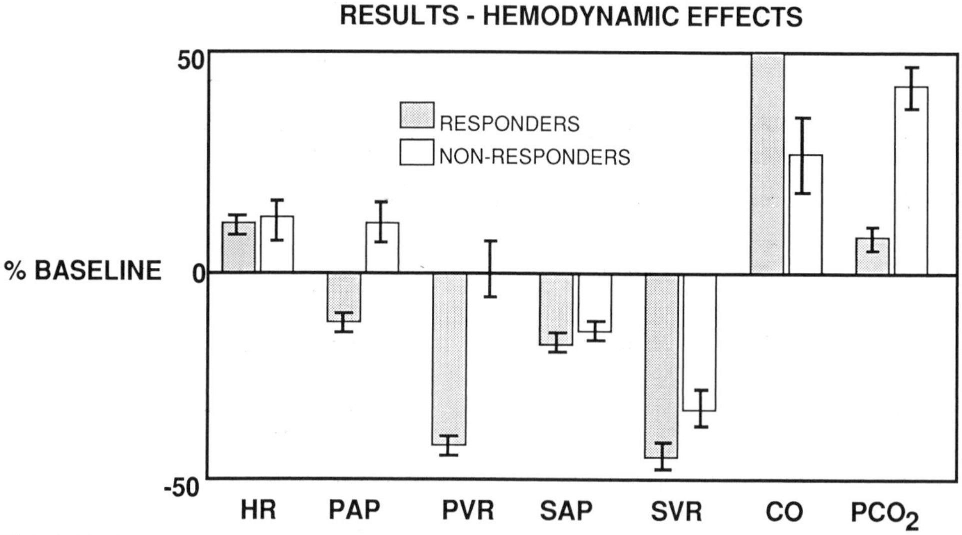

FIG. 8.10. Pulmonary vasodilating effects of drug X in primary pulmonary hypertension.

- Increases and decreases from baseline are readily apparent in this graph.
- Scaling is inadequate because CO value for responders is off the scale. This limits our knowledge of the true value and its variability.

Illustrates a method of displaying individual patient data so that clinically significant changes are easily identified.

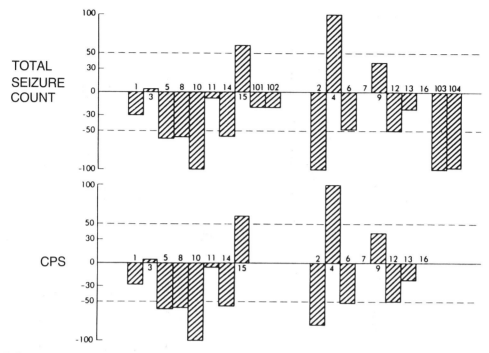

FIG. 8.11. Percentage modification (+, increase; −, decrease) in total seizures (**top**) and in complex partial seizures (CPS) (**bottom**) during the verum period as compared with the placebo period. Each bar represents an individual patient. Broken lines indicate ± 50% changes. Reprinted from Loiseau et al. (1983) with permission.

• Changes of at least 50% are defined as clinically significant in this presentation.

• The reason why no bar appears for patients numbered 101 to 104 in the bottom graph could be noted in the legend.

Illustrates a presentation to display subjective responses.

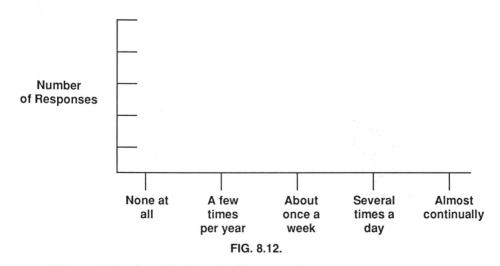

FIG. 8.12.

• This graph is often filled in with histogram bars.

Illustrates responses to individual survey questions using histograms.

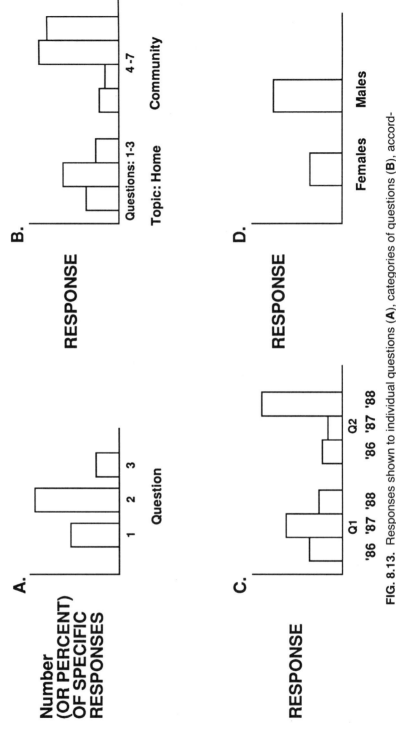

FIG. 8.13. Responses shown to individual questions (**A**), categories of questions (**B**), according to year (**C**), or to any specific factor such as gender (**D**). Many other types of comparisons are possible and data may be transformed.

Illustrates using a vertical stack of four displays to facilitate a comparison between four different groups on different parameters.

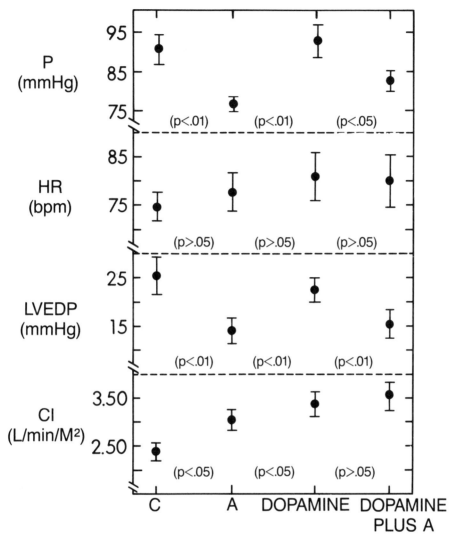

FIG. 8.14. Effect of drug A, dopamine, and the combination of drug A with dopamine on (1) mean systemic arterial pressure (P), (2) heart rate (HR), (3) left ventricular end-diastolic pressure (LVEDP), and (4) cardiac index (CI). C, control. Points are mean ± SE.

• Easy to detect clinical and statistical differences.

Illustrates how to get a large amount of data into a single graph.

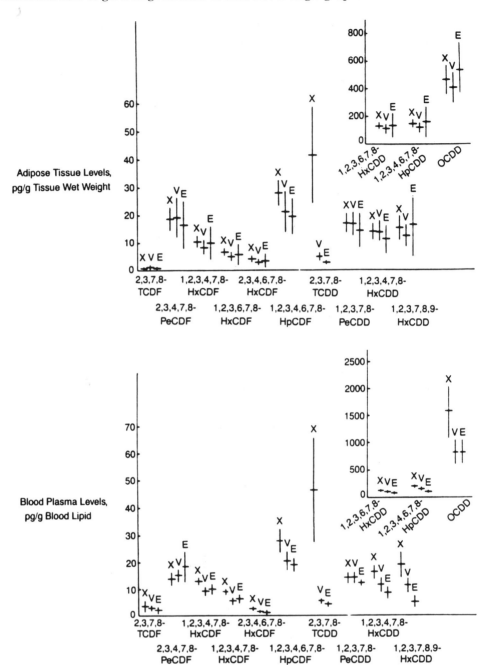

FIG. 8.15. Mean (± SE) for all 13 congeners found in adipose tissue (**top**) and blood plasma (**bottom**). Insets contain three compounds graphed with an ordinate that differs from that of the other 10 compounds. **X** indicates exposed subjects (10); **V**, Vietnam control subjects (10); **E**, era control subjects (7); **HxCDD**, hexachlorodibenzo-*p*-dioxin; **HpCDD**, heptachlorodibenzo-*p*-dioxin; **OCDD**, octachlorodibenzo-*p*-dioxin; **TCDF**, tetrachlorodibenzofuran; **PeCDF**, pentachlorodibenzofuran; **HxCDF**, hexachlorodibenzofuran; **HpCDF**, heptachlorodibenzofuran; **TCDD**, tetrachlorodibenzo-*p*-dioxin; and **PeCDD**, pentachlorodibenzo-*p*-dioxin. Reprinted from Kahn et al. (1988) with permission.

• Confusing at first, but worth the effort to plow through.

Illustrates placing study design information on a graph to help interpret efficacy data.

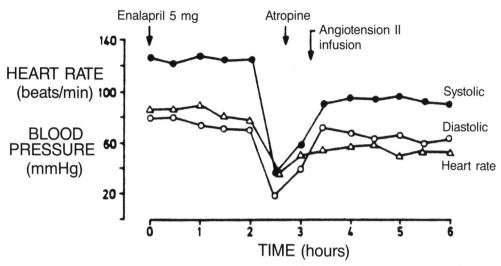

FIG. 8.16. Changes in systolic (●) and diastolic (○) blood pressure and heart rate (Δ) after 5 mg enalapril by mouth. Reprinted from Cleland et al. (1985) with permission.

- It is easy to see the effect of drug on responses.
- This is a situation where vital sign data are a direct measure of efficacy.
- Using the same scale on the same axis to represent both mmHg for blood pressure and beats/minute for heart rate is unusual.

Illustrates two scales on right and two others on left. Single patient's data.

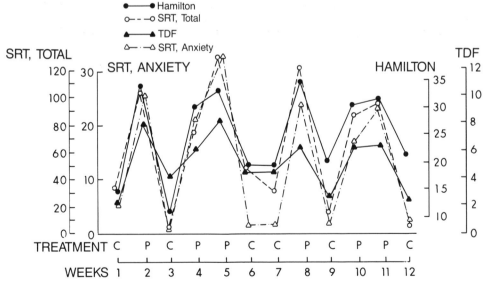

FIG. 8.17. Patient 3 showed conspicuous response to chlordiazepoxide (C) compared to placebo (P), as measured on total distress and anxiety scores of the Symptom Rating Test (SRT), Hamilton Anxiety Rating Scale, and thinking disturbance factor (TDF) of Brief Psychiatric Rating Scale. Reprinted from Kellner et al. (1975) with permission.

Illustrates that half an error bar is adequate and that p values may be stated on a graph for each comparison.

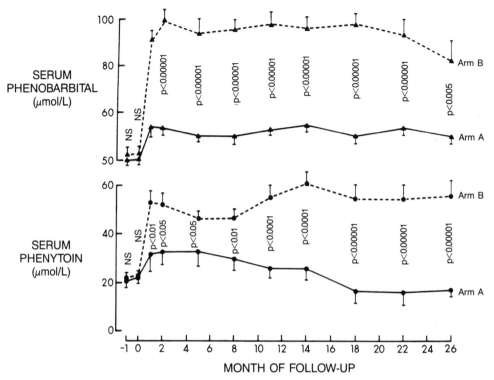

FIG. 8.18. The mean serum antiepileptic drug levels in the two study arms at different intervals of follow-up: −1 and 0 month values represented the two serum levels taken 1 month apart prior to entry. Bar = SE. The two study arms showed a significant difference in serum levels at all intervals of follow-up, whether for phenytoin or phenobarbital. Reprinted from Woo et al. (1988) with permission.

• Different symbols for different p values would make the graph cleaner.

Illustrates that putting the same scale at two sides of a graph (e.g., top and bottom) may make it easier to read.

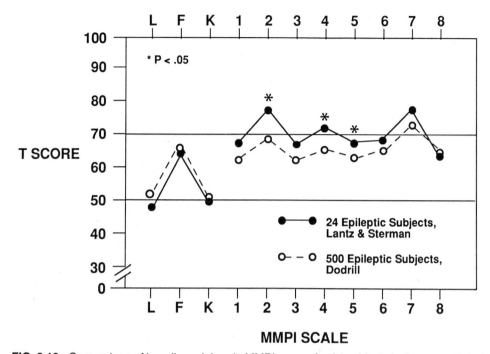

FIG. 8.19. Comparison of baseline mini-mult. MMPI scores for 24 subjects in the present study with long form MMPI scores for a larger independent sample of subjects with epilepsy. Reprinted from Lantz and Sterman (1988) with permission.

Illustrates data from multiple cohorts on a single graph.

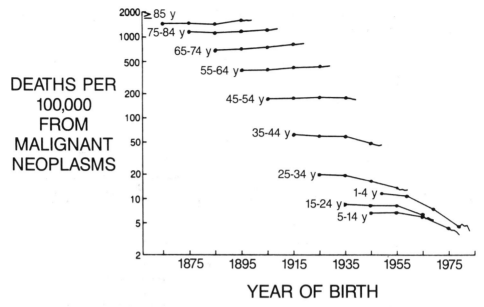

FIG. 8.20. Cohort age contours for mortality from malignant neoplasms, 1950 through 1984. Four points plotted within each contour indicate mortality rate for 1950, 1960, 1970, and 1980, respectively. Each contour represents different 10-year age group. Reprinted from Breslow and Cumberland (1988) with permission.

• Ordinate should state whether deaths are per 100,000 people, people years of exposure, or another parameter.

Illustrates a common method to show variability and statistical significance on a graph.

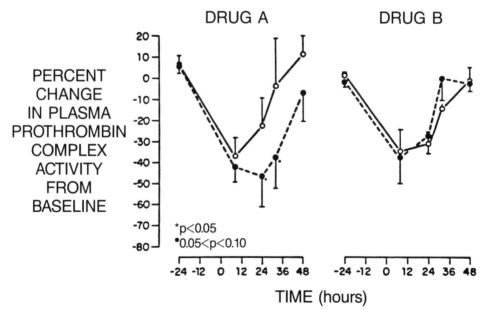

FIG. 8.21. Time course of percent change in plasma prothrombin complex activity from baseline value for two different drugs during the control period (○) and the drug treatment period (●).

Illustrates using study design information to display time course of graph.

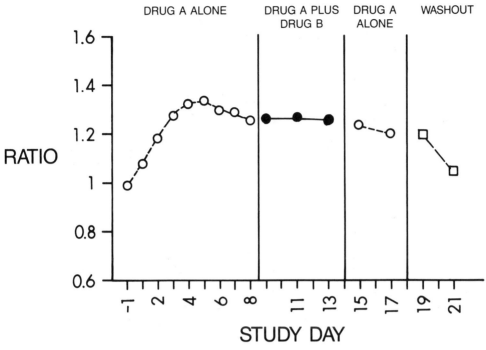

FIG. 8.22. Mean prothrombin time ratios, by study day for different drug regimens.

• Study days along the x-axis would be easier to read if rotated 90°.

Illustrates a comparison between two treatment regimens over time, with variability and significance values.

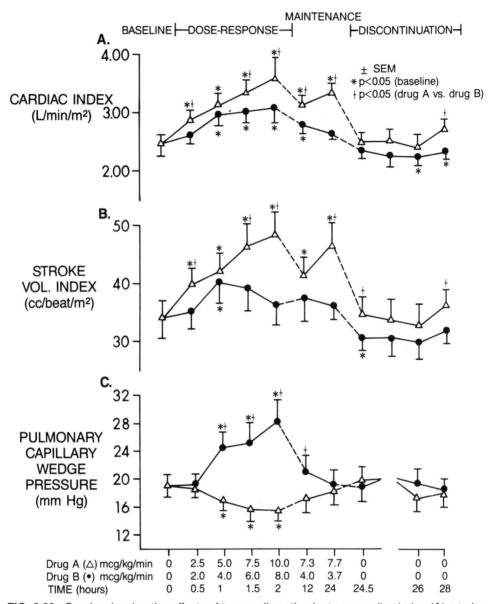

FIG. 8.23. Graphs showing the effects of two cardiac stimulants on cardiac index (**A**), stroke volume index (**B**), and pulmonary capillary wedge pressure (**C**).

Illustrates time to onset of action.

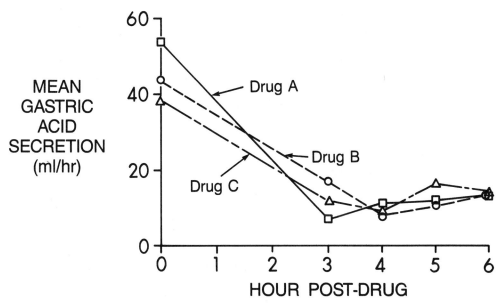

FIG. 8.24. Onset of action of three drugs affecting gastric acid secretion.

• More data points during the first 3 hr are needed to better define the characteristics of onset.

• A key or legend may be placed inside the body of the graph to indicate (1) identity of the groups presented, (2) specific values of the curves shown, or (3) any derived data from the curves for different parameters.

Illustrates individual patient data before and during drug administration for three related parameters. Others could be shown.

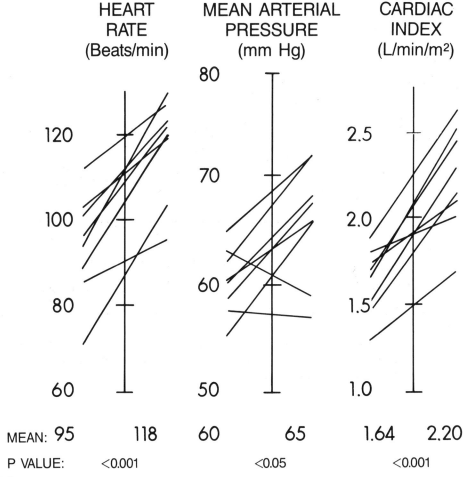

FIG. 8.25. Effect of dopamine on hemodynamic status. Results in individual patients are shown prior to and during dopamine infusion.

• Mean values could also be shown on the graph itself for before and after states for each parameter.

Illustrates effects of four infusion rates on three parameters; illustrates a dose-response.

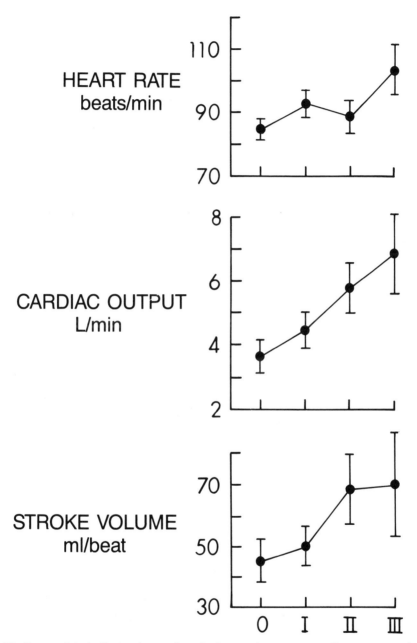

FIG. 8.26. Dose-related effects of a cardiotonic drug on heart rate, cardiac output, and stroke volume. Each dose-response curve represents the mean values and standard error for the group at a control state (0) and following infusion rates of 1(I), 5(II), and 10 μg per kilogram per min (III).

Illustrates how two treatments can be compared by only showing differences from baseline.

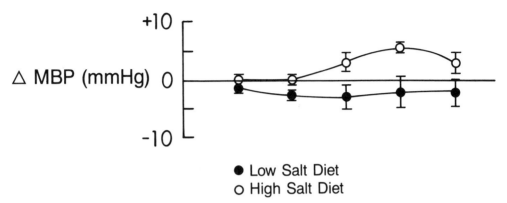

FIG. 8.27. Dose-response relationships for drug X at two sodium loads in normals. The dosages are 10 ng/kg/min IV for the first point, 30 for the second, 100 for the third, 300 for the fourth, and 1,000 for the last. MBP, mean blood pressure.

Illustrates change in volume after drug compared with a saline control.

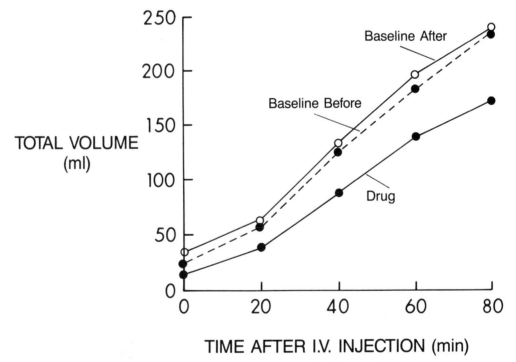

FIG. 8.28. Mean cumulative volume (ml) of duodenal juice.

• Baseline values after drug are a valuable procedure to demonstrate return to predrug control levels.

Illustrates changes in four treatment groups over time.

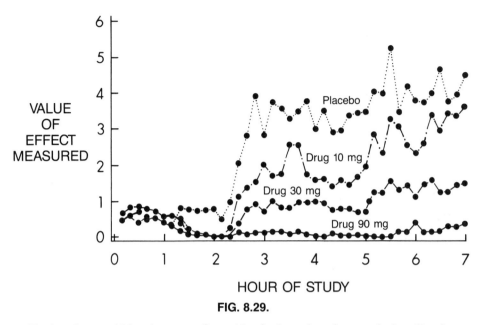

FIG. 8.29.

- Each point could be the mean for a 10-min (or other time period) collection.
- Error bars could be shown for selected (or all) values.

Illustrates changes in rates of hospitalization over time for a specific disease in several patient populations using different line patterns for each group.

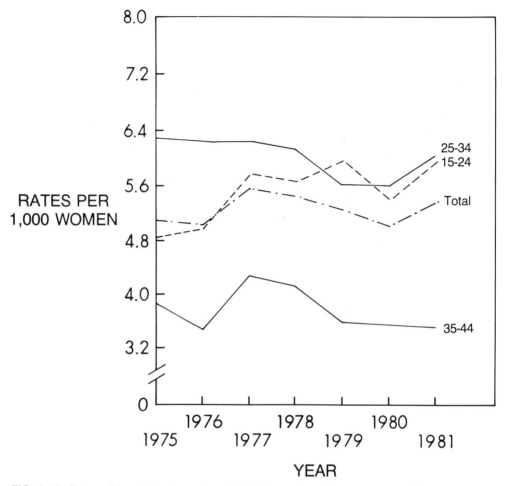

FIG. 8.30. Rates of hospitalizations for pelvic inflammatory disease among all women aged 15 to 44 years in United States during 1975 to 1981. Reprinted from Washington et al. (1984) with permission.

• Rates of hospitalization and a relative risk of hospitalization (compared with index group with lowest rate) may also be graphed.

Illustrates three ways of showing mortality data.

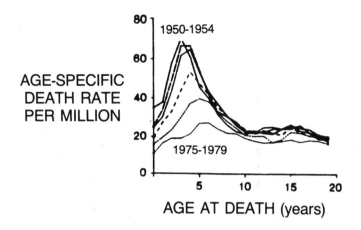

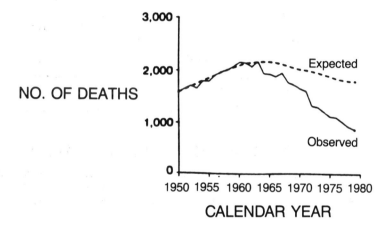

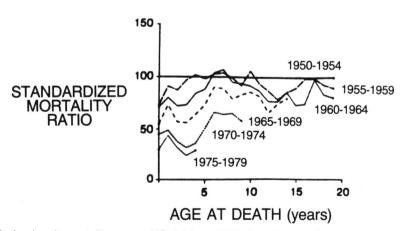

FIG. 8.31. Leukemia mortality among US children, 1950 through 1979: **Top**, mortality by single year of age, and 5-year calendar intervals; **Center**, observed vs. expected numbers among persons younger than 15 years at the 1950 rate by calendar year; **Bottom**, standardized mortality ratios for 5-year cohorts, 1950 through 1979, using 1950 through 1954 as the standard. Reprinted from Miller and McKay (1984) with permission.

Illustrates results of subgroup analyses along with results from the main population.

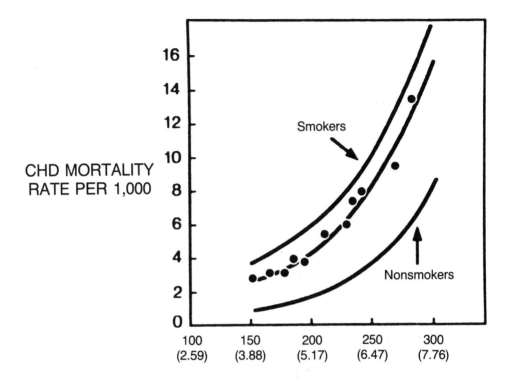

FIG. 8.32. Yearly coronary mortality rates (per 1,000) vs. plasma cholesterol level for normotensive smokers and nonsmokers among Multiple Risk Factor Intervention Trial participants. Intermediate curve is that for whole population. Reprinted from Grundy (1986) with permission.

Illustrates superimposing a reference line on data displayed by a histogram.

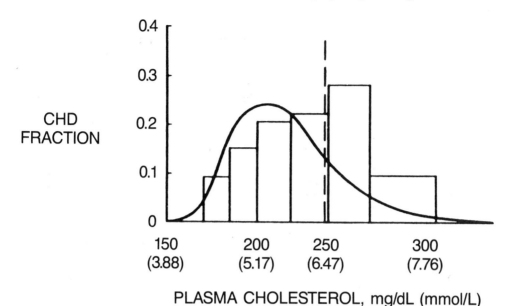

FIG. 8.33. Fraction of total population dying of coronary heart disease (CHD) among Multiple Risk Factor Intervention Trial participants who had different levels of plasma cholesterol at screening. Current distribution of plasma cholesterol values for American adults is superimposed. Approximately 38% of those dying of CHD had cholesterol levels greater than 245 mg/dL (6.34 mmol/L) at screening. Reprinted from Grundy (1986) with permission.

- Although vertical reference lines are usually helpful, this one is less so because it does not come at a boundary of the bars.
- Different bar widths should be explained in the legend.

Illustrates comparing two groups (e.g., high-dose and low-dose) by summarizing many parameters.

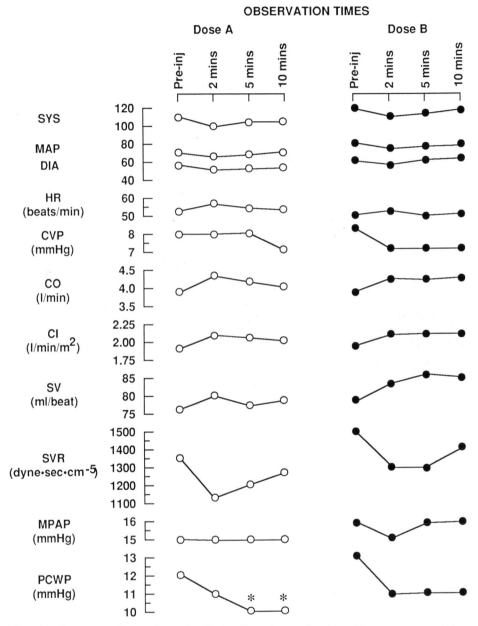

FIG. 8.34. Summary of hemodynamic effects of two doses of a drug at four assessment times. Mean values of hemodynamic parameters in coronary artery bypass graft patients receiving dose A (N = 8 patients, open symbols) or dose B (N = 8 patients, solid symbols). Values are reported prior to injection (Pre-inj) and at 2, 5, and 10 min after injection. An asterisk (*) indicates a statistically significant difference (p≤0.05) from pre-injection value.

• Many other parameters could be shown similarly.

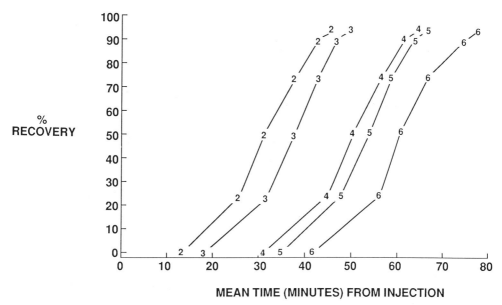

FIG. 8.35. Recovery from neuromuscular blockade after each of five doses of drug X.

Illustrates two major methods for graphing dose-response data.

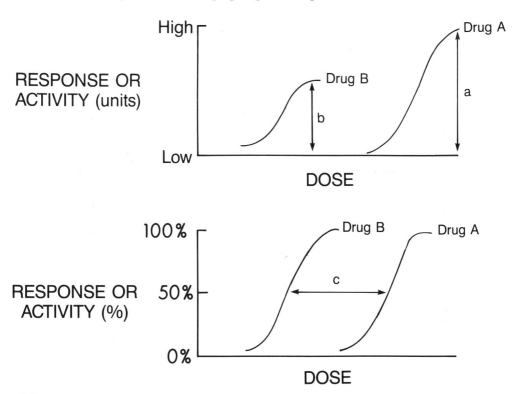

FIG. 8.36. Measuring activity and potency of drugs through use of dose-response curves. In the upper graphs the activity of each drug is noted by the vertical arrow. In the lower graph the comparative potency is shown by the horizontal arrow, such that at 50% response drug B is more potent than drug A by the magnitude C. Reprinted from Spilker (1987) with permission.

Illustrates natural history of a disease.

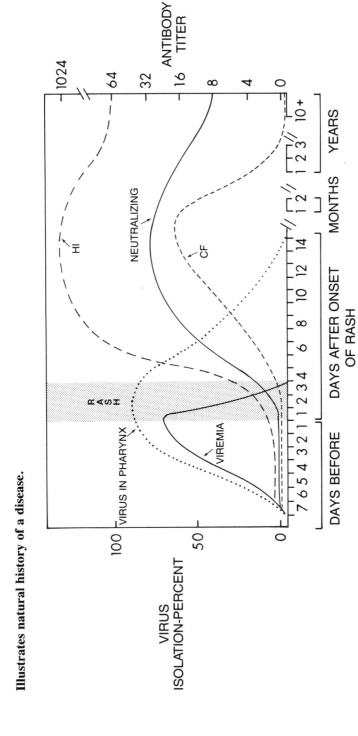

FIG. 8.37. Natural history of postnatal rubella. Pattern of virus excretion and antibody response. Reprinted from Krugman and Ward (1973) with permission.

Illustrates a means of comparing healing versus relapses for two drugs.

ULCER HEALING

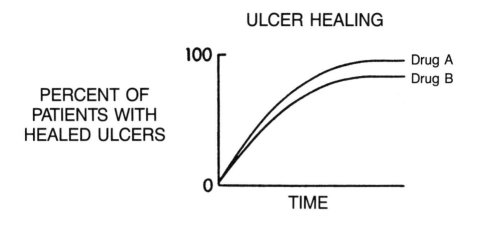

PERCENT OF
PATIENTS WITH
HEALED ULCERS

ULCER RELAPSES

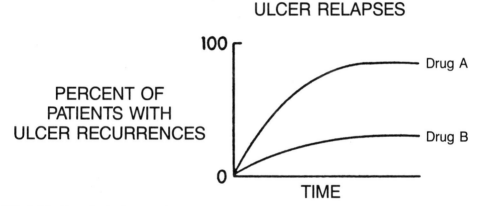

PERCENT OF
PATIENTS WITH
ULCER RECURRENCES

FIG. 8.38. Hypothetical rates of ulcer healing for two drugs (upper graph) and recurrence of disease (i.e., relapses) after drug treatment is discontinued for the same two drugs (lower graph). Reprinted from Spilker (1987) with permission.

Illustrates rate of recurrence of disease which occurs after treatment cessation.

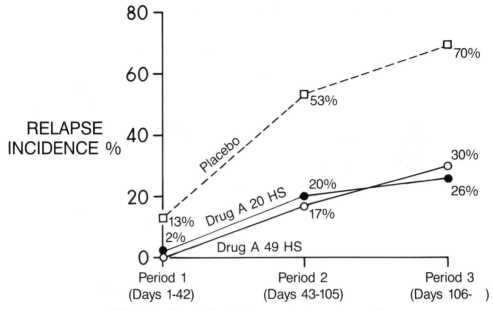

FIG. 8.39. Cumulative incidence of relapse (percent).

Illustrates using a vertical line to demarcate a change in the frequency of assessments (daily on left of line and weekly on right of line).

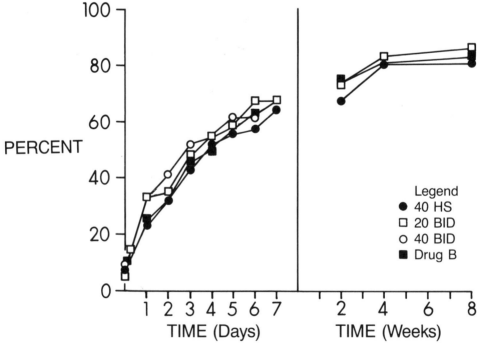

FIG. 8.40. Percentage of patients with no pain.

• Alternatively, one could divide the graph to illustrate day pain and night pain.

Illustrates how shading can accentuate a changing difference between two groups.

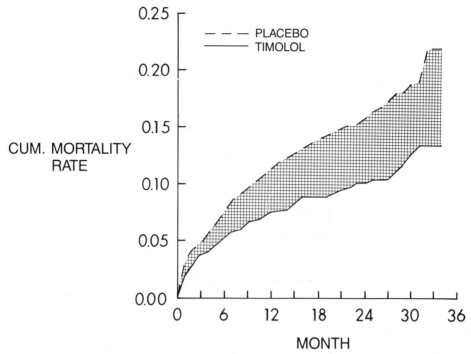

FIG. 8.41. Life table based on cumulative rates for total death (intention-to-treat approach).

• Other related parameters could be graphed similarly (e.g., nonfatal reinfarction).

• Shading can emphasize differences between two trends (e.g., the area or zone between trends may be shaded after one line crosses the other).

Illustrates effect of plotting doses of a drug required to yield a specified clinical response versus severity of disease.

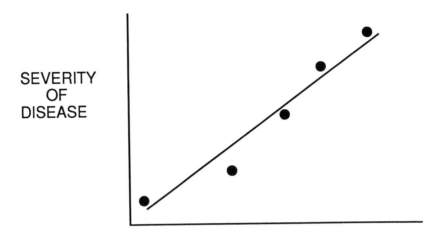

DOSE OF DRUG REQUIRED TO YIELD A
SPECIFIED CLINICAL RESPONSE

FIG. 8.42. The y-axis may either be a continuous scale or discontinuous (i.e., divided into mild, marked, severe).

• Other parameters may be plotted on the y-axis (e.g., age of patient, duration of prior treatment with other drugs).

Illustrates that an index of clinical state may be shown to change over time.

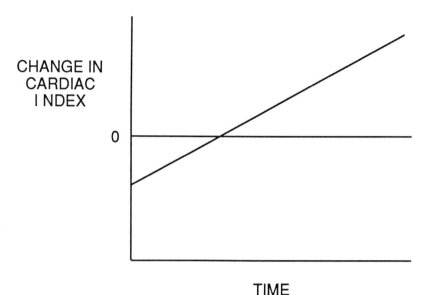

FIG. 8.43.

• The time axis may illustrate only effects after treatment is initiated or both pre- and posttreatment effects may be shown.

• Other parameters may be plotted on the x-axis (e.g., dose of drug, doses of numerous drugs showing multiple curves).

• A percent change in index may be used instead of units change.

• Almost any disease may be measured with an index (weighted or unweighted) that combines two or more parameters.

Illustrates a classic presentation of data using drug dose versus time.

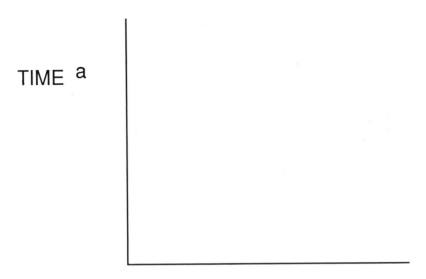

TIME ª

DOSE ᵇ

FIG. 8.44. Graph of dose versus time. Selected characteristics of each that may be plotted are: ªTime to onset of effect, time to X% peak effect, time to maximal effect, time to recovery after drug infusion stopped, time to X% recovery after drug infusion stopped, time of total effect. ᵇDose may be expressed in terms of fixed mg, mg/kg, mg/m² body surface area, ED_{50}, ED_{95}, ID_{50}, or various other measures. The axes may be reversed.

Illustrates single patient data for alternating ABAB pattern of baseline/drug.

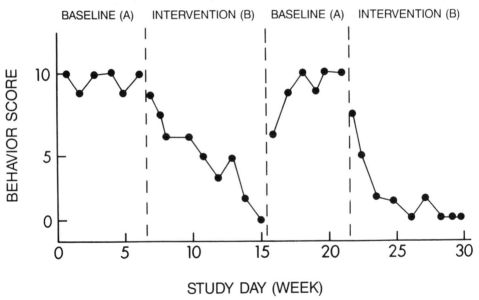

BASELINE (A)   INTERVENTION (B)   BASELINE (A)   INTERVENTION (B)

BEHAVIOR SCORE

STUDY DAY (WEEK)

FIG. 8.45. Behavior scores for an intervention alternating with a baseline. Reprinted from Dattilo and Nelson (1986) with permission.

Illustrates a presentation of a three-patient study design using multiple baselines.

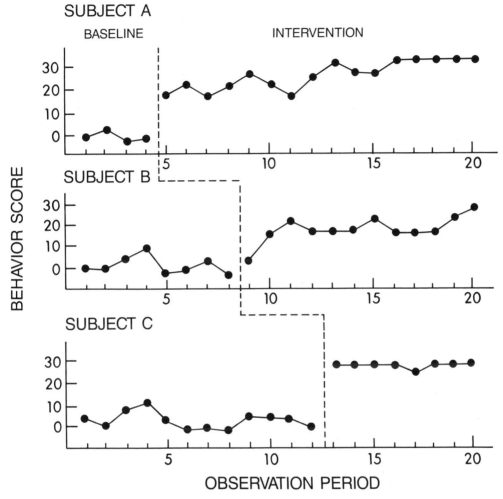

FIG. 8.46. Reprinted from Dattilo and Nelson (1986) with permission.

Illustrates 12 types of single-patient data patterns with one change from baseline to treatment.

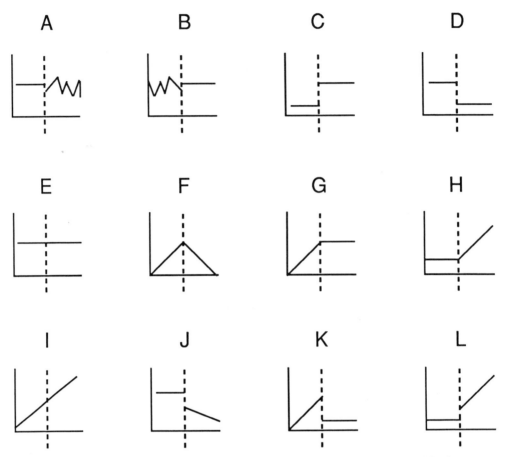

FIG. 8.47. The three characteristics of data shown in these 12 figures are trend in data, stability of data, and level of data. Reprinted from Wolery and Harris (1982) with permission.

- Interpretations are based on the pattern observed.
- The ordinate is a measure of response and the abscissa is a measure of time.
- Delays in response after change of treatment could be illustrated.
- Although these figures represent an AB study design (i.e., baseline then treatment, or treatment then baseline), more sophisticated designs have the potential to yield stronger interpretations.

Illustrates relationship of two efficacy parameters.

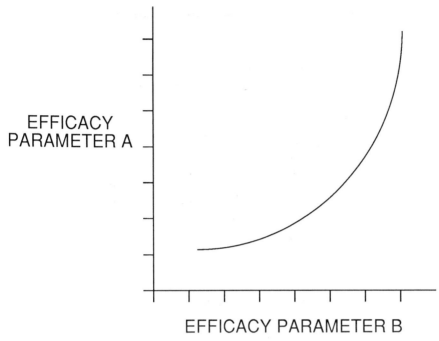

FIG. 8.48. Graph of parameter A versus parameter B.

• One may plot raw units versus raw units, percent of maximal response versus percent of maximal response, percent change from baseline versus percent change from baseline, etc.

• Various relationships (linear or nonlinear) may be shown for one or more groups of patients.

• It is possible that a single drug will yield a single point on this graph. In that situation different drugs, drug and placebo, or drug and combination drugs may be compared statistically.

• Care must be taken if different types of data transformations are plotted versus each other. Plots must make inherent sense.

Illustrates a completely filled in line graph changing over time.

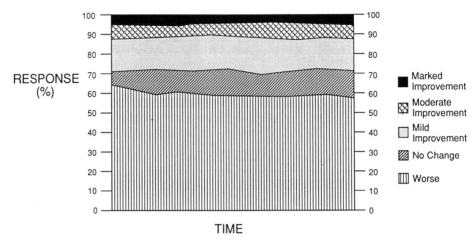

FIG. 8.49. Changes in patients status over time.

Illustrates line graph of percent of maximal response.

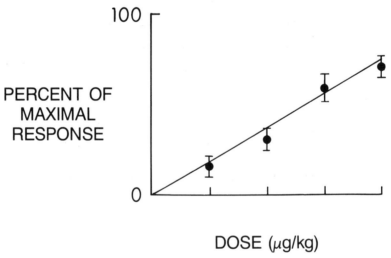

FIG. 8.50. Dose-response curve.

• Maximal response may be defined based on maximal response to a standard drug or to the drug being studied.

• Maximal response may refer to the mean value for the patient or group being studied or it may refer to a historical value.

Illustrates a scattergram of results from different studies.

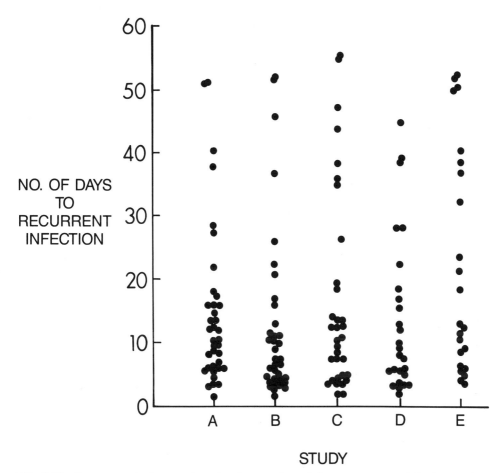

FIG. 8.51. Responses in five studies showing number of days to recurrent infections in individual patients.

Illustrates comparison of number of episodes during baseline versus during placebo treatment for individual patients.

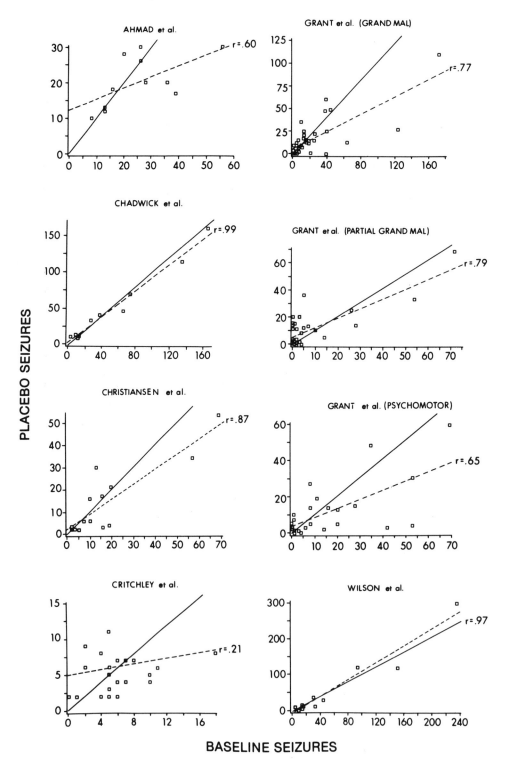

FIG. 8.52. Total number of seizures during baseline and placebo treatment for eight clinical studies. Each patient is denoted by a single mark on the plot. The solid line is the line of equivalence (45°), and the dotted line is the least-squares regression line. The product-moment correlation coefficient is indicated on each of the eight plots. Reprinted from Spilker and Segreti (1984) with permission.

Illustrates comparison of rank orders of a parameter during baseline versus during placebo treatment for individual patients.

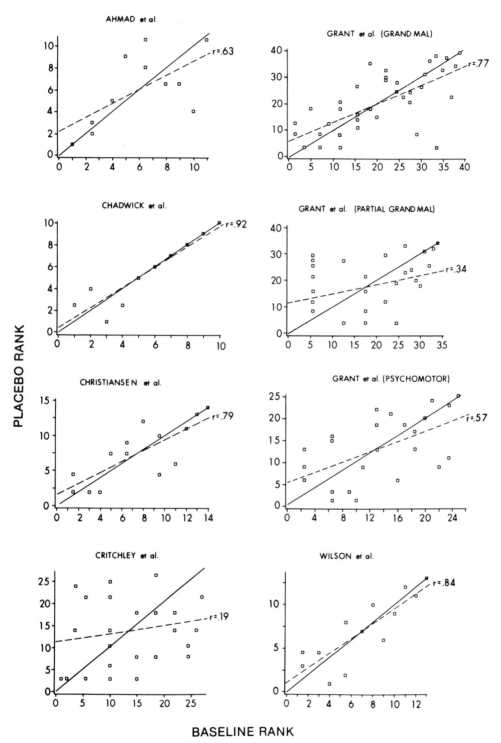

FIG. 8.53. Ranks of total seizures during placebo and baseline periods for patients in the eight clinical studies. Each patient is denoted by a single mark on the plot. The solid line is the line of equivalence (45°), and the dotted line is the least-squares line. The rank correlation coefficient is indicated on each of the eight plots. Reprinted from Spilker and Segreti (1984) with permission.

Illustrates fitting a straight line (linear) relationship to data from three groups of patients.

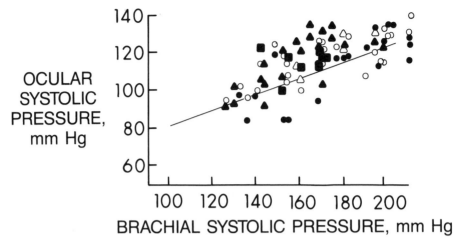

FIG. 8.54. Graph of ocular pneumoplethysmography data for patients with stroke alone, transient ischemic attack (TIA) alone, and stroke preceded by TIA. Closed and open **circles** indicate right- and left-sided stroke, respectively (N = 29); closed and open **triangles**, right- and left-sided TIAs, respectively (N = 12); and closed and open **squares**, right- and left-sided stroke/TIA, respectively (N = 4). Reprinted from Meissner et al. (1987) with permission.

• It is hard to compare different groups of symbols, but it is easy to see that most are clustered near the line of best fit.

Illustrates a means of comparing results at different sites when many sites are involved in a study. (Each site is represented by a single point.)

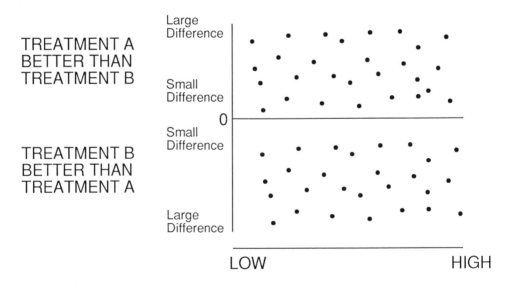

FIG. 8.55. If treatment A is better than B at a site, it is shown with points above the midline, whereas points below the line mean that treatment B is better than A.

Illustrates a scattergram for individual patients or centers on two related parameters.

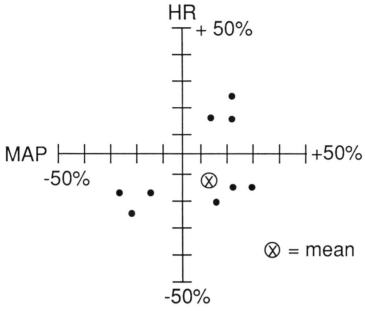

FIG. 8.56. Comparison of heart rate and blood pressure for individual patients.

- Hatch marks along the axes may be deleted.
- Other parameters may be used.
- Multiple graphs may be placed next to each other to illustrate multiple doses, groups, or other parameters.

Illustrates individual patients who stopped an activity for varying periods of time versus a level measured.

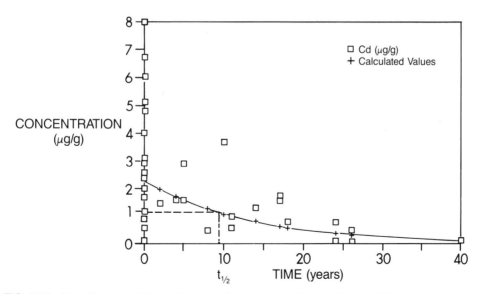

FIG. 8.57. Negative correlation between pulmonary cadmium content and time since stopping smoking. Reprinted from Pääkkö et al. (1988) with permission.

Illustrates annotating a scatterplot with linear regression line and statistics describing the parameters of that regression line.

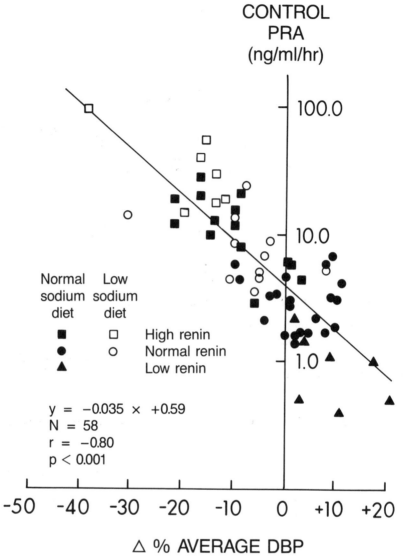

FIG. 8.58. Relationship between plasma renin activity and blood pressure response to drug X (10 μg/kg/min) in hypertensive patients under two different sodium loads.

Illustrates use of letters as symbols instead of dots or other symbols to show points on a graph.

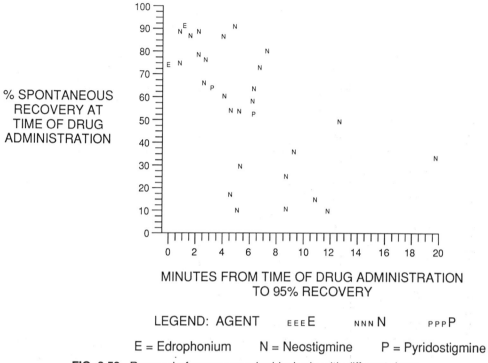

FIG. 8.59. Reversal of neuromuscular blockade with different drugs.

• A similar graph could illustrate results, with a single drug at multiple study sites identified with different letters or symbols.

Illustrates natural history of a disease.

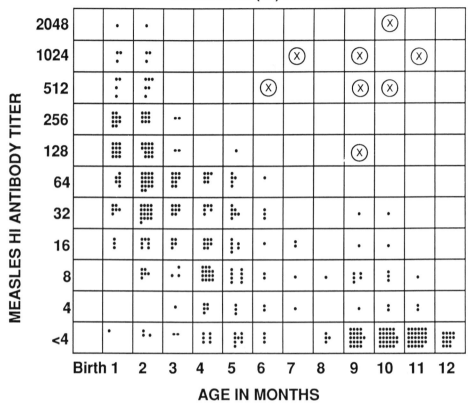

SERIAL DETERMINATIONS OF HEMAGGLUTINATION-INHIBITION (HI) ANTIBODY

(X) = > 4 fold rise in titer after measles infection

FIG. 8.60. Measles antibody during the first year of life—a longitudinal study of 107 infants. Note the disappearance of passive antibody by 12 months of age and the occurrence of eight cases of measles from 6 to 11 months of age. Reprinted from Krugman and Ward (1973) with permission.

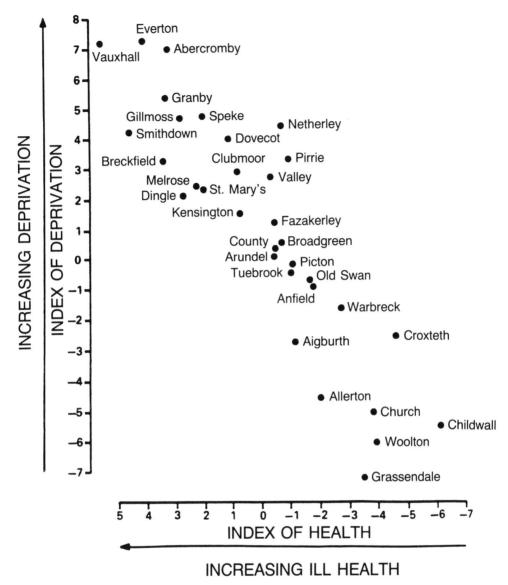

FIG. 8.61. Relation between deprivation and health for Liverpool's 33 wards. The health index combines standardized mortality ratios for the under 65s and figures for permanent sickness and low birth weight. The deprivation index covers unemployment, car ownership, overcrowding, and owner occupation. The gap between the most and least deprived areas in Liverpool is growing, as is that between Liverpool and more affluent parts of the country. Reprinted from Delamothe (1988b) with permission.

- Plotting geographical areas on two scales allows easy comparison.
- This is an unusual ordering of scales because the vertical scale improves as one approaches the origin, whereas the horizontal scale worsens as one approaches the origin.
- Each town or geographical area may be plotted on a scattergram that compares actual versus predicted values (e.g., actual versus predicted mortality rates overall, or for a specific disease).
- Another means of explicitly identifying each point on a scatterplot is to place numbers by each point that refer to a legend or text.

**Illustrates a means of comparing responses of a combination drug to its components
and to placebo.**

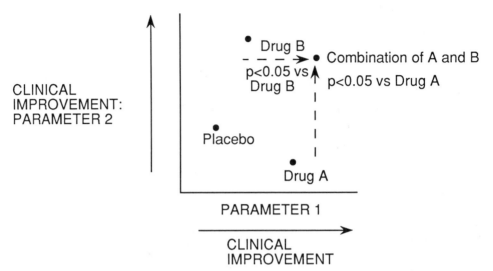

FIG. 8.62. Plot of two clinical parameters to demonstrate that a combination drug is superior
to its components or to a placebo.

   • The arrows are only included for illustrative purposes.
   • The arrows with dotted lines illustrate the comparison of the combination drug
with each of its components.

Illustrates using data for both a scattergram and curve.

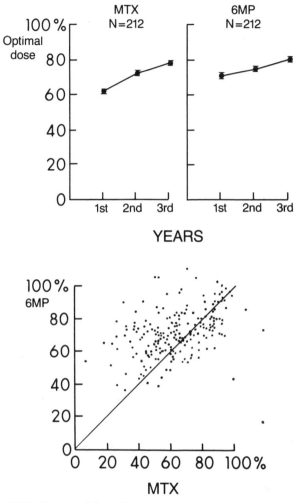

FIG. 8.63. Reprinted from Peeters et al. (1988) with permission.

• Note the 45° line of equivalence in the scattergram.

Illustrates an individual patient's serum values of a drug in relation to therapeutic ranges for two doses.

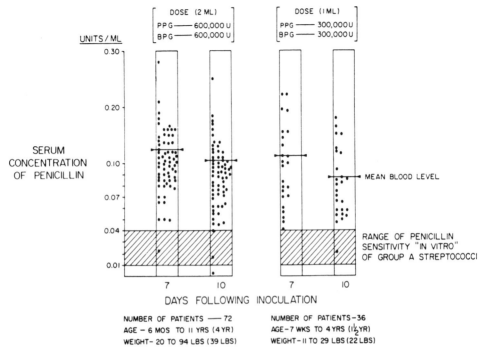

FIG. 8.64. Penicillin blood levels 7 and 10 days after a single injection of a mixture of aqueous procaine penicillin G and benzathine penicillin G (BPG). Each black dot represents one blood level determination. From Krugman and Ward (1973) with permission.

• Note the line through each bar of the scattergram. This represents the mean blood level and greatly aids the interpretability of the graph.

Illustrates a scattergram plot with a 95% confidence interval at each point.

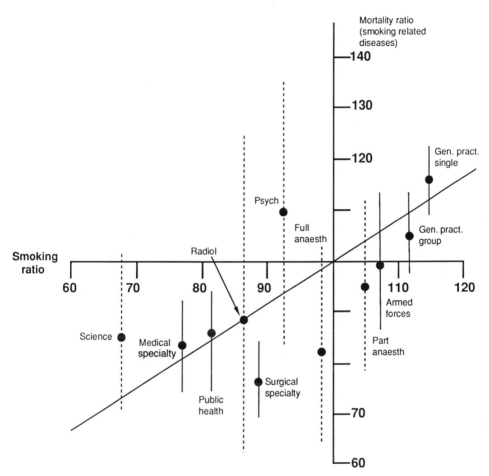

FIG. 8.65. Standardized mortality ratio (SMR) (with 95% confidence interval) for mortality from main smoking-related diseases against smoking ratio for each of 11 specialties, together with regression line of SMR on smoking ratio. Longer confidence intervals corresponding to groups with fewer deaths are given by broken lines only to emphasize visually that they are unreliable and that attention should be directed chiefly to shorter solid lines, which describe more reliable SMRs. Reprinted from Doll and Peto (1977) with permission.

Illustrates a life survival type graph.

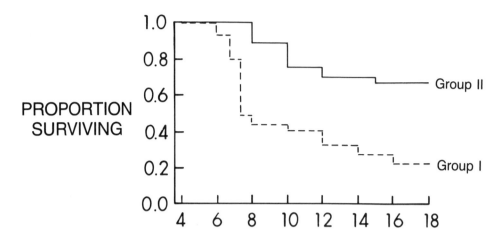

DAYS (months) SINCE START OF THERAPY

FIG. 8.66. Proportion of patients surviving in two treatment groups.

• This is also referred to as a life expectancy graph.

• The horizontal axis should begin at the start of therapy rather than four "units" later. Time is often expressed in years.

• The number surviving at X years (e.g., five) is often quoted for different treatments or cohorts.

• Without any treatment, the graph illustrates the natural history of the disease.

• Instead of death, one may plot the percentage of patients with their first recurrence of symptoms or signs after being treated.

• Many groups may be compared as well as numerous subgroup analyses (e.g., males versus females, high risk versus low risk groups, patients with a laboratory value above a set point versus those with a laboratory value below that point).

• The ordinate could illustrate the percent of patients with an adverse reaction (i.e., a cumulative probability of an event or events).

Illustrates data from a life table analysis for seven cohorts given different doses.

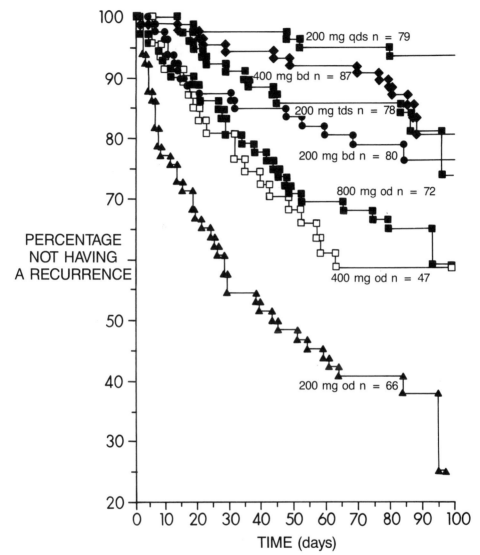

FIG. 8.67. Percentage of patients treated with acyclovir not having a recurrence. Reprinted from Mindel et al. (1988) with permission.

Illustrates data from a life table for different cohorts diagnosed at different times.

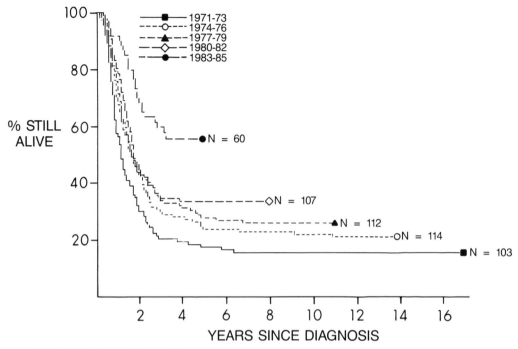

FIG. 8.68. Survival for children with osteosarcoma diagnosed in 1971–85. Reprinted from Stiller (1988) with permission.

• Cumulative data may also be shown as a continuous curve.

Illustrates a novel means of presenting seasonal data.

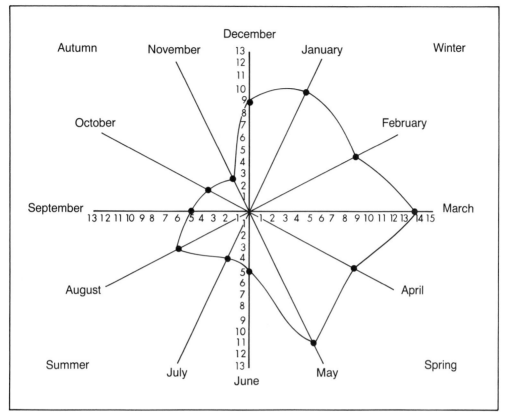

FIG. 8.69. Distribution of bathtub-related electrocutions by month, United States, 1979 to 1982. Reprinted from Budnick (1984) with permission.

• This is an example of a circular line graph, although it is not presented in a circular format.

• The excellent, clear display shows seasonality of events.

• A circle around the origin would indicate no seasonal effect.

• "Filling in" each quadrant of the polygon with different hatch marks or design would emphasize the seasonality of the results.

• For this type of display to be correctly presented, the horizontal and vertical axes must use the same scale.

Illustrates anatomical location of lesions with drawings as well as showing the degree of activity.

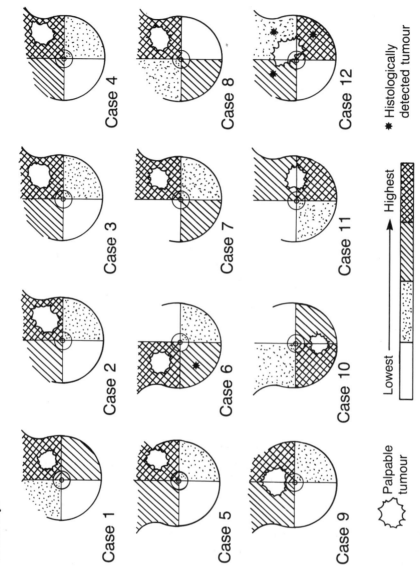

FIG. 8.70. Aromatase activity in adipose tissue from breast quadrants in relation to site of tumor detected clinically and pathologically in 12 patients. Activity was ranked as shown on scale and quadrants shaded accordingly. Reprinted from O'Neill et al. (1988) with permission.

Illustrates individual patient differences and similarities using filled in or empty squares.

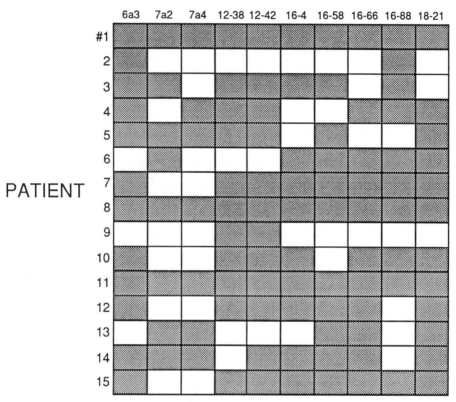

FIG. 8.71. Distribution of antigens in paraffin sections of colorectal tumors. Reprinted from Oldham (1987) with permission.

Illustrates filled-in boxes to convey a large amount of data.

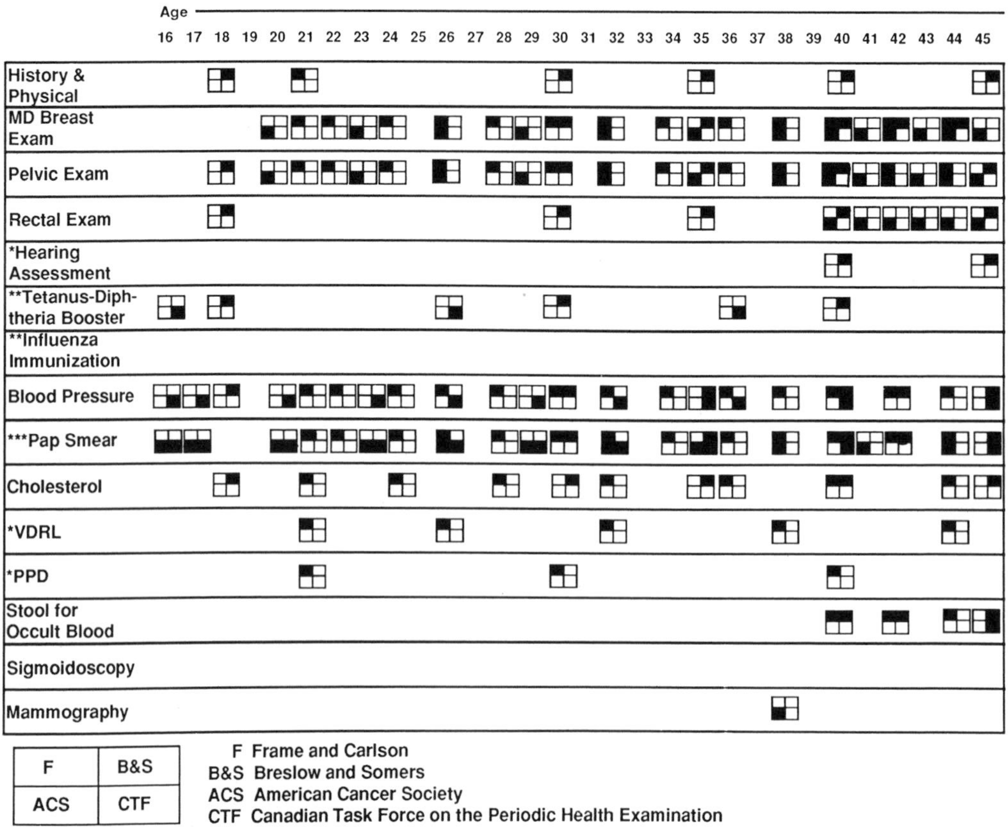

FIG. 8.72. Summary of recommendations of four major studies. A blackened square indicates that a study has considered the maneuver and recommends it. Squares left empty do not necessarily indicate that the study considered but did not recommend the maneuver. Reprinted from Council on Scientific Affairs (1983) with permission. Only half of the original figure is shown.

Illustrates the box plot method of showing data.

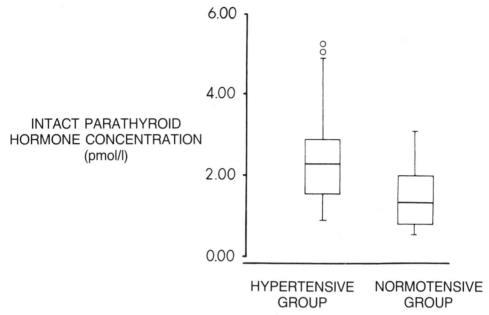

FIG. 8.73. Box plot of plasma intact parathyroid hormone concentration in young hypertensive and normotensive subjects. Top and bottom lines of each box show 75th and 25th centiles, and middle line shows 50th centile (median value). Vertical bars extend to upper and lower adjacent values, points outside this range being indicated by open circles (hypertensive group only). Adjacent values are equivalent to the outlier cut-off values. Outliers are defined as larger than Q3 + 2/3 (Q3–Q1) and smaller than Q1–2/3 (Q3–Q1). For a Gaussian distribution 0.7% of the population is outside the outlier cut-off values. Thus the population outlier cut off values contain ±99.3% of the distribution. Reprinted from Grobbee et al. (1988) with permission.

Illustrates histological section—could show a photograph from a light microscope, electron microscope, scanning electron microscope, or others.

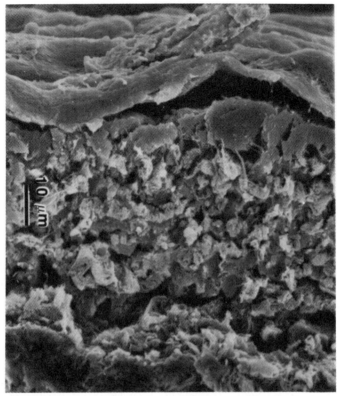

A

FIG. 8.74. Photographs of histological section viewed under light microscopy (A) and scanning electron microscopy (B).

• Bars of known measurement may be placed in the photos (e.g., in A above).
• Labels of specific areas or spots may be noted with symbols (e.g., letters, arrows), words, or in another manner (e.g., in B).

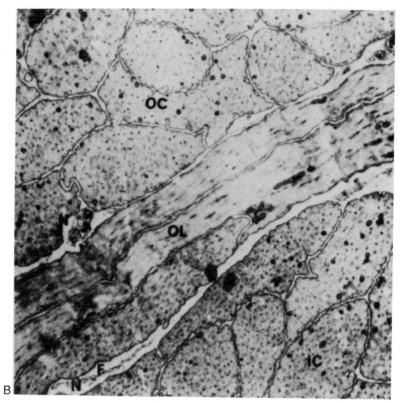

FIG. 8.74. *Continued*

Illustrates patient exposure to drug using a Venn diagram. Could be used to illustrate patient preference for one or more drugs in a complete study.

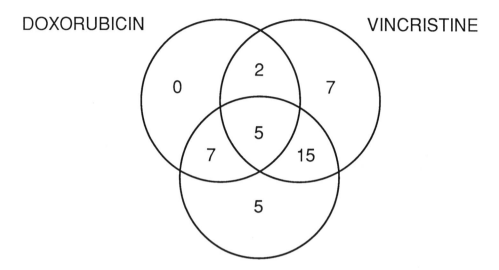

FIG. 8.75. Diagram of occupational exposure to antineoplastic drugs. Forty-one nurses reported exposure to antineoplastic drugs. Of the 14 (34.1 percent) exposed to doxorubicin, none were free of exposure to the other two drugs. Of the 32 (78.0 percent) exposed to cyclophosphamide, 5 (16.1 percent) were not exposed to the other drugs, and of the 29 (70.7 percent) exposed to vincristine, 7 (24.1 percent) were not exposed to the other drugs. Reprinted from Selevan et al. (1985) with permission.

- This can be used to illustrate drug preference in crossover studies.
- Venn diagrams are sometimes defined as including the total universe of possibilities of sets (e.g., Fig. 1.69) shown with a circle or box around the entire diagram.
- Fig. 8.75 does not show the entire universe, but uses circle diagrams, often called Euler diagrams after the 18th century Swiss mathematician, Leonhard Euler.

Illustrates physiological raw data and graph of the data.

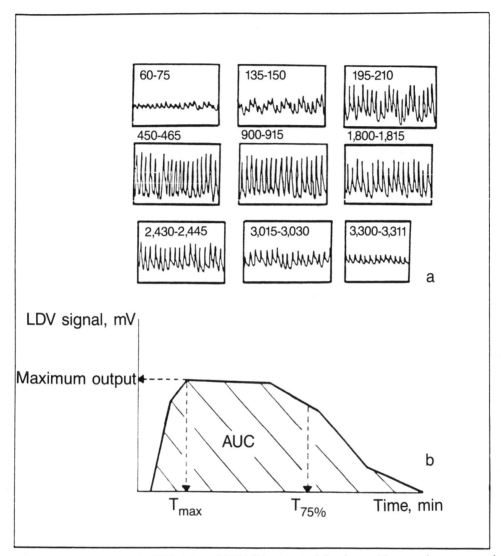

FIG. 8.76. Characteristic PPG (**a**) and LDV (**b**) outputs following a 15-second exposure of ventral forearm skin to an aqueous solution of drug (150 mM). The figures above the PPG recordings are the time ranges in seconds postdrug application. Reprinted from Stevenson et al. (1987) with permission.

Illustrates metabolic pathway (hypothesized or proven).

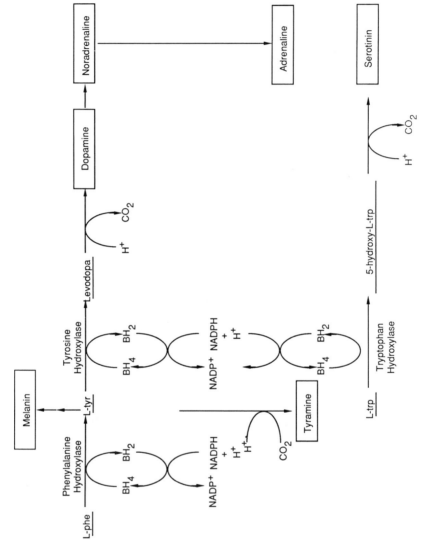

FIG. 8.77. Normal metabolic pathway of aromatic amino acids. All three aromatic amino acid hydroxylases use tetrahydrobiopterin (BH_4) as a cofactor, which is converted to dihydrobiopterin (BH_2). BH_2 is reconverted back to BH_4 by enzyme dihydropteridin reductase using NADPH as energy source. Reprinted from Woo et al. (1984) with permission.

Illustrates method of preparing material to study.

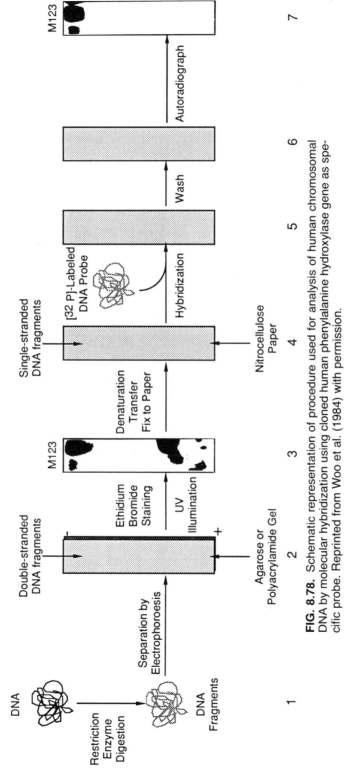

FIG. 8.78. Schematic representation of procedure used for analysis of human chromosomal DNA by molecular hybridization using cloned human phenylalanine hydroxylase gene as specific probe. Reprinted from Woo et al. (1984) with permission.

Illustrates natural life of a disease.

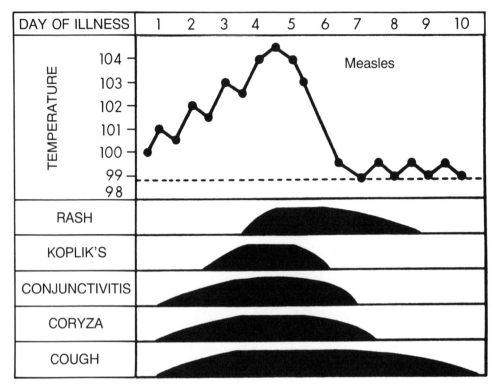

FIG. 8.79. Schematic diagram of clinical course of typical case of measles. The rash appears 3 to 4 days after onset of fever, conjunctivitis, coryza, and cough. Koplik's spots usually develop 2 days before the rash. Reprinted from Krugman and Ward (1973) with permission.

• This graph and the next 2 contain examples of silhouette charts.

Illustrates natural history of a disease.

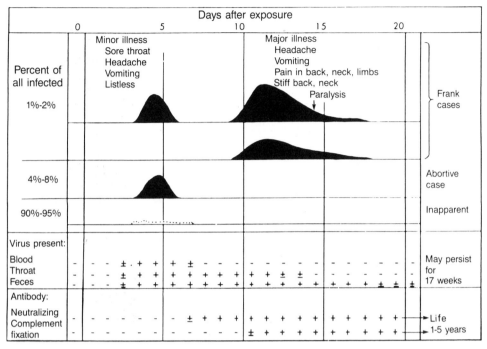

	Days after exposure				
	0	5	10	15	20

Virus present:

Blood	−	− − ± . + +	+ ± − − −	− − − − −	− − − − −	− May persist
Throat	−	− − ± + +	+ + + + +	+ + ± ± −	− − − − −	− for
Feces	−	− − ± + +	+ + + + +	+ + ± ±	+ + ± ± ±	± 17 weeks

Antibody:

Neutralizing Complement	−	− − − − −	− ± + + +	+ + + + +	+ + + + +	→Life
fixation	−	− − − − −	− − − − −	± + + + +	+ + + + +	→1-5 years

FIG. 8.80. Schematic diagrams of the clinical and subclinical forms of poliomyelitis, showing presence of virus and antibodies in relation to the development and subsidence of the infection. Black areas denote febrile periods. Reprinted from Krugman and Ward (1973) with permission.

Illustrates natural history of a disease.

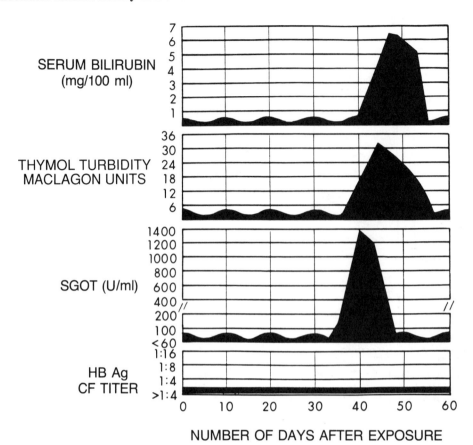

NUMBER OF DAYS AFTER EXPOSURE

FIG. 8.81. Schematic illustration of a typical case of viral hepatitis type A. Note that (1) the incubation period is relatively short—35 days from exposure to first evidence of abnormal SGOT levels and 40 days to first evidence of jaundice; (2) the period of abnormal serum transaminase activity is relatively short and jaundice appears when SGOT peaks; (3) thymol turbidity is abnormal; and (4) hepatitis B antigen (HG Ag) is not present. Reprinted from Krugman and Ward (1973) with permission.

Illustrates use of shading to accentuate graphs, especially where both upper and lower bounds are important.

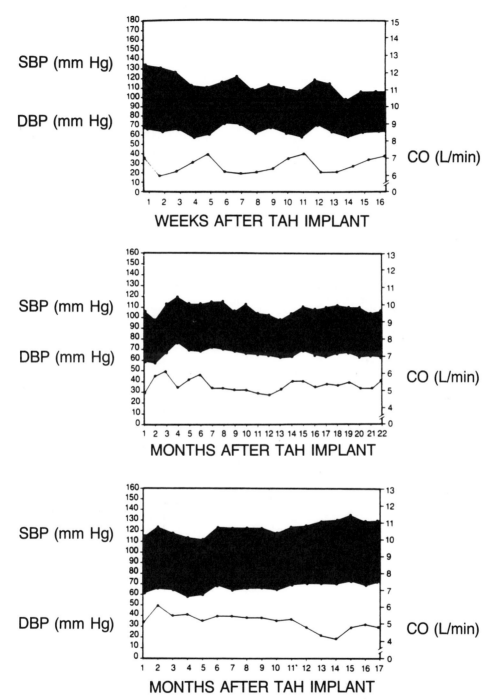

FIG. 8.82. Mean arterial blood pressure (systolic and diastolic blood pressures [SBP and DBP]) and cardiac outputs (CO) for each long-term recipient (weekly or monthly as indicated). TAH indicates total artificial heart. **Top**, Patient 1 (B.C.), arterial blood pressure SE range, 1.0 to 5.5 mm Hg; CO SE range, 0.06 to 0.25 L/min. **Center**, Patient 2 (W.S.), arterial blood pressure SE range, 0.5 to 1.9 mm Hg; CO SE range, 0.04 to 0.17 L/min. **Bottom**, Patient 3 (M.H.), arterial blood pressure SE range, 0.4 to 1.8 mm Hg; CO SE range, 0.05 to 0.13 L/min. Reprinted from DeVries (1988) with permission.

404

Illustrates prototype physiological tracings for descriptive purposes.

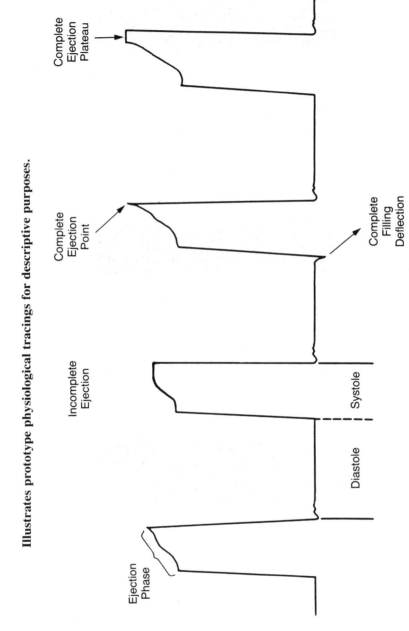

FIG. 8.83. Various ejection patterns seen on drive-pressure waveforms. Reprinted from Mays et al. (1988) with permission.

Illustrates a patient's case history focusing on infections and drugs used to treat them.

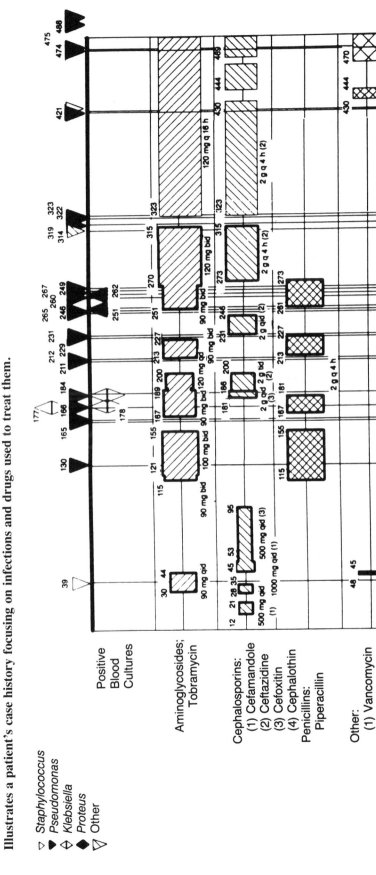

FIG. 8.84. Episodes of bacteremia and use of antimicrobial agents in case 2 (M.H.). **Numbers** indicate number of days following implantation of artificial heart; **symbols**, days that bacteremia with various organisms was noted. Reprinted from Kunin et al. (1988) with permission.

Illustrates clinical change of specific patients by using their clinical class or stage as a starting point and final outcome.

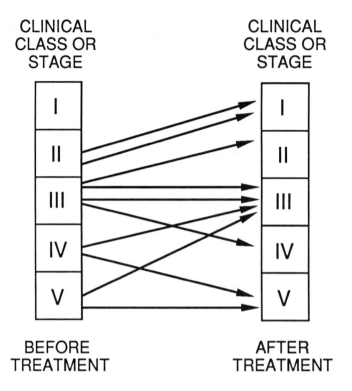

N = 10 patients in a study

FIG. 8.85. Classification of disease before and after treatment.

Illustrates comparison of two methods for diagnosing a disease by focusing on the agreement between the methods.

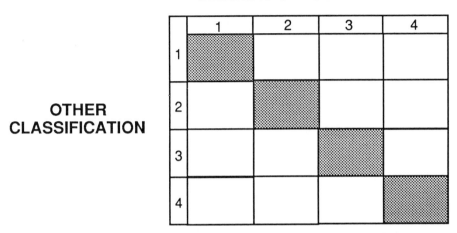

FIG. 8.86. Comparison of two methods used to diagnose a disease.

• Numbers in the hatched squares should account for most, if not all, patients if the two methods agree. Other squares should be zero or near zero.
• This scenario occurs rather commonly in antiinfective studies when one wants to compare clinical and bacteriological responses.

Illustrates a classic 2 × 2 table of predicted versus actual results.

		Actual		
		No Return	Return	
PREDICTED	NO RETURN (HEAVY PHYSICAL ACTIVITY AND <12 Y OF EDUCATION)	27	31	58
	RETURN (LIGHT OR MODERATE PHYSICAL ACTIVITY AND ⩾ 12 Y OF EDUCATION)	15	78	93
		42	109	151

FIG. 8.87. Reprinted from Smith and O'Rourke (1988) with permission.

9
Pharmacokinetics

There is probably greater agreement about how to present pharmacokinetic data than any other type of clinical data. This is probably a result of the generally standardized study designs used in most clinical evaluations, and the limited number of study objectives pursued. A majority of pharmacokinetic studies are crossover studies conducted in up to approximately 24 to 30 male volunteers. Blood samples usually are taken immediately prior to dosing and then at prespecified time points during the subsequent 24 hr to several days (i.e., up to at least five half-lives of the drug). Most data obtained are quantitative and are generally combined across patients (i.e., volunteers) relatively easily.

Tables 9.1 to 9.4 are prototype tables for listing and summarizing individual sample plasma drug levels, whereas Tables 9.5 to 9.14 provide formats for listing and summarizing pharmacokinetic parameters and for evaluating bioavailability and bioequivalence. The remaining tables in this chapter (Tables 9.15 to 9.27) are suggested presentations for other pharmacokinetic considerations (e.g., metabolism, elimination, and absorption).

Most of the figures in this chapter present prototypes for various ways of presenting plasma drug concentration data. A few figures (e.g., 9.23) are directed toward other components or summaries of pharmacokinetic investigations.

Illustrates listing of individual patient plasma concentrations (individual patient data, single site or study).

TABLE 9.1. Plasma Concentrations of Drug (μg/ml) in Study Patients on IV (or oral) Administration[a]

Time[b] (hour)	Patient numbers													
	01	02	03	04	05	06	07	08	10	11	12	13	14	16
0														
0.30														
0.75														
1.00														
1.25														
1.50														
2.00														
2.50														
3.00														
4.00														
6.00														
8.00														
10.00														
12.00														
18.00														
24.00														
30.00														
36.00														
48.00														

[a]Values may be after 1st, 2nd, or nth dose of drug.
[b]Scheduled time; exact times may differ slightly.

• Footnotes may be used to denote points where no sample was collected or analyzable, or where no plasma drug concentrations were detected.

• This table is often accompanied by plots (one for each patient) of plasma concentration versus time.

• This table is usually accompanied by a table stating the actual times of blood sampling, because pharmacokinetic parameters (e.g., area under the curve, half-life) are calculated based on plasma drug concentration at the actual sampling times.

Illustrates summary statistics for plasma concentrations (group data, single site or study).

TABLE 9.2. Basic Pharmacokinetic Table Summarizing Plasma Levels for Treatment A

Minutes postdose	Number of patients	Mean plasma level (ng/ml)	SD	Range[a]	Coefficient of variation (%)
0					
5					
10					
15					
20					
45					
60					
. . .					
n					

[a]Minimum value and maximum value headings may be used.

• A "separate table" is presented for each treatment group.

• Gives overview of plasma data—treatment groups are usually *not* compared at each sampling point.

• Observed mean C_{max} (maximum plasma concentration) is easy to see.

• A "good guess" of mean T_{max} (time of maximum plasma concentration) is easy to obtain.

• Table is usually accompanied by a figure in which mean concentration versus time is plotted.

Illustrates assessing bioequivalence at the individual sampling points (group data, single site or study).

TABLE 9.3. Comparison (ANOVA) of Treatment A and Reference Standard (Treatment B) with Respect to Plasma Concentrations

Minutes postdose	Mean diff.[a]	SD	Range	p value	Power[b]	95% CI[c]
5						
10						
20						
60						
120						
180						
240						
360						

[a]Treatment A minus Treatment B (reference standard) value.
[b]Power to detect a difference equal to 20% of the mean value of the reference standard.
[c]95% confidence interval centered at the (observed) mean value in the reference standard.

• Most statisticians and clinicians (although not necessarily all regulatory agencies) argue against the utility of statistical comparisons at each time point.

• If statistical testing is done, it is extremely important that this table includes the power of the test so that results may be properly interpreted.

• Sample size (N) must be stated somewhere. N should be the same at all time points (otherwise some strange events may appear in analyses) and hence need not be included in each row of the table.

• This common table is of limited utility unless expanded to report the mean values in the reference standard group.

Illustrates a contemporary approach to assessing bioequivalence at the individual sampling points (group data, single site or study).

TABLE 9.4. Comparison of Treatment A and Reference Standard with Respect to Plasma Concentrations[a]

Time postdose	Mean concentration of test product	Mean concentration of reference drug	Ratio of test product / reference	p value	Power	90% CI[b]

[a]This table is a more contemporary approach than is Table 9.3.
[b]Confidence intervals based on two one-sided t-tests. This approach to evaluating bioequivalence is currently recommended by the Food and Drug Administration.

Illustrates a presentation to demonstrate bioequivalence between two formulations (group data, single site or study).

TABLE 9.5. Bioequivalence Between 20 mg Tablet and Other 20 mg Formulation in 16 Subjects (Mean ± SD)[a]

	Tablet	Other formulation
Peak plasma level (ng/ml)	68.1 ± 21.8	66.9 ± 16.7
T_{max} (hours)	2.0 ± 0.7	2.5 ± 0.6
AUC (0–∞), (ng-hr/ml)	395.1[b]	381[b]
Total urinary recovery (% of dose)	33.8[c]	30.5[c]
Renal clearance (ml/min)	255 ± 70	250 ± 102
Relative bioavailability (F)	1.054[d]	—

[a]Other comparisons (e.g., drug A vs. drug B; drug with and without food) could be made.
[b]Geometric mean.
[c]Based on actual assayed content of the test medication. SD values could be given.
[d]Relative to other formulation, geometric mean.

• Statistical comparison and resulting p-values, power computations, and ranges would enhance presentation.

Illustrates concept of within-subject ratios for addressing bioequivalence (single patient data, single site or study).

TABLE 9.6. Area Under the Curve (AUC) Calculations for Drug X

Subject	AUC 20 mg dose	AUC[a] 40 mg dose	Ratio
1			
2			
3			
4			
5			
6			
7			
8			
9			
10			
11			
12			
13			
14			
15			
Mean			
SD			

[a]Normalized to the 20 mg dose.

Illustrates summary of differences of pharmacokinetic parameters for two treatments (group data, single site or study).

TABLE 9.7. Comparison of Treatment A and Reference Standard with Respect to Pharmacokinetic Parameters

Parameter	Mean diff.[a]	SD	Range	p value	Power[b]	95% CI[c]	75/75[d] Rule
AUC							
C_{max}							
T_{max}							
$T_{1/2}$							
K_{el}							
V_d/F							
Cl/F							

[a]Treatment A minus reference standard value.
[b]Power to detect a difference equal to 20% of the mean value of the reference standard.
[c]A 95% confidence interval centered at the (observed) mean value in the reference standard.
[d]This is a regulatory "rule" that was often applied in the past by some regulatory officials. It has recently been dropped because of lack of statistical validity.

- The sample size (N) needs to be mentioned somewhere.
- Both model-dependent and model-independent parameters should be displayed. This may be done in one or more tables.
- The power column is extremely important.
- The table would be more informative if it included a column reporting mean values in the reference group.
- Results of the 75/75 rule are not always given. When these results are included, a footnote explaining the rule must be added. Attention has recently been directed at performing two one-sided t-tests for each parameter.

Illustrates a summary of pharmacokinetic parameters under different conditions (group data, single site or study).[a]

TABLE 9.8. Pharmacokinetic Parameters of Drug X Under Three Treatment Conditions

Parameters[b]	Treatment coadministration			Power to detect 20% difference A or B vs. C
	Drug A	Drug B	No drugs (C)	
V_1 (l/kg)	0.21 ± 0.06	0.24 ± 0.05	0.26 ± 0.14	0.29
Vd_β (l/kg)	1.08 ± 0.36	1.16 ± 0.37	1.17 ± 0.38	0.87
$T_{1/2}$ (hr)	52.6 ± 25.5	72.2 ± 31.8[c]	54.7 ± 21.48	0.78
AUC (mg/hr/ml)	9.45 ± 3.96	11.76 ± 3.08[c]	9.78 ± 4.11	0.88
Cl (ml/min/kg)	0.277 ± 0.11	0.201 ± 0.054[c]	0.27 ± 0.138	0.65

[a]These data could also come from multiple studies.
[b]V_1, volume of distribution in the central compartment; Vd_β, dose divided by (AUC times k_{el}); $T_{1/2}$, half-life; AUC, area under the curve; Cl, clearance.
[c]$p < 0.05$.

- Vd_{ss} = volume of distribution of central plus peripheral compartments at steady state.
- A drug that only distributes in one compartment has only one volume of distribution (i.e., Vd).
- Various abbreviations are used for many pharmacokinetic parameters. The particular abbreviations must therefore be defined in each table, graph, or figure.

Illustrates a summary of pharmacokinetic parameters under different conditions (group data, single site or study).

TABLE 9.9. Pharmacokinetic Parameters of Drug X Under Three Conditions

	Treatment A 40 mg drug X alone	Treatment B 40 mg drug X with antacid	Treatment C 40 mg drug X with food
Peak plasma level (ng/ml)	81.09 ± 54.15	60.83 ± 21.62[a]	81.55 ± 29.60
Time to peak plasma level (hour)	2.62 ± 1.19	2.24 ± 0.79	2.44 ± 0.63
AUC (ng-hour/ml)	443.3 ± 249.2	355.0 ± 125.1	434.8 ± 145.9
Urine recovery			
(mg)	9.87 ± 4.29	8.81 ± 2.91	11.34 ± 2.99[a]
(% dose)	24.82 ± 10.79	22.1 ± 7.31	28.52 ± 7.51[a]
Half-life (hour)			
Renal clearance (l/hour)	25.8 ± 10.5	27.8 ± 11.6	28.5 ± 11.6
Rel. bioavailability (geom. mean)	—	0.900	1.141
95% CI	—	0.703, 1.151	0.932, 1.396

[a]Significantly different from drug X alone, $p < 0.05$. All other parameters were not significantly different. Data could be recalculated excluding Subject 212 and 416 as outliers.

• Variations would include (1) data before and during drug treatment, plus change and its level of significance; (2) same as above for one drug in presence and absence of a second drug.

• This table could present data separately for single or multiple doses.

Illustrates data on bioequivalence and dose proportionality (individual patient data, single site or study).

TABLE 9.10. Bioavailability of the 20 mg and the 40 mg Tablets and the 20 mg Dry-Filled Capsule in 16 Subjects[a]

Volunteer	40 mg Tablet	20 mg Tablet	20 mg Capsule
1			
2			
3			
4			
5			
6			
7			
8			
9			
10			
11			
12			
13			
14			
15			
16			
Mean:			
SD:			
95% CI:			

[a]Data presented in this table could be area under the curve or relative bioavailability.

Illustrates pharmacokinetic parameters for two routes of administration (individual and group data, single site or study).

TABLE 9.11. Parameters and Absolute Oral Bioavailabilities Derived from Plasma Level Data[a]

Patient no.	Intravenous				Oral							
	C_T (μg/ml)	AUC (μg hr/ml)	MRT_{IV} (hr)	$t_{1/2}$ (hr)	t_0 (min)	t_{max} (hr)	C_{max} (μg/ml)	AUC (μg hr/ml)	MRT_{po} (hr)	MAT (hr)	$t_{1/2}$ (hr)	F (%)
01												
02												
03												
04												
05												
06												
07												
08												
10												
11												
12												
13												
14												
16												
Median												
Range												

[a] C_T, plasma drug concentration at a particular time (T); MRT, mean residence time; MAT, mean absorption time; t_0, lag time for absorption; F, bioavailability.

Illustrates summary of major pharmacokinetic parameters for two treatments (individual patient data, single site or study).

TABLE 9.12. Summary of Pharmacokinetic Parameters

Treatment	Parameters	Pt 1 . . . Pt N[a]	N	Mean	SD	Minimum value	Maximum value	Coefficient of variation (%)
A	C_{max} (μg/ml)							
	T_{max} (hour)							
	AUC (μg·hr/ml)							
	$T_{1/2}$ (hour)							
	K_{el} (hour^{-1})							
B[b]	C_{max} (μg/ml)							
	T_{max} (hour)							
	AUC (μg·hr/ml)							
	$T_{1/2}$ (hour)							
	K_{el} (hour^{-1})							

[a]If N is relatively large it may be necessary to reverse the rows and columns. Pt, patient.
[b]A separate table may be made for each treatment studied.

• From the viewpoint of bioavailability and bioequivalence, the most important parameters are AUC, C_{max}, and T_{max}.

• Individual patient data are listed in this table. Often only summary statistics are included, and individual patient data are listed elsewhere.

• There can be both a model-dependent and a model-independent set of pharmacokinetic parameters. Both sets are summarized in the same manner. Recently, some pharmacokineticists have preferred to use compartmental versus noncompartmental parameters to be more specific.

Illustrates pharmacokinetic parameters in a dose-proportionality study (group data, single study).

TABLE 9.13. Summary of Dose-Proportionality Study (Mean ± SD)

	Drug dose (mg)			
	5	10	20	40
Peak plasma level (ng/ml)	14.0 ± 5.7	32.7 ± 11.0	43.4 ± 17.7	75.5 ± 28.6
Peak time (hours)	2.3 ± 1	1.9 ± 0.7	2.3 ± 0.9	1.9 ± 0.8
Total AUC (ng-hr/ml)	69.9 ± 42.6	183.3 ± 86.3	281.2 ± 125.3	482.3 ± 181.2
Urinary recovery (% of dose)	27.4 ± 13.6	27.7 ± 8.5	23.7 ± 6.7	19.5 ± 5.3
Renal clearance (l/hr)	294	227	276	263
Terminal half-life (hr)	—[a]	2.5 ± 1.0	2.6 ± 0.8	2.6 ± 0.9
Bioavailability[b]	1.21		1.17	—

[a]Not determined, data not amenable to analysis.
[b]Relative to the 40 mg dose; geometric mean.

- Various treatment groups and their numbers could be given.

Illustrates demonstration of power results (group data, single site or study).

TABLE 9.14. Power to Detect a 20 Percent Difference[a]

Percentage difference	A vs. B	A vs. C	B vs. C
10	0.24	0.16	0.21
15	0.49	0.31	0.43
20	0.76	0.52	0.69
25	0.93	0.74	0.88
30	0.99	0.89	0.98

[a]A, 20 mg capsule; B, 20 mg tablet; C, 20 mg tablet. The two tablets have different formulations.

- The significance level of test should be given.

Illustrates listing of clearance values (single patient data, multiple sites or studies).

TABLE 9.15. Individual Creatinine Clearance and Drug X Plasma Half-Life Reported in Study Number 66 (16 Healthy Patients) and Number 55 (8 Elderly Patients)

Patient number	Creatinine CL[a] (ml/min)	Drug X pharmacokinetic parameters				
		Renal CL (ml/min)	Half-life (hours)	Plasma CL (ml/min)	Nonrenal CL (ml/min)	Urinary recovery (% of dose)
(Healthy)						
1						
2						
3						
4						
5						
6						
7						
8						
9						
10						
11						
12						
13						
14						
15						
16						
(Elderly)						
1						
2						
3						
4						
5						
6						
7						
8						

[a]Creatinine clearance adjusted to 1.73 m^2. Patients could be ordered in descending order of creatinine clearance. CL, creatinine clearance.

Illustrates summary of clearance values (group values, single site or study).

TABLE 9.16. Renal Insufficiency Study[a]

Group	Creatinine clearance (ml/min)	Half-life (hours)	Plasma clearance[b] (l/hour)	Renal clearance (l/hour)
I	98.9	2.6	22.7	16.6
II	73.8	3.0	21.4	14.7
III	49.2	4.5	13.7	8.9
IV	10.3	11.7	4.5	1.0
V	0	13.7	6.3	—
V[c]	4.9	13.0	4.3	0.6

[a]All values are group mean values.
[b] There are occasions when it is also relevant to list plasma clearances in ml/min/kg (e.g., for neuromuscular blocking drugs).
[c]These patients are receiving dialysis.

• Some measure of variability should generally be incorporated into this type of presentation.

Illustrates excretory pathways, metabolic fate (if the drug is extensively metabolized) and mass balance (individual patients, single site or study).

TABLE 9.17. Elimination Pathways of Individual Subjects

	Subject:	1	2	3	. . .	N	Mean ± SD
Percent of the dose excreted							
A. Radioactive Methods (^{14}C)							
Urine (0 to 120 hr)[a]							
Feces (0 to 96 hr)							
Ratio of unchanged drug/total							
radioactivity excreted[b]							
B. Cold Methods (e.g., HPLC)							
Urine unchanged drug (0–24 hr)							
Urine parent and conjugates							
Feces (0 to 96 hr)							
parent drug							

[a]Each of these periods could be subdivided into 24-hr or other segments.
[b]Total radioactivity excreted would be in terms of unchanged drug plus metabolites and conjugates.

• These data could be divided into several tables, particularly if many patients were studied.
• Rows and columns should be reversed for more than 8 or 10 subjects.

Illustrates ability of three drugs to affect the kinetics of antipyrene (group data, single site or study).

TABLE 9.18. Effect of Single-Dose Receptor Antagonists ($476 \pm$ moles/kg i.p. at -30 min) on the Kinetics of Antipyrine (Mean $\pm$ SD)

Drug treatment	Half-life (min)	Volume of distribution (ml/kg)	Clearance (ml/min/kg)
Drug A			
No Treatment	135 ± 156	745 ± 39	4.31 ± 1.39
With Treatment	131 ± 24	849 ± 78^a	4.16 ± 0.33
Drug B			
No Treatment	155 ± 33	749 ± 80	3.46 ± 0.72
With Treatment	176 ± 58	738 ± 86	3.30 ± 1.51
Drug C			
No Treatment	149 ± 34	881 ± 93	4.33 ± 1.29
With Treatment	379 ± 99^b	679 ± 66^c	1.29 ± 0.21^b

[a]Significantly different from control (no treatment), $p<0.05$.
[b]Significantly different from control (no treatment), $p<0.01$.
[c]Significantly different from control (no treatment), $p<0.02$.

Illustrates a comparison of plasma level and urinary recovery (group data, single site or study).

TABLE 9.19. Plasma Levels and Urinary Recoveries of Drug X on Day 1 and Day 8 (Mean $\pm$ SD) of Six Subjects Following Repeated Administration (20 mg bid at 8:00 am and 5:00 pm for 15 Doses) of IV Drug

Day	Time (hr)	Plasma level (ng/ml)	Day	Time (hr)	Recovery in urine (% of dose)
1	0	0	1	0–2	55.70 ± 8.90
	0.17	368.19 ± 68.07		2–4	13.10 ± 1.60
	0.33	221.37 ± 53.05		4–6	7.00 ± 0.95
	0.5	175.41 ± 53.00		6–9	4.60 ± 1.30
	1	126.69 ± 32.20		9–24	79.20 ± 7.85
	2	96.34 ± 19.02			
	4	63.25 ± 13.89			
	6	31.17 ± 10.47			
	9	14.34 ± 12.87			
3	0	5.83 ± 5.56			
	9	16.43 ± 16.88			
6	0	6.44 ± 6.14			
	9	16.21 ± 16.76			
8	0	5.43 ± 5.80	8	0–2	64.10 ± 7.75
	0.17	388.12 ± 148.71		2–4	15.40 ± 3.30
	0.33	266.61 ± 35.30		4–6	6.35 ± 2.80
	0.5	207.89 ± 82.72		6–9	6.90 ± 4.35
	1	180.20 ± 55.66		9–24	5.85 ± 1.55
	2	128.00 ± 40.82			
	4	69.17 ± 28.01			
	6	35.26 ± 14.45			
	9	18.19 ± 11.34			

• Separate columns for different doses could be used.

Illustrates urine concentrations, volumes and amounts in patients treated with drug (individual patient data, single site or study).

TABLE 9.20. Urine Drug Concentrations (μg/ml), Volumes and Amounts in Study Patients on IV (or oral) Administration

Time (hour)	01	02	03	04	05	06	07	08	...	16	Mean	SD
				Urine drug concentration in patients numbered								
0												
0–4												
4–8												
8–12												
12–24												
24–36												
36–48												

Urine volumes (ml) in patients numbered as above

Time (hour)												
0												
0–4												
4–8												
8–12												
12–24												
24–36												
36–48												

Total amounts (drug concentration times urine volume) in patients numbered as above

Time (hour)												
0												
0–4												
4–8												
8–12												
12–24												
24–36												
36–48												

Illustrates a presentation of metabolite recovery in urine (group data, single site or study).

TABLE 9.21. Recovery of Metabolite X in Selected Urine Samples Relative to the Total Urinary Excretion in Human Subjects

Dose (mg)	Route	Regimen	No. of subjects	Time (hour)	Metabolite X (% of dose)
20	IV	single dose	2	0–2 (Day 1)	8.0
10	IV	bid for 3 days	2	0–2 (Day 1)	9.1
				0–2 (Day 3)	5.9
80	PO	single dose	1	0–2 (Day 1)	14.1
			1	6–8 (Day 1)	20.8
160	PO	single dose	2	2–4 (Day 1)	8.5
20	PO	bid for 5 days	3	0–10 (Day 1)	11.0
				10–24 (Day 5)	10.9
40	PO	bid for 5 days	3	0–10 (Day 1)	18.2
				10–24 (Day 5)	16.3

Illustrates a presentation of protein binding (individual patient data, single site or study).

TABLE 9.22. Protein Binding of Drug X in Human Plasma[a]

	Drug X concentration (ng/ml)	SD	Bound fraction (%)	SD
Pooled plasma:				
Individual plasma:				
Subject 1				
Subject 2				
Subject 3				
Subject 4				
Subject 5				

[a]Whole plasma was used, but the values could have been determined in a plasma ultrafiltrate.

Illustrates excretion of drug and its metabolite (group data, single site or study).

TABLE 9.23. Excretion of Parent Drug and a Metabolite

	Amount				Metabolite A
	Parent drug		Metabolite A		Metabolite A
Biological sample[a]	(μg)	(% total)	(μg)	(% total)	Parent drug
Urine					
Feces					
Bile					
Tissue A					
Tissue B					

[a]To calculate the amount of parent drug or metabolite in μg the total volumes divided by weights must be known. For urine and feces, the volumes divided by weights may be measured or estimated. For tissues, the weights or volumes must be measured if it is ethically acceptable to take a biopsy.

Illustrates radioactivity levels after injection of labeled drug (group data, single site or study).

TABLE 9.24. Plasma Level of Total Radioactivity and Drug X (Mean ± SD) Following Oral Administration of 20 mg (Containing 20 μCi ^{14}C-Drug X) to Four Healthy Subjects

Time (hr)	Drug X (ng/ml)	Total radioactivity (ng-eq/ml)
0	0	0
0.33	20 ± 21	19 ± 15
0.67	33 ± 16	42 ± 19
1	53 ± 30	60 ± 24
1.5	59 ± 17	58 ± 19
2	56 ± 30	58 ± 20
3	56 ± 23	54 ± 22
4	49 ± 22	49 ± 21
5	38 ± 16	45 ± 18
6	26 ± 13	35 ± 12
8	18 ± 10	22 ± 8
10	10 ± 3	21 ± 10
12	4 ± 4	11 ± 4
24	0	4 ± 1

Illustrates effect of an investigational drug on standard drugs (individual patient data, single site or study).

TABLE 9.25. Effect of Drug X (40 mg bid for 7 Days) on the Elimination Half-Life of Antipyrine and Aminopyrine in Healthy Subjects

	Antipyrine half-life (hr)			Aminopyrine half-life (hr)		
Subject	Baseline	Day 7	% Change	Baseline	Day 7	% Change
1						
2						
3						
4						
5						
6						
7						
8						
Median						

Illustrates changes in plasma metabolite concentrations over time (group data, single site or study).

TABLE 9.26. Illustrating Relative Changes in Plasma Metabolite Concentrations

Time after drug (min)	Metabolite number						
	1	2	3	4	5	. . .	N
0	1[a]	1	1	1	1		1
A							
B							
C							
D							
. . .							
N							

[a]All values are normalized to 1.

- This table clearly shows relative changes.
- Metabolite concentration could be shown for whole blood.

Illustrates one means of presenting trough and peak drug levels.

TABLE 9.27. Serum Levels of Drug X in Patients Receiving 120 mg Every 8 Hours

		Mean levels (mg/l) and range	
Initial prescribed dose	N	Trough	Peak
Less than nomogram dose	16	1.4 (0.4–4.3)	4.6 (2.5–8.1)
Nomogram dose	14	3.0 (1.3–4.7)	7.8 (6.1–9.6)
More than nomogram dose	7	6.1 (4.1–8.5)	10.6 (7.8–14.6)
Unable to calculate nomogram dose	5	1.7 (1.6–2.1)	6.9 (5.4–8.1)

Illustrates using different colored, shaded, or otherwise distinguishable bars to visually compare between subject results.

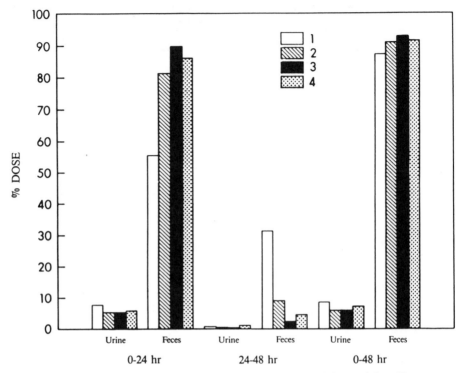

FIG. 9.1. Excretion of radioactivity after a single oral dose of drug X.

• 1, 2, 3, 4 represent individual subjects.

Illustrates putting lines indicating variability at top of bars of a histogram.

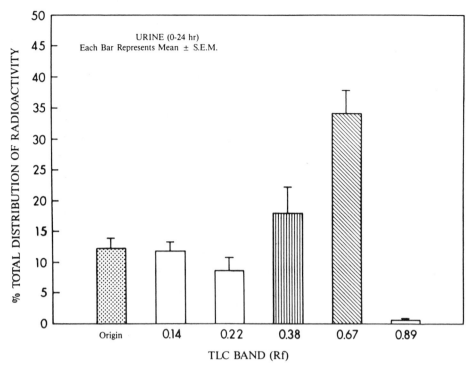

FIG. 9.2. The profile of drug X and metabolites in urine.

• Individual subject data may be shown.
• The framing effect of the upper and right side line may be eliminated.
• The ordinate's label may be placed horizontally for ease of reading.
• The ordinate's mark indicating values should usually be placed outside the y-axis rather than inside the y-axis.
• A similar graph may be shown for distribution of radioactivity for various metabolites in feces.

Illustrates using a histogram to show individual patient data (single site or study).

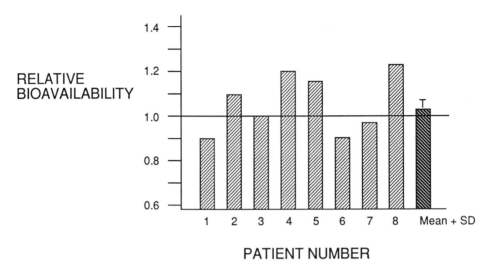

FIG. 9.3. Relative bioavailability data of eight patients.

- Different parameters could be illustrated similarly.
- Different studies or sites could be illustrated similarly.
- Note that the last bar displays summary data (mean ± SD) of the individual patient data presented by the other bars. The different shading used in the last bar emphasizes its uniqueness.

Illustrates using a three-dimensional block chart to compare formulations of two drugs.

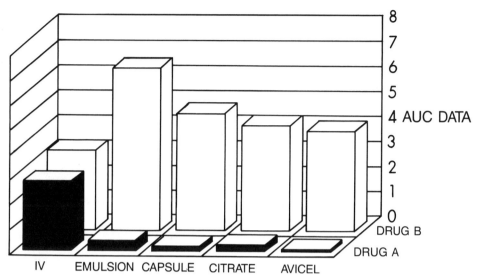

FIG. 9.4. Comparison of various formulations of two drugs.

• This three-dimensional display allows the reader to simultaneously compare five formulations of two drugs.

• One may immediately notice that there is little difference in AUC for the IV formulations, but there are relatively large differences for the oral formulations.

• One may immediately notice that within each drug the AUC is heavily dependent upon formulation.

• The y-axis needs to have units added for proper interpretation.

• The "boxing in" (i.e., series of horizontal lines—one at each value of y-axis) is extremely helpful in reading the graph.

Illustrates superimposing reference points for toxicity and efficacy on plasma concentration plots.

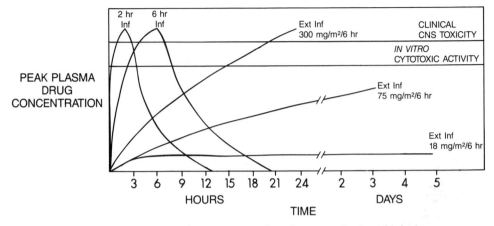

FIG. 9.5. Peak plasma drug concentrations for several rates of infusion.

• Although most time-concentration displays are not designed to explicitly identify toxicity levels, they add valuable information.

• Note the change in scale of x-axis from hours to days.

Illustrates escalating doses infused during several regimens to identify the maximal tolerated dose.

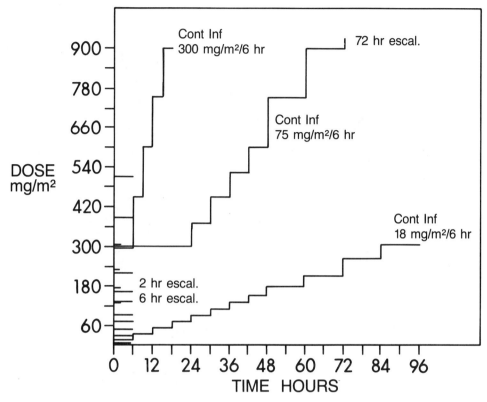

FIG. 9.6. Dose (mg/m²) versus time.

• An additional graph showing clinical efficacy or response versus time, dose, or concentration would be informative.

Illustrates peaks and troughs of plasma concentrations after and immediately following multiple doses.

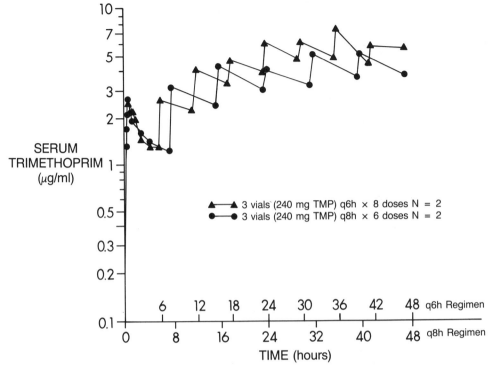

FIG. 9.7. Pharmacokinetics of multiple doses of trimethoprim in adult volunteers. TMP, trimethoprim.

• Similar curves may be simulated prior to a clinical study.

Illustrates plasma concentrations as a function of time for multiple products.

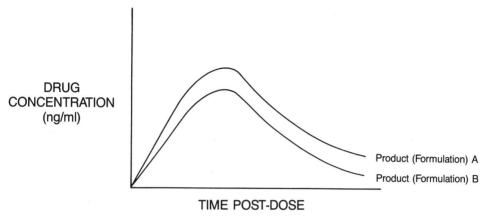

FIG. 9.8. Plot of plasma concentration vs. time.

- Each product (formulation) is represented by a "line" on the plot.
- Confidence bars (giving 95% or another confidence interval) can be added.
- Display allows immediate easy comparison of all treatments with respect to hourly concentrations, C_{max}, and T_{max}. One can also get a reasonable estimate of AUC (area under the curve) from this figure.
- Display is sometimes accompanied (usually in an appendix) by individual patient concentration versus time plots. These plots are identical in format to this mean plot.
- A partial or entire chemical structure may be placed next to each curve if they represent the parent drug or metabolites.
- The graphs could be labeled with arrows or symbols to designate C_{max}, T_{max}, or other pharmacokinetic parameters.

Illustrates placing models of compartments on plasma level versus time curves (single patient, single site or study).

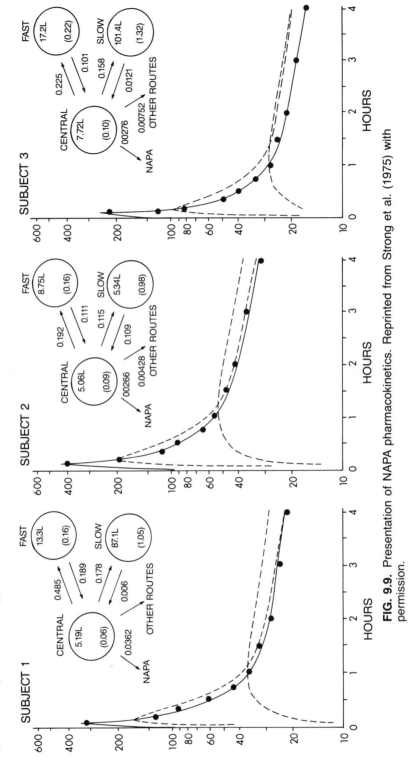

FIG. 9.9. Presentation of NAPA pharmacokinetics. Reprinted from Strong et al. (1975) with permission.

Illustrates using a vertical sequence of plots to vividly display the effect of increasing dose.

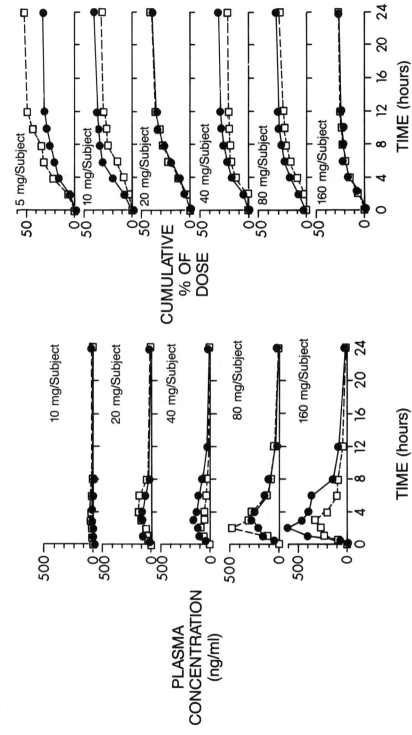

FIG. 9.10. Bioavailability of single oral doses (**left**) and urinary excretion of single oral doses (**right**). The symbols represent two subjects.

• Similar sequence of data from each patient in a dose escalation study would be informative. Mean data with variability bars should also be shown for study results in separate graphs.

Illustrates plasma concentrations on a logarithmic scale.

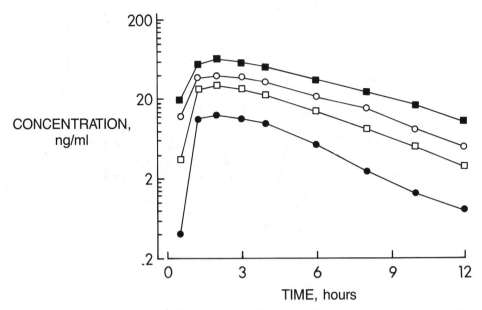

FIG. 9.11. Mean plasma level profiles of drug X following oral dose administration of dry-filled capsules to 15 young healthy subjects at various dose levels. Key: ● = 5 mg; □ = 10 mg; ○ = 20 mg; ■ = 40 mg.

• Use of this transformation provides more insight into what happens during the elimination phase.
  • An arithmetic scale may be used for the ordinate.
  • Similar graphs may be used to illustrate results of
    a. Different formulations.
    b. Different ingredients of a combination drug product.
    c. Different patient populations.
    d. First dose versus n^{th} dose.
    e. Different patients (i.e., individual patient data).
    f. Interaction with food (i.e., with and without food).
    g. Other drugs (i.e., results in presence and absence of another drug).
    h. Total radioactivity.

Illustrates use of multiple breaks in horizontal axis.

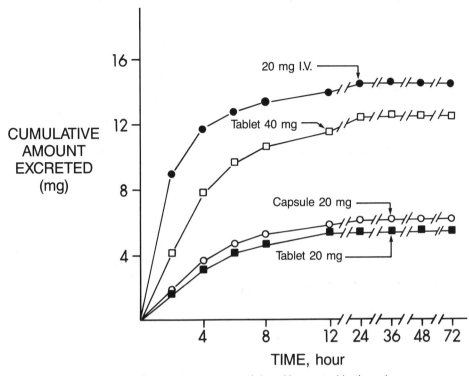

FIG. 9.12. Cumulative amount of drug X excreted in the urine.

• Indicating the break in the lines of the plot, as well as on the axis, is helpful, although it is often preferable to use a logarithmic scale for other parameters than time.

Illustrates vertically stacked plots to show effect of increasing dose—also illustrates a way of indicating the range of observed values by a "band" around the mean line.

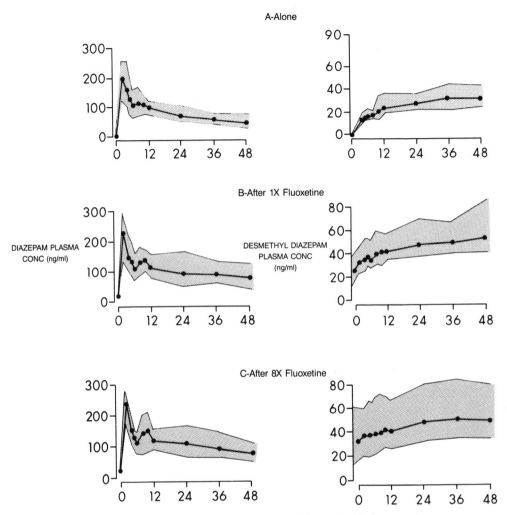

FIG. 9.13. Mean and range (N = 6) of diazepam and *N*-desmethyldiazepam plasma concentration observed after the administration of diazepam (10 mg) alone (A), diazepam (10 mg) after single-dose fluoxetine (60 mg) (B), and diazepam (10 mg) after multiple-dose fluoxetine (8 days at 60 mg/day) (C). Abscissa is in hours. Reprinted from Stuck et al. (1988) with permission.

Illustrates plotting creatinine clearance versus plasma clearance.

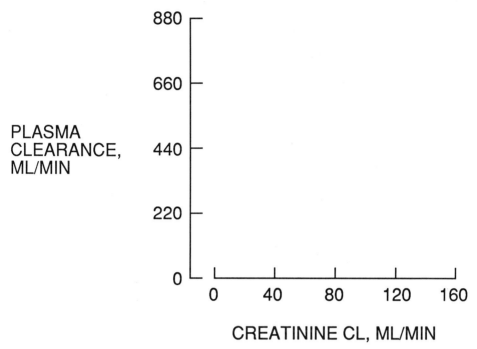

FIG. 9.14. Effect of creatinine clearance on drug X's plasma clearance.

• Alternate parameters for y-axis include urinary recovery (percent of dose administered), renal clearance (ml/min), and plasma half-life (hr).

Illustrates superimposing individual subject plasma concentration plots using one set of axes.

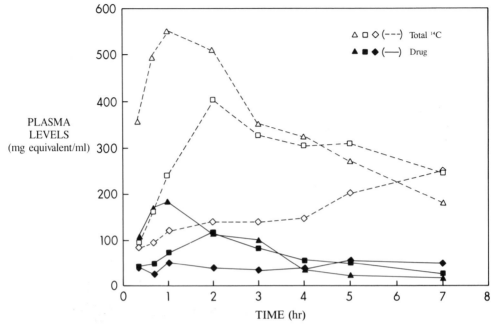

FIG. 9.15. Plasma concentrations of total radioactivity and drug X in individual males after an oral dose of drug X (5 mg/kg).

• Vividly illustrates significant betweeen-subject variability.

Illustrates superimposing (only when appropriate) the linear regression line on a scatterplot.

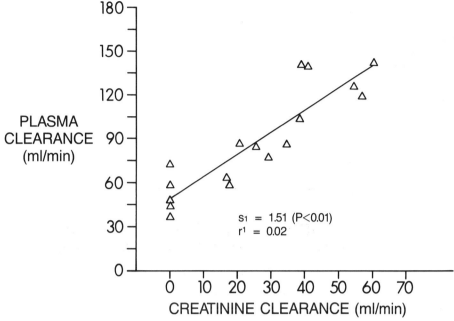

FIG. 9.16. Renal function and plasma clearance of drug X in renal impaired patients.

• Renal function versus total area under the curve or versus renal clearance also could be illustrated.

• If multiple graphs relating one variable (renal function) to others (e.g., renal clearance, area under the curve, and plasma half-life) are placed on a single page, the reader can obtain a better perspective.

• A set of graphs similar to those described above would help evaluate the importance of intact renal function in excreting the drug, if data were obtained in patients with normal renal function.

• Presentation is enhanced by printing the regression coefficient and its corresponding p value on the scatterplots with the regression lines.

Illustrates converting longitudinal data to a single point.

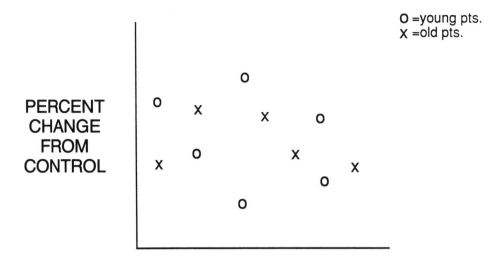

AREA UNDER CURVE FOR DRUG X (ng•min/ml)
or DRUG X CONCENTRATION (ng/ml)

FIG. 9.17. Area under the curve for an investigational drug as a percent of control.

• Scatterplot could use percent of control rather than percent change from control on the vertical axis.
• Showing only one quadrant implies that change from control must be positive, which is often invalid.

Illustrates how a scatterplot may be used to show a relationship (half-life versus creatinine clearance) both within and between three distinct patient populations.

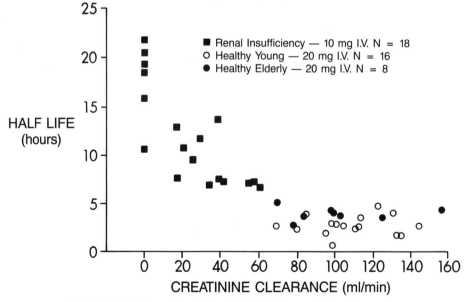

FIG. 9.18. Relationship of drug X half-life to creatinine clearance.

Illustrates appearance of a "typical" thin layer chromatography (TLC)/ autoradiograph.

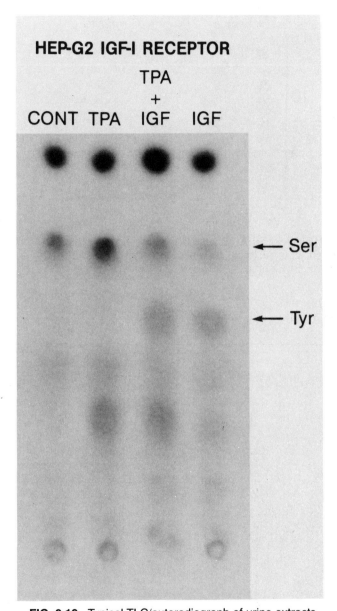

FIG. 9.19. Typical TLC/autoradiograph of urine extracts.

Illustrates presenting pharmacokinetic data with a scattergram.

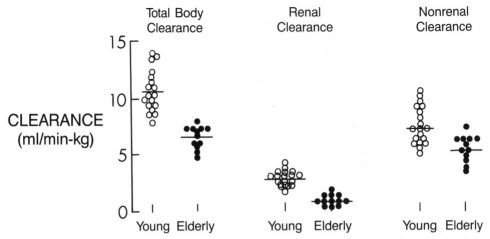

FIG. 9.20. Plasma clearances of unbound prednisolone in young (open symbols) and elderly (closed symbols) subjects. All three clearance values were lower (p<0.001) in the elderly subjects. Reprinted from Stuck et al. (1988) with permission.

Illustrates using a picture of a human to indicate drug disposition.

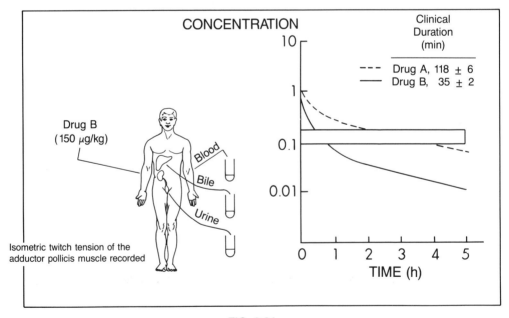

FIG. 9.21.

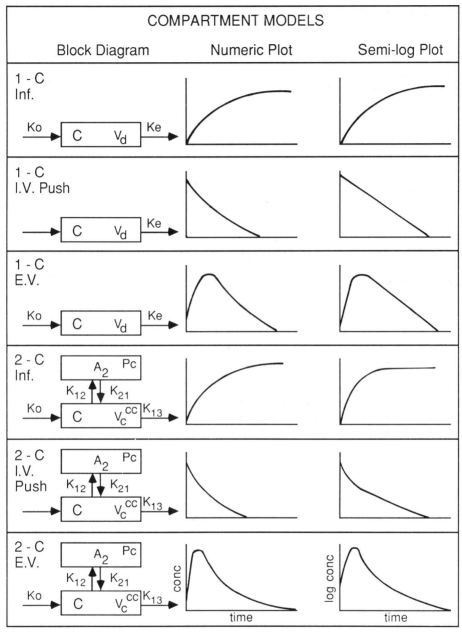

FIG. 9.22. Schematic representation of pharmacokinetic models in form of block diagrams (**left column**); and blood level–time curves as numeric (**middle column**); and semilog plots (**right column**) for intravenous infusion, IV administration, and extravascular administration according to the open one-compartment model and open two-compartment model. k_0, zero-order infusion rate; C(t), drug concentration in blood; V_d, apparent volume of distribution; k_e, overall elimination rate constant; k_a, absorption rate constant; k_{12}, distribution rate constant from the central to the peripheral compartment; k_{21}, distribution rate constant from the peripheral to the central compartment; CC, central compartment (blood and any organ or tissue which is in immediate equilibrium with the drug concentration in blood); k_{13}, elimination rate constant for loss of drug from the central compartment; A_2, drug amount in peripheral compartment; 1-C, open one-compartment model; 2-C, open two-compartment model; I.V., intravascular; E.V., extravascular; V_c, central compartment volume of distribution; PC, peripheral compartment. Reprinted from Ritschel (1984) with permission.

Illustrates the metabolic path of a drug in humans.

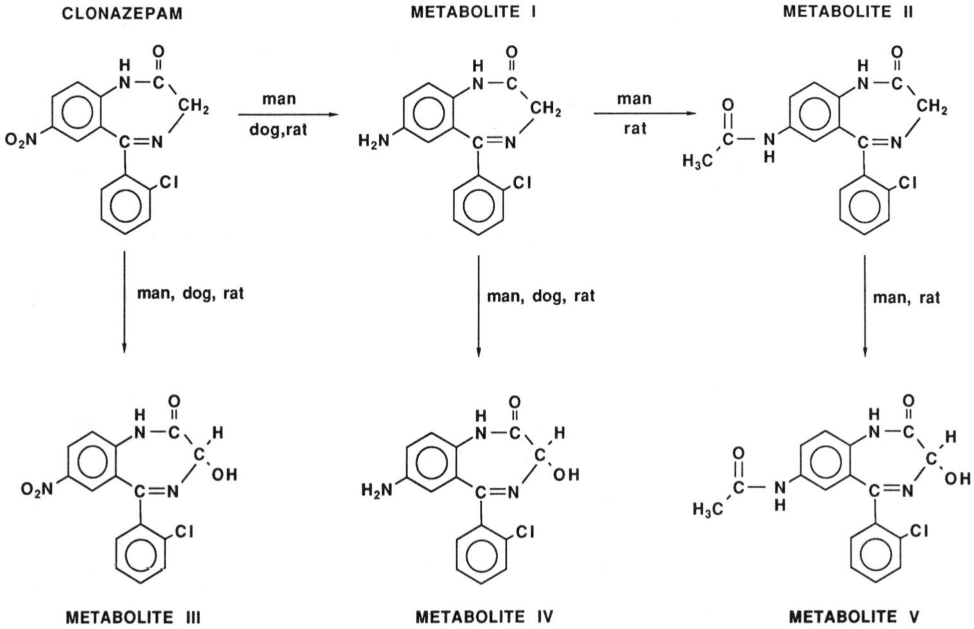

FIG. 9.23. Metabolism of clonazepam in humans. Reprinted from Eschenhof (1973) with permission.

• Other characteristics of each metabolite may be listed on the schematic (e.g., biological properties, amounts produced after a certain period, amounts produced by a specific organ [e.g., liver], physicochemical properties).

10
Quality of Life

Quality of life considerations are becoming increasingly important each year, and this trend is expected to continue for many years. Clinical treatments chosen for use in the future will undoubtedly be heavily influenced by quality of life issues. These issues are especially relevant in the current era of cost containment where many major purchasing decisions are based to a large degree on quality of life considerations.

The universe of quality of life studies is extremely broad and includes studies that are based in disciplines other than medicine (e.g., sociology, psychology, economics). This book is concerned with medical studies and includes predominantly tables and figures that focus on medical aspects. Cost-effectiveness data are presented in Chapter 11.

Separate studies may be conducted to evaluate quality of life factors just as safety, efficacy, and pharmacokinetic factors may be evaluated in separate studies. Any two or more of these categories may also be evaluated in a single study. In fact, safety considerations are present in virtually all clinical studies even when safety is not a primary objective.

For the most part, quality of life variables are displayed and analyzed similarly to efficacy data and readers are referred to Chapter 8. Since there is as yet no single definition of quality of life, each presentation should include a definition of the variables utilized. Readers interested in more information are referred to *Quality of Life Assessments in Clinical Trials* (Spilker, 1990).

The tables and figures illustrate results of representative tests and scales used to measure quality of life, and show means of presenting data.

Illustrates an example of a battery of tests used to evaluate quality of life.

TABLE 10.1. Measures Used to Assess Quality of Life in Publication of Croog et al. (1986)

1. The General Well-Being Adjustment Scale
2. The Physical Symptoms Distress Index
3. The Sleep Dysfunction Scale
4. The Sexual Symptoms Distress Index
5. The Positive Symptoms Index
6. The Wechsler Memory Scale
7. The Reitan Trail Making Test
8. The Life Satisfaction Index

[a]Each of these scales may be described in the table.

Illustrates summarizing baseline status and documenting comparability of treatment groups (group data, single site or study).

TABLE 10.2. Composite Scores at Baseline by Treatment Group[a]

	Placebo (N = 149)	Auranofin (N = 154)	p value
Clinical composite	-1.6 ± 0.05[b]	-1.5 ± 0.04	0.37
Functional composite	0.96 ± 0.08	0.98 ± 0.07	0.90
Pain composite	-0.63 ± 0.07	-0.72 ± 0.07	0.40
Global assessments composite	3.6 ± 0.06	3.5 ± 0.06	0.64

[a]Reprinted from Bombardier et al. (1986) with permission.
[b]Means $\pm$ SE.

• The footnote should identify the statistical test used, and whether the test was one or two sided.

Illustrates classification of patients as improved, no change or worsened (group data, single site or study).

TABLE 10.3. Changes in Quality-of-Life Measures in the Three Treatment Groups[a]

Quality-of-life measure	Percent of patients			p value[b]
	Improvement	None	Worsening	
General well-being				
Captopril (N = 181)	51.4	17.7	30.9	
Methyldopa (N = 143)[c]	39.2	9.8	51.0	p<0.01
Propranolol (N = 161)[c]	39.1	15.5	45.4	
Physical symptoms				
Captopril (N = 181)	29.3	45.3	25.4	
Methyldopa (N = 142)[c]	19.7	43.4	36.6	p<0.05
Propranolol (N = 160)[c]	17.5	45.6	36.9	
Sexual dysfunction				
Captopril (N = 181)	18.2	63.0	18.8	
Methyldopa (N = 141)[c]	9.2	66.7	24.1	p<0.05
Propranolol (N = 160)[c]	8.8	65.6	25.6	

[a]Reprinted from Croog et al. (1986) with permission.
[b]P value based on chi-square test (3 × 3) for independence with 4 degrees of freedom.
[c]Variations in the numbers of patients in the methyldopa and propranolol treatment groups are due to incomplete responses to the assessment measures.

Illustrates changes from baseline for different symptoms (group data, single site or study).

TABLE 10.4. Mean Changes in Reported Physical Symptoms from Baseline to Week 24, According to Differences in Scores from Baseline (N = 486)[a]

Symptom	Treatment group[b]			Significance of difference between groups[c]
	Captopril (N = 181)	Methyldopa (N = 143)	Propranolol (N = 162)	
Feeling worn out	− 1	+ 15	+ 6	
Feeling faint or lightheaded	+ 6	+ 14	+ 6	
Skin rash	+ 7	− 6	+ 1	
Tiredness or fatigue	− 6	+ 17	+ 16	AB, AC
Slow heart beat	− 1	− 4	+ 13	AC, BC
Shortness of breath	− 8	+ 1	+ 16	AC, BC
Hands sensitive to cold	− 5	− 10	− 3	
Numbness or tingling of hands	− 2	+ 1	+ 3	
Swelling of ankles	− 6	− 4	− 1	
Nightmares	+ 6	+ 6	+ 1	
Dry mouth	− 1	+ 39	− 1	AB, BC
Loss of taste	+ 3	+ 8	+ 2	
Blurred vision	− 4	+ 12	+ 10	AB

[a]The results for each physical symptom were based on a 5-point scale (0–4). A unit change on the table represents a unit change of 1 percent on the scale. Reprinted from Croog et al. (1986) with permission.
[b]Minus signs indicate improvement as a reduction in symptom score; plus signs indicate worsening as an increase in symptom score.
[c]All comparisons shown are significant at p<0.05.

• Footnote *c* should say "All *indicated* comparisons. . .". Otherwise the casual reader might read the footnote and assume that all possible comparisons were statistically significant.

• The table should indicate how statistical comparisons were made and if an adjustment for multiple comparisons was used.

Illustrates within-treatment summary and between-treatment comparisons (group data, single site or study).

TABLE 10.5. Effect of ICU Illness on Quality of Life[a]

	ICU group (N = 59)		Controls (N = 109)		Difference
Sickness Impact Profile					
Ambulation	9.0	± 1.6	9.1	± 1.3	NS
Mobility	5.9	± 1.6	5.6	± 1.1	NS
Body care and movement	3.2	± 0.9	3.5	± 0.7	NS
Social interaction	6.5	± 1.3	4.9	± 0.8	NS
Communication	2.7	± 0.9	3.3	± 0.8	NS
Alertness	10.8	± 2.3	7.0	± 1.5	NS
Emotion	4.6	± 1.2	2.4	± 0.7	NS
Sleep and rest	12.2	± 2.0	8.8	± 1.1	NS
Eating	2.0	± 0.4	2.4	± 0.4	NS
Work	22.4	± 4.2	3.5	± 1.3	$p < .001$
Home maintenance	12.7	± 2.7	1.4	± 0.3	$p < .001$
Recreation	14.4	± 2.6	10.1	± 1.4	NS
Physical subscore	5.3	± 1.1	5.2	± 0.8	NS
Psychosocial subscore	6.3	± 1.1	4.5	± 0.7	NS
Total SIP score	7.4	± 1.0	4.8	± 0.6	$p < .001$
Adjusted SIP score[b]	6.3	± 1.0	4.7	± 1.1	NS
Uniscale	8.09 ± 0.36		8.58 ± 0.20		NS

[a]Reprinted from Sage et al. (1987) with permission.
[b]Does not include work category.
ICU, intensive care unit; NS, not significant; SIP, Sickness Impact Profile.

• Listing actual p values rather than "NS" for those instances when $p > .05$ would be more informative.

Illustrates interrelationships of the quality of life variables (group data, single site or study).

TABLE 10.6. Correlations Between PAIS Sections[a]

Section	I	II	III	IV	VI	
I						Health care orientation
II	0.330					Vocational environment
III	0.387	0.531				Domestic environment
IV	0.251	0.406	0.534			Sexual relationship
VI	0.301	0.519	0.563	0.507		Social environment
VII	0.485	0.558	0.597	0.499	0.398	Psychological distress

[a]Reprinted from Kaplan De-Nour (1982) with permission.

• Many quality of life studies concentrate on the correlation between various quality of life measurement scales.
• Data are often displayed by presenting the correlation matrix.
• This "unique" display nicely indicates the types of scales being correlated.

Illustrates summary of changes and between-treatment analyses (group data, single site or study).

TABLE 10.7. Changes in Clinical and Health Status Measures and Composite Scores Between Baseline and Sixth Month by Treatment Group (N = 303)[a]

	Possible range (worst to best)	Change from baseline		Treatment effect (p value)[b]
		Placebo (N = 149)	Auranofin (N = 154)	
Clinical measures				
Number of tender joints		− 4.5 ± 0.9[c]	− 7.3 ± 1.0	0.01
Number of swollen joints		− 3.6 ± 0.7	− 5.5 ± 0.7	0.01
50-foot walk time (sec)		+ 0.61 ± 0.66	− 0.74 ± 0.40	0.11
Duration of morning stiffness (min)		− 12 ± 13	− 28 ± 12	0.1
Grip strength adjusted (mm Hg)		− 2 ± 8	+ 13 ± 8	0.02
Composite score		0.16 ± 0.05	0.35 ± 0.05	0.003
Function measures				
Health Assessment Questionnaire	3–0	− 0.17 ± 0.04	− 0.31 ± 0.05	0.01
Keitel Assessment	98–0	+ 1.7 ± 1.0	− 1.5 ± 0.9	0.003
Quality of Well-Being Questionnaire	0–1	− 0.001 ± 0.007	+ 0.023 ± 0.007	0.005
Composite score		0.05 ± 0.05	0.28 ± 0.05	0.001
Pain measures				
McGill Pain Questionnaire	78–0	− 5.6 ± 1.0	− 8.0 ± 1.1	0.02
Pain ladder scale (6-day mean)	0–10	+ 0.61 ± 0.13	+ 0.96 ± 0.18	0.09
10-centimeter pain line	10–0	− 0.91 ± 0.18	− 1.44 ± 0.17	0.01
Composite score		0.48 ± 0.07	0.74 ± 0.08	0.021
Global impression measures				
Arthritis				
Categorical scale	1–5	+ 0.31 ± 0.07	+ 0.65 ± 0.08	<0.001
Ladder scale (6-day mean)	0–10	+ 0.59 ± 0.14	+ 0.98 ± 0.18	0.11
Overall health				
Ladder scale, current	0–10	+ 0.39 ± 0.14	+ 0.65 ± 0.15	0.19
Ladder scale, 6-day mean	0–10	+ 0.35 ± 0.12	+ 0.87 ± 0.15	0.007
RAND Current Health Assessment	9–45	+ 0.51 ± 0.47	+ 1.82 ± 0.49	0.01
10-centimeter line, by patient	0–10	+ 0.51 ± 0.13	+ 0.89 ± 0.16	0.1
10-centimeter line, by physician	0–10	+ 0.46 ± 0.12	+ 0.58 ± 0.13	0.2
Composite score		0.27 ± 0.05	0.50 ± 0.07	0.007

[a]Reprinted from Bombardier et al. (1986) with permission.
[b]Significance level of the treatment effect determined by analysis of covariance adjusting for baseline values of age, sex, clinic, functional class, and the variable tested.
[c]Mean changes ± SE.

- Inclusion of the range for each scale is helpful.
- One analyzes the change in each scale, not the absolute value. Thus, the reader does not know what part of the scale contains results. This missing information is crucial for a meaningful interpretation.
- Note the helpful grouping of the scales.

Illustrates summarization of change and between-treatment analyses (group data, single site or study).

TABLE 10.8. Results of Utility and Other Measures[a]

	Possible range (worst to best)	Placebo		Auranofin		Treatment effect (p value)
		Value or Change[a]	Number of patients	Value or Change[a]	Number of patients	
Utility measures						
Patient Utility Measurement Set (derived change score)[b]	0–100	9.9 ± 2.2	117	20.9 ± 2.6	122	0.002[c]
Standard gamble (percent change of death)[d]	100–0	30 ± 3	124	23 ± 2	119	0.07[c]
Willingness-to-pay (percent of income)[d]	100–0	23 ± 1	105	21 ± 1	112	0.79[c]
Other measures						
NIMH Depression Questionnaire[e]	60–0	− 4.1 ± 0.8	149	− 3.3 ± 1.1	154	0.54[g]
RAND General Health Perceptions Questionnaire[e]	0–110	− 0.07 ± 0.75	149	+ 0.52 ± 0.79	154	0.32[g]
Clinical and functional measures not included in composites						
Erythrocyte sedimentation rate (mm/hr)[e]		+ 0.57 ± 1.68	149	− 4.31 ± 1.65	154	0.02[g]
Toronto Activities of Daily Living Questionnaire (perceived change score)[f]	4–1	0.00 ± 0.006	149	0.00 ± 0.007	154	0.02[c]

[a]Reprinted from Bombardier et al. (1986) with permission. Values are means ± SE.
[b]No value obtained at baseline: derived retrospectively at 5th month from patient's comparisons of baseline and current states.
[c]Significance level of treatment effect determined by analysis of covariance adjusting for baseline values of age, sex, clinic, and functional class but not the variable tested.
[d]No value obtained at baseline: not a change score.
[e]Values obtained at baseline and 6th month.
[f]No value obtained at baseline; recorded retrospectively at 6th month.
[g]Significance level of treatment effect determined by analysis of covariance adjusting for baseline values of age, sex, clinic, functional class, and the variable tested.

- It would be easy to add a within-treatment analysis.

Illustrates summary and between-treatment comparisons of QOL variables (group data, single site or study).

TABLE 10.9. Quality-of-Life Scales at Baseline and During Active Therapy (24 Weeks) for Patients with Complete 24-Week Follow-up Who Were Receiving Captopril (N = 181), Methyldopa (N = 143), or Propranolol (N = 162); Means ± SE

Scale[a]	Baseline[b]			24 Weeks[b]			Comparisons between groups in changes from baseline[c]
	Captopril (A)	Methyldopa (B)	Propranolol (C)	Captopril (A)	Methyldopa (B)	Propranolol (C)	
General well-being (+)	103.4 ± 1.0	105.0 ± 1.1	104.0 ± 1.1	105.6 ± 1.1[d]	103.4 ± 1.2	103.7 ± 1.1	AB[d] AC[d]
Physical symptoms (−)	5.0 ± 1.0	4.9 ± 0.4	4.9 ± 0.4	4.8 ± 0.3	5.8 ± 0.4[e]	5.5 ± 0.4[e]	AB[e] AC[e]
Sexual dysfunction (−)	2.3 ± 0.3	2.3 ± 0.3	1.9 ± 0.3	2.5 ± 0.3	2.9 ± 0.3[e]	2.7 ± 0.3[e]	AC[e]
Work performance (−)	16.8 ± 0.5	17.2 ± 0.6	17.8 ± 0.5	15.9 ± 0.5[e]	18.2 ± 0.7	17.6 ± 0.6	AB[d] BC[e,f]
Sleep dysfunction (−)	7.9 ± 0.3	7.7 ± 0.3	7.5 ± 0.3	7.7 ± 0.3	7.5 ± 0.3	7.6 ± 0.3	AB[e]
Cognitive function (−) (Trail Making B)	97.4 ± 3.5	93.8 ± 4.0	97.1 ± 3.7	78.4 ± 2.3	82.9 ± 3.3[d]	80.2 ± 2.7[d]	AB[e]
Life satisfaction (−)	28.4 ± 0.3	28.2 ± 0.4	28.1 ± 0.4	28.9 ± 0.4	29.5 ± 0.4[d]	28.8 ± 0.4[e]	AB[e]
Social participation (−)	11.9 ± 0.2	12.1 ± 0.2	12.5 ± 0.2	11.6 ± 0.2	11.9 ± 0.2	11.9 ± 0.2[d]	

[a]Plus sign denotes improvement with an increasing score, and minus signs denote improvement with a decreasing score. (Reprinted from Croog et al. [1986] with permission.)
[b]Symbols in the body of the table indicate p values comparing 24-week levels with baseline levels, based on the mean difference and t-statistic.
[c]Univariate contrasts of rates of change between groups within pairs, determined with the F-statistic.
[d]p of difference <0.01.
[e]p of difference <0.05.
[f]A univariate contrast is reported, although in overall multivariate analysis. B versus C was not significant.

Illustrates the effect of a third variable (age) on quality of life (group data, single site or study).

TABLE 10.10. Effect of Age on Quality of Life

	ICU patients		Non-ICU patients		
	Age 65–75 (N = 39)	Age ≥ 76 (N = 20)	Age 65–75 (N = 43)	Age 76–85 (N = 44)	Age ≥ 86 (N = 22)
Sickness Impact Profile (SIP)					
Physical score	3.6 ± 0.8	8.7 ± 2.6	1.5 ± 0.4[a]	5.3 ± 1.0[a]	12.3 ± 2.7[a]
Psychosocial score	5.3 ± 1.3	8.3 ± 2.1	2.9 ± 1.0	5.4 ± 0.8	8.7 ± 2.4
Total SIP score	5.6 ± 1.1[a]	11.0 ± 2.0[a]	2.3 ± 0.6[a]	4.9 ± 0.8[a]	9.4 ± 2.0[a]
Adjusted SIP score[b]	4.8 ± 1.0[a]	9.1 ± 2.0	2.2 ± 0.5[a]	4.8 ± 0.8[a]	9.3 ± 2.0[a]
Uniscale	8.13 ± 0.45[a]	8.00 ± 0.57	9.05 ± 0.24[a]	8.25 ± 0.31	8.32 ± 2.0

[a]Group differs significantly ($p < .05$) from all other groups.
[b]Does not include work category. Reprinted from Sage et al. (1987) with permission.

• Compares ICU (Intensive Care Unit) and non-ICU patients with respect to various quality of life measures.

• The exact nature of the values are not stated, but are presumed to be mean ± standard error. However, this should be made clear in the table.

• Readers are not told if statistical tests were one- or two-sided.

• The range of scales measured are not shown. It is also desirable to know if large or small values of the scales are clinically desirable.

Illustrates adverse reactions as indicators of quality of life (group data, single site or study).

TABLE 10.11. Adverse Events by Treatment Groups (N = 309)[a]

	Placebo (N = 152)		Auranofin (N = 157)		
	Number	Percent	Number	Percent	p value
Diarrhea	29	19	93	59	<0.0001
Rash	31	20	37	24	0.50
Digestive[b]	37	24	48	31	0.22
Abdominal pain	16	11	33	21	0.01
Oral ulcers/stomatitis	18	12	17	11	0.78
Pruritus	10	7	20	13	0.07
Headache, general	10	7	19	12	0.10
Proteinuria[c]	1	0.7	5	3.2	0.22
Anemia[d]	1	0.7	1	0.6	1.00
Leukopenia[e]	3	2.0	1	0.6	0.37
Thrombocytopenia[f]	1	0.7	2	1.3	1.00
Serum glutamic oxaloacetic transaminase increase[g]	1	0.7	6	3.8	0.12
Alkaline phosphatase increase[g]	0	0.0	4	2.6	0.12
Blood urea nitrogen increase[h]	2	1.3	6	3.8	0.28

[a]Includes adverse reactions that led to patient withdrawal. Reprinted from Bombardier et al. (1986) with permission.

[b]Includes nausea, vomiting, gastrointestinal disorder (general).

[c]2+ or higher by dipstick, or 1 g per 24 hr.

[d]Hemoglobin more than 10 percent below investigator's lower limit of normal, or at least 3 g/dl drop from baseline.

[e]Less than 3,000/mm^3.

[f]Less than 100,00/mm^3.

[g]More than twice investigator's upper limit or normal.

[h]At least 20 percent above investigator's upper limit of normal, or at least 30 mg/dl.

Illustrates using a bar chart to represent the preevent and postevent distribution of a quality of life variable.

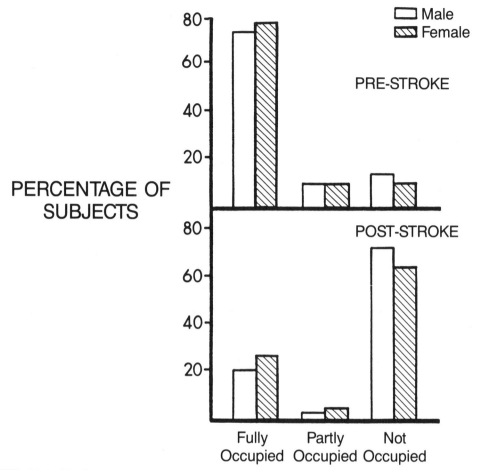

FIG. 10.1. Distribution of occupational status before stroke, as compared with the situation 3 years after the event in 45 patients. "Fully occupied" includes housework for a family, in the case of women; "not occupied" includes those people capable of self-care but with no responsibility outside self-care. Reprinted from Lawrence and Christie (1979) with permission.

• Separate displays for males and females readily show that there is no difference between the sexes.

• Presenting prestroke data immediately above poststroke data vividly emphasizes the effect of the stroke.

• It is important that the same vertical scale be used for both the prestroke and poststroke graphs.

Illustrates breaking the bars of the bar chart in order to indicate a break in the vertical axis. Also illustrates printing sample size numbers within the bars of the graph.

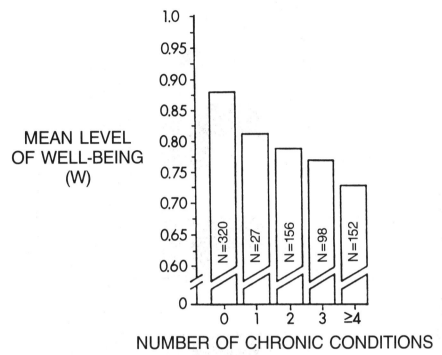

FIG. 10.2. Mean symptom-standardized level of well-being (W) for groups of persons reporting specific numbers of chronic conditions (weighted Pearson's r = −0.96). Reprinted from Kaplan et al. (1976) with permission.

• Note that the break in the y-axis is indicated by a "broken" axis. A novel addition is the corresponding break in each of the bars. This adds emphasis to the break and is helpful to the reader.

• Note the sample sizes printed inside each bar.

• Including the value of the correlation coefficient in the legend is helpful in interpreting the strength of the relationship.

458

Illustrates using different shading patterns within each bar of the histogram in order to present the distribution of a second variable.

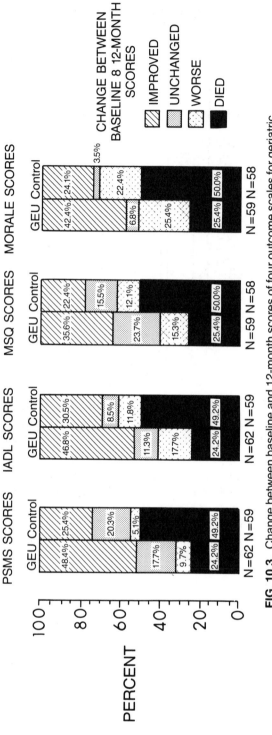

FIG. 10.3. Change between baseline and 12-month scores of four outcome scales for geriatric evaluation unit (GEU) and control patients. The four scales are the Personal Self-Maintenance Scale (PSMS), Instrumental Activities of Daily Living (IADL), Mental-Status Questionnaire (MSQ), and Lawton Morale Scale. Reprinted from Rubenstein et al. (1984) with permission.

• This displays disease progression. Shading an area emphasizes the changing severity.

• Printing the percentages in the bars of the histogram is helpful.

• It is important that the ordering of categories within the bars is sensible and the same in all bars.

Illustrates using off-set and different shaded bars in a histogram to make treatment group comparisons.

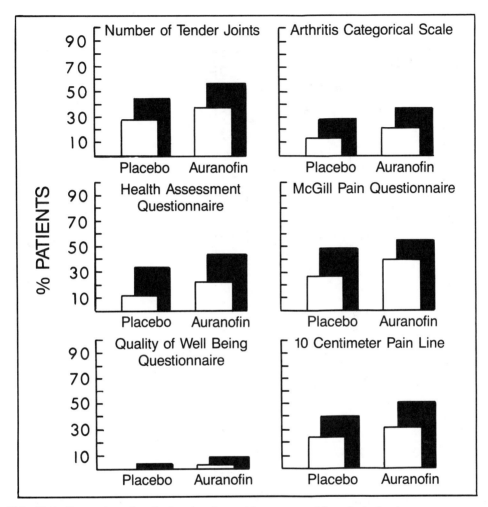

FIG. 10.4. Proportion of patients who showed improvement in selected outcome measures, by treatment group. Moderate improvement is a change of more than 25 percent from baseline value (shaded bars), and substantial improvement is a change of more than 50 percent from baseline value (open bars). Reprinted from Bombardier et al. (1986) with permission.

• Use of shaded and open bars allows for two comparisons in a single chart.

• Within each treatment group, a comparison of the heights of the shaded and open bars evaluates the "difference" between moderate and substantial improvement.

• The marked overlap of bars is a clear and dramatic presentation.

Illustrates grouping line graphs together on a single page in order to make simultaneous treatment group comparisons and get a view of the "overall picture."

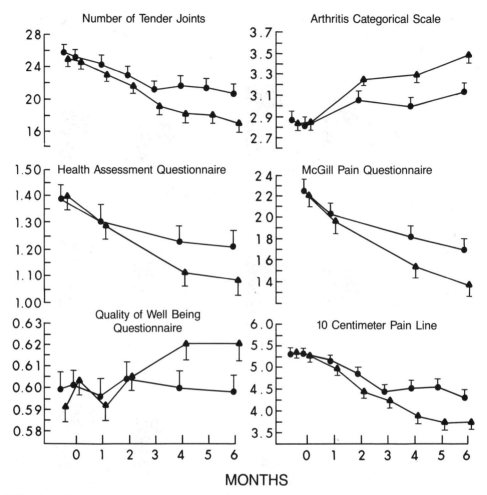

FIG. 10.5. Changes in selected outcome measures during the trial, by treatment group. These outcome measures illustrate representative changes in the clinical measures (tender joint count); in the functional measures (Health Assessment Questionnaire and Quality of Well-Being Questionnaire); in the global measures (Arthritis Categorical Scale); and in the pain measures (McGill Pain Questionnaire and 10-Centimeter Pain Line). **Each point** represents a specific assessment ± SE. **Solid triangles** indicate values for the auranofin group, and **solid circles** indicate values for the placebo group. Reprinted from Bombardier et al. (1986) with permission.

• For each quality of life variable, plotting both treatment groups allows for rapid interpretation.

• Note that error bars for triangles are minus standard error regardless of whether the values are above or below the line connecting solid circles.

Illustrates the use of utility curves to evaluate the effect of an intervention strategy on quality of life.

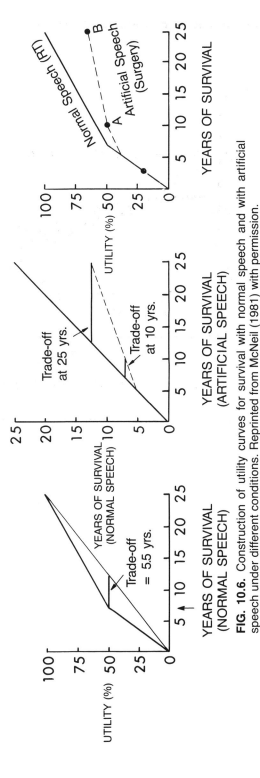

FIG. 10.6. Construction of utility curves for survival with normal speech and with artificial speech under different conditions. Reprinted from McNeil (1981) with permission.

Illustrates the use of shading to emphasize the difference between two curves being compared.

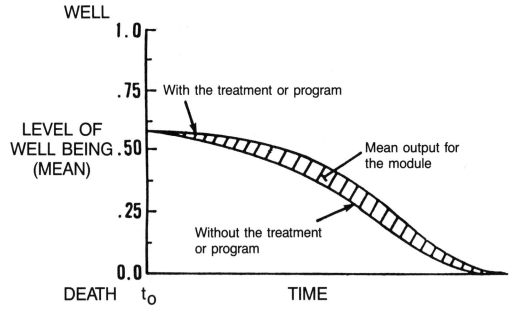

FIG. 10.7. Level of well being over time with and without a program. Reprinted from Kaplan (1982) with permission.

• Area between lines (highlighted by slanted lines) represents the improvement attributable to the treatment.

Illustrates grouping several scattergrams together to compare effect of an intervention on multiple quality of life variables.

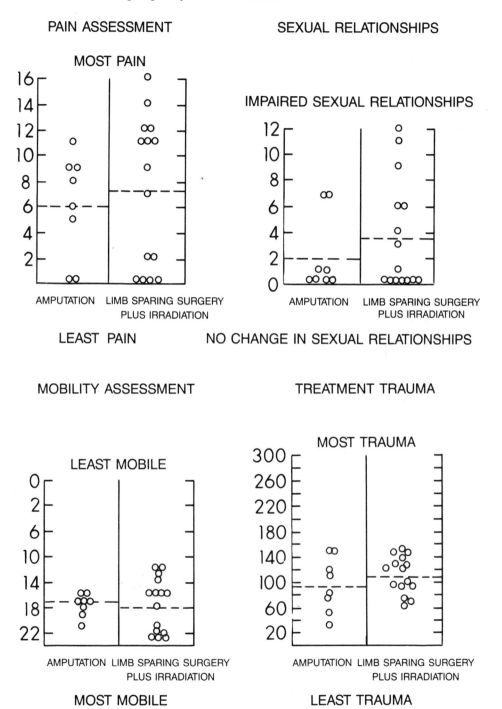

FIG. 10.8. Clinical tests to specifically link treatment consequences with quality of life. Reprinted from Sugarbaker et al. (1982) with permission.

Illustrates influence of various medical events on quality of life in a diagrammatic manner.

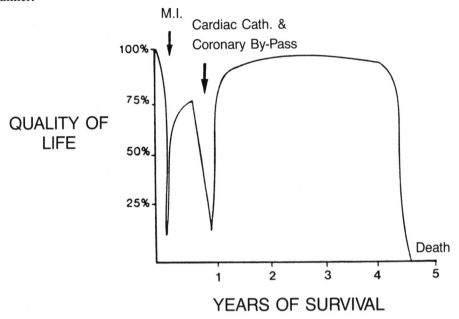

FIG. 10.9. "Vitagram" showing quality of life in patient who had coronary artery bypass graft following myocardial infarction (MI). Cath., catheterization. Length of life for this patient after MI was 4.5 years. Reprinted from Eiseman (1981) with permission.

Illustrates a schematic or qualitative approach to illustrating a patient's quality of life.

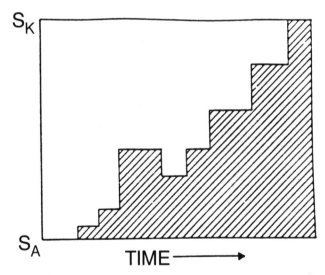

FIG. 10.10. Severity of a chronic progressive illness over time. The y-axis of S_A to S_K represents increasing severity of disease. In comparing outcomes, it is essential to consider both cumulative dysfunction and the pattern of such dysfunction. Outcomes of equivalent total dysfunction over time may be manifest according to different patterns. Reprinted from Schipper and Levitt (1985) with permission.

• Different patterns of illness (e.g., episodic illness, complete recovery) are shown in this diagrammatic way by Schipper and Levitt (1985).

Illustrates how individual patient's quality of life is associated with changes in an important efficacy parameter.

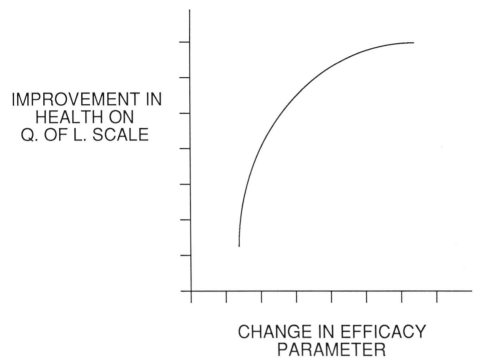

FIG. 10.11. Improvement in health as a function of change in efficacy parameters. Q. of L., quality of life.

11

Compliance, Concomitant Therapy, and Cost-Effectiveness

COMPLIANCE

Compliance usually refers to how closely patients follow instructions specified in the protocol and by the investigator. Although primarily thought of in terms of how well patients adhere to the dosage regimen, compliance also includes cooperation and adherence to other aspects of the protocol. These other aspects may involve (1) adherence to a specific diet, (2) following an exercise program, (3) avoiding alcohol, or (4) another factor.

Compliance may also be used to describe adherence of the investigator and staff to a protocol. One of the reasons for measuring compliance in a study is to exclude patients from efficacy analyses if compliance is below a predefined standard. On the other hand, even when a patient's compliance is below a minimal standard defined prior to a study, it is often unacceptable to delete the patient's data from the primary efficacy analyses. This is because of the "intention to treat" concept. For this reason, some studies support two efficacy analyses; one on an efficacy-defined population and the other one on the intent-to-treat population. Although patients entered in a study who are later found not to meet entry criteria are sometimes excluded from efficacy analyses, they should never be excluded from safety analyses.

Measuring Compliance

Methods of measuring (and presenting) data on compliance include:

1. *Pill counts* May be expressed (a) as percent expected, (b) as acceptable or unacceptable, or (c) in another related manner.
2. *Urine levels of drug or metabolite* May be expressed as (a) acceptable or unacceptable, (b) actual concentrations, (c) percent of dose excreted, (d) whether values are or are not within a given range, or (e) ratio of urine to plasma value.
3. *Urine levels of a biological marker* May be expressed as above.
4. *Asking patients about their compliance* A general nonthreatening question is often effective. Data may be presented as number of doses forgotten per week, or a different scale may be used (e.g., patient takes 100% of doses, 90 to 99%, 80 to 89%, etc.).
5. *Physician's assessment of patient compliance* May be expressed as a number or percent of patients with adequate compliance. Alternatively, a three or greater

point scale could be used (e.g., excellent, good, fair, poor). This assessment is based on patient interviews and/or other factors.

Other measures of compliance plus a discussion of the topic are presented in Chapter 18 of *Guide to Clinical Studies and Developing Protocols* (Spilker, 1984).

Noncompliance

Noncompliance may be expressed in numerous ways, including:

1. Number of patients who were noncompliant with any part of the study.
2. Number of patients who were noncompliant with a specific part of the study.
3. Listing of patient numbers, initials, or other identifiers of those patients who are in category one or two above.
4. Complete list of reasons and criteria why patients could be considered as non-compliers.
5. Number of patients who were noncompliant for each of the reasons listed in point four.
6. Listing of patient numbers, initials, or other identifiers and the reasons for their noncompliance.
7. Quantitative measures of the degree of noncompliance. These may be graphed or put in a table for individual patients and/or groups of patients.

Illustrates overall summary of compliance—addresses the "bottom line" of what patients are excluded due to compliance issues (individual patient data, single site or study).

TABLE 11.1. Listing of Noncompliant Patients

Treatment	Patient no.	Criteria violated	Analyses excluded from
Placebo	104	Insufficient drug taken	
	117		
Study drug	231		

- Common criteria that may be violated are the following:

1. Use of study medication (e.g., patient may have used too much or too little).
2. Remain in a specified locale (e.g., in [seasonal] allergic rhinitis studies patients often are told to remain outside during a specified study period).
3. Follow behavioral requests (e.g., patients are often told to avoid alcohol or food during a specified period).
4. Use self-administered doses of other drugs.
5. Failure to complete assessments in a patient diary.

- If a "sufficient" number of patients violate any one criteria, then a summary similar to that of concomitant medications (Table 11.3) might be generated.
- Although use of concomitant therapies (drug or nondrug) may be included in this table, those areas of compliance are usually discussed separately. This table is usually limited to criteria that cause exclusion from one or more analyses.

Illustrates amount of drug actually ingested during study (group data, single site or study).

TABLE 11.2. Dose Administered by Treatment Week—Combined Centers[a]

Week[b]	Study drug			Placebo		
	Mean	Median	Range	Mean	Median	Range
6						
7						
8						
9						
10						
11						
12						
13						
14						
15						
16						
17						
18						
19						
20						
21						
22						
23						
24						
25						
26						

[a]Values are expressed in mg/kg/day. Separate tables could be constructed for each study site.
[b]Weeks 1 to 5 are baseline, 6 to 11 are dose ascension, 12 to 22 treatment, and 23 to 26 taper and posttreatment.

  • This table may be considered as compliance, since it presents the amount (summaries) of drug that was actually ingested. The table may also be considered and used as a "first table" in the efficacy section of a study report. In the latter context it is used to help interpret the efficacy data.

  • Source(s) of these data should be mentioned—e.g., diaries, physician and/or hospital records.

  • "Type" of data (e.g., based on assigned dosing or actual dosing) should also be indicated.

  • Footnote *b* adds relevant information concerning study design. In particular, it explains why weeks 1–5 are not included in the table.

CONCOMITANT THERAPY

Because of the usually straightforward approaches to presenting data on concomitant therapy, only a few tables are included here. Major parameters for medications include drugs taken, prohibited drugs taken, dosages taken, duration of dosage, plus patient demographics and characteristics of those who used concomitant medications. In some cases, it may be relevant to compare patients who used concomitant medications with those who did not. Nondrug therapies may be similarly presented.

Illustrates summary of the extent of usage of concomitant therapy (group data, single site or study).

TABLE 11.3. Concomitant Therapy

| | Treatment group | | | |
	Placebo		Drug	
Total at study start	168		176	
Patients in time range	168		176	
Patients with the following therapy	N	%	N	%
Diet, low carbohydrate	2	(1.2)	1	(0.6)
Hydrochlorothiazide	1	(0.6)		
Diet, low cholesterol	5	(3.0)	7	(4.0)
Thyroxine			1	(0.6)
Allopurinol	7	(4.2)	3	(1.7)
Diet, other	1	(0.6)	1	(0.6)
Dalmane	1	(0.6)	1	(0.6)
Diet, low calorie	20	(11.9)	20	(11.4)
Diet, low fat	1	(0.6)	1	(0.6)
Ampicillin	2	(1.2)	2	(1.1)

• Concomitant therapy could be divided into categories (e.g., drug, nondrug) or listed from most common to least common.

• If only a small number of patients are in the study or only a few patients used concomitant therapy, then concomitant therapy may be listed by patient.

• If some concomitant medications were allowed by protocol and others were not, then the display should indicate this. A possible improvement would be to have two displays, one of allowable medications and the other of prohibited medications.

• Concomitant therapy used to treat the primary disease may be differentiated from other concomitant therapy.

• Concomitant therapy used to treat adverse reactions should be differentiated from other concomitant therapy.

• Since patients may be counted more than once, a separate table could be presented of the number of patients with one, two, etc. types of concomitant therapy, perhaps specifying the exact combinations.

• A deficiency of this presentation is that one cannot "add down" the columns to determine the number of patients using a concomitant medication. A row giving the total number of patients using any (prohibited) concomitant medication could be added to the table.

• One cannot determine the number of patients who used more than one of the listed concomitant medications.

• If sufficient numbers of patients use a medication, then treatment groups could be compared with respect to the proportions who use those medications.

• An enhancement of this table would be to indicate the duration of use of concomitant medications—possibly the minimum number of days for each medication.

Summary of Use of Concomitant Nondrug Therapy

• Displays would be similar to use of concomitant medications.
• Nondrug therapies could be combined with concomitant medications. However, the authors feel that they should usually be presented separately.
• If any concomitant therapy (drug or nondrug) causes a patient to be excluded from an analysis, then this should be indicated, probably via a footnote to the appropriate row of the table. The information would also be included in the summary of compliance (Table 11.1).

Illustrates identification of concomitant drug therapy used to treat disease under study (individual patient data, single site or study).

TABLE 11.4. The Clinical Data of 11 Patients with Complex Partial Seizures (CPS) or Simple Partial Seizures (SPS), and Generalized Tonic-Clonic Seizures (GTC)[a]

Patient	Age	Classification of seizures	Seizures per month in the 6 months prior to the trial	Daily dosage of progabide (mg)	Concomitant drug therapy (mg)	
1	26	CPS, GTC	16.1	1,500	Carbamazepine	1,100
2	44	CPS, GTC	57.0	2,100	Phenytoin	475
3	37	CPS	10.0	1,500	Phenobarbital	200
					Phenytoin	400
					Keto-carbamazepine	300
4	43	CPS, GTC	52.0	1,800	Phenytoin	375
					Clobazam	10
5	37	CPS, GTC	10.3	1,200	Keto-carbamazepine	300
6	76	CPS	1.5	1,200	Phenobarbital	200
					Phenytoin	275
					Carbamazepine	200
7	31	SPS, GTC	5.3	4,200	Phenobarbital	300
8	38	CPS	17.3	1,800	Phenobarbital	200
9	31	CPS, GTC	6.3	1,800	Carbamazepine	1,200
10	34	CPS, SPS, GTC	6.4	3,000	Carbamazepine	1,100
					Valproic acid	1,500
11	44	CPS, SPS, GTC	24.8	3,000	Carbamazepine	1,200

[a]Reprinted from Loiseau et al. (1983) with permission.

• The inclusion of age and seizure history help data interpretation.
• The table would have been more readily interpretable if patients had been ordered in terms of increasing daily dosage of progabide.
• Since some patients require more than one row, clarity would be improved if a blank line was inserted between patients.

Illustrates extent of usage of a concomitant medication that would most probably affect the primary efficacy variable (group data, single site or study).

TABLE 11.5. Antacid Consumption by Treatment Groups[a]

Treatment group	N	Week 1	N	Week 2	N	Week 4	N	Week 8
				Mean number of antacid tablets				
Placebo	98	2.2	95	2.1	70	1.7	37	1.4
40 mg/hs	92	1.7^b	87	1.4^b	56	1.0^b	21	1.2
20 mg/bid	84	1.9	80	1.2^b	45	1.0^b	18	0.7^b
40 mg/bid	93	1.5^b	84	0.9^b	51	0.6^b	12	0.3^c
				Mean days of antacid therapy				
Placebo	98	4.1	95	3.6	70	3.3	37	2.8
40 mg/hs	92	3.3	87	2.7^b	56	2.2^b	21	2.9
20 mg/bid	84	3.5	80	2.5^b	45	1.9^b	18	1.0^c
40 mg/bid	93	2.9^b	84	2.0^b	51	1.3^b	12	0.8^b

[a]Standard deviations or other measures of variability could also be given in the table.
[b,c]Significantly different from placebo p < 0.01, p < 0.05, respectively.

• An additional footnote should indicate duration of the study. This is necessary to interpret the effect of antacid usage.

Illustrates individual patient use of prohibited drugs during a study (individual patient data, single site or study).

TABLE 11.6. Use of Prohibited Drugs[a]

Patient	Treatment	Medication	Start date	End date	Study days used	Daily dose
1004	A	Sine-off	01/05/85	01/05/85	−1	2 capsules
1020	B	Afrin nose drops	01/22/85	01/24/85	6 to 8	1–2/nostril
		Otrivin ped nasal drops	01/24/85	01/29/85	8 to 13	4 qhs^b
		Dristan nasal spray	02/01/85	02/08/85	16 to 20	bid^b
1025	B	Sinus Tylenol	01/20/85	01/20/85	−1	1 caplet
1030	C	Benadryl	01/21/85	01/21/85	0	1 inj.
1031	C	Chlor-trimeton	01/20/85	01/20/85	−1	1 tablet
1051	A	Benadryl	01/13/85	02/14/85	16 to 17	150 mg
1057	A	Comtrex	02/03/85	02/03/85	5	3 doses
1060	C	Duration spray	01/29/85	01/30/85	−1 to 0	2x/day
2003	A	Chlor-trimeton				12 mg
2005	C	Dristan	01/03/85	01/03/85	−1	8 pills
2010	C	Entex	01/16/85	01/16/85	12	1 tablet
		Entex LA	01/23/85	01/23/85	19	1 tablet
2020	B	Comtrex	01/26/85	01/27/85	19 to 20	2 ounce
2021	C	Marax	01/19/85	01/19/85	12	½ tablet
		Marax	01/24/85	01/24/85	17	½ tablet
2035	B	Chlor-trimeton				1 qd^b
		Chlor-trimeton				1 qd
		Chlor-trimeton				1 qd
2054	C	Nyquil	02/04/85	02/04/85	19	½ dose
2055	A	Novahistamine	12/01/84		prior to baseline to ?	
3003	C	Trinalin	01/21/85	01/22/85	prior to baseline	2 tablets qd
3007	A	Contac	01/23/85		−2 to ?	1 capsule

[a]Data obtained from patient diaries.
[b]qhs, each night at bedtime; bid, twice a day; qd, once a day.

COST-EFFECTIVENESS

Cost-effectiveness data are usually presented in a series of tables. Representative examples are illustrated in the following group. Choice of formats depends on the particular study parameters measured and evaluations desired. Figures could be used to illustrate these data, particularly histograms (e.g., Fig. 1.25). Various treatments are sometimes compared based on cost per quality-adjusted life year (QALY).

Illustrates base, best, and worst cases relating to clinical assumptions.

TABLE 11.7. Clinical Assumptions[a]

Variables	Base case	Best case	Worst case	References[b]
Prevalence (per 1,000 participants) of abnormal Papanicolaou test results	13.5	21.4	5.6	9, 18, 23, 26–28, 30
Progression rate, %				
CIN to CIS	80	90	60	24, 29, 31–33
CIS to ICC	100	100	80	31–33
Papanicolaou test false-positive rate, % (1-specificity)	10	10	20	19, 29, 34
Transition time, y				
Between CIN and CIS	1	1	3	
Between CIS and ICC stage 1	1	1	3	19, 24, 25, 31, 37–40
Between ICC stage 1 and stages 2 through 4	1	1	3	
ICC stage of diagnosis in absence of screening, %				
Stage 1	25	13	34	22, 23, 35, 36
Stages 2 through 4	75	87	66	

[a]All calculations are based on an "average" patient, i.e., a 70-year-old black woman (shorter life expectancies than white women). Program personnel consisted of full-time equivalent physicians and nurse-practitioners (0.7), based on a 49-hour work week. CIN, cervical intraepithelial neoplasia; CIS, carcinoma *in situ*; and ICC, invasive cervical cancer. Reprinted from Mandelblatt and Fahs (1988) with permission.

[b]Reference numbers refer to original article.

Illustrates base, best, and worst cases relating to costs.

TABLE 11.8. Cost-Effectiveness of Papanicolaou Test Screening[a]

	Case[b]		
	Base (actual)	Best	Worst
Cost of screening program (includes diagnosis, treatment, and follow-up) ($)	59,733	76,925	40,003
Cost of averted treatment ($)	107,936	191,845	19,191
LYS	30.33	54.14	5.59
Quality-adjusted life years saved	36.77	—	—
Cost of added years of life ($)	135,378	241,628	24,948
Cost (savings)/100 Papanicolaou tests ($)	(5907)	(14,083)	2,550
LYS/100 Papanicolaou tests	3.7	6.63	0.69
Cost (savings)/year of life saved ($)	(1,589)	(2,123)	3,723
Cost (savings)/quality-adjusted LYS ($)	(1,311)	—	—
Cost/year of life, including cost of added years of life ($)	2,874	2,340	8,186

[a]Quality adjustments are only calculated for the base case. LYS indicates life-years saved. Reprinted from Mandelblatt and Fahs (1988) with permission.
[b]Values for all cases are determined at a 5% discount rate.

Illustrates a presentation of various types of medical care costs.

TABLE 11.9. Medical Care Costs[a]

	Dollars
Outpatient screening costs[b]	
Staff[c]	
Physician (1 session/wk)	4,907
Nurse-practitioner (7 sessions/wk)	20,379
Office space: 100 sq. ft., 8 sessions/wk (direct costs: $17.70/sq ft/yr)	1,475
Equipment	
Speculums (disposable)	600
Laboratory	
Papanicolaou cytology, 816 tests at $3.25/test	2,652
Procedures[d]	
8 colposcopies at $79/colposcopy	632
Subtotal	30,645
Treatment costs[e]	23,239
5-yr follow-up[f]	5,849
Total	59,733

[a]1985 US dollars. Reprinted from Mandelblatt and Fahs (1988) with permission.
[b]Screening costs were adjusted to the 10-month period of the actual program.
[c]Values are determined from the salary and benefit formula of the New York City Health and Hospital Corp.
[d]Actual cost estimates from the municipal hospital are used. When not available, these costs are approximated by the New York City Health and Hospital Corp. Reimbursement Consulting Charge Structure or Medicare (area B) rates.
[e]Unit costs are $459 at the municipal hospital and $486 at the tertiary care hospital. Unit costs are for fiscal year 1985 and include medical education costs but exclude fixed capital costs.
[f]Future follow-up discounted at a rate of 5% and adjusted to include year-to-year survival probabilities.

Illustrates a comparison of time spent on different medical functions.

TABLE 11.10. Personnel Time (mean no. of min per dose) for the Three Major Work Elements: Reconstitution and Preparation, Drug Administration, and Follow-up[a]

Hospital	Reconstitution and preparation			Drug administration			Follow-up			Total time[b]
	Pharmacy	Nurses' station	Weighted total	Burette	Piggyback	Weighted total	Continuous IV line	Heparin lock	Weighted total	
A	—	2.28	2.28	2.41	—	2.41	0.23	1.60	0.68	5.37 ± 1.96
B	0.67	—	0.67	1.88	2.05	2.02	0.70	1.05	0.74	3.43 ± 0.28
C	1.34	2.28	1.45	—	1.92	1.92	0.57	1.66	1.10	4.47 ± 1.28
D	—	2.67	2.67	—	2.27	2.27	0.00	1.55	0.87	5.81 ± 0.18
Weighted mean[c]	0.83	2.33	1.67	2.35	2.05	2.21	0.44	1.53	0.76	4.64 ± 1.21

[a]Reprinted from Eisenberg et al. (1984) with permission.
[b]Numbers are mean ± SD expressed in decimal minutes.
[c]Weighted by percentage of drug use at each hospital: hospital A, 47.8%; hospital B, 33.5%; hospital C, 11.9%; and hospital D, 6.9%.

Illustrates comparison of different costs for specific work elements.

TABLE 11.11. Comparisons Among the Total Standard Variable Costs (mean dollars per dose) for Methods of Preparing and Administering Cephalosporin Antibiotic[a]

Work element	Methods compared (cost)	p value
Reconstitution and preparation	Pharmacy ($1.58) vs. Nurses' station ($1.01)	<.001
Drug administration	Burette ($0.59) vs. Piggyback ($0.92)	<.001
Follow-up	Continuous IV ($0.10) vs. Heparin lock ($0.56)	<.001

[a]Reprinted from Eisenberg et al. (1984) with permission.

Illustrates potential savings expressed in different ways.

TABLE 11.12. Potential Savings with Use of Once-Daily Administration of Cefonicid for Each Hospital that Participated in the Study[a]

Hospital	Total standard variable cost per dose ($)	Differential dose frequency[b]	Savings per patient day ($)	Patient days per year[c]	Savings per bed per year ($)
A	1.66	2.24	3.72	25,942	139
B	2.88	2.51	7.23	17,046	179
C	2.50	2.79	6.98	5,593	213
D	2.65	2.53	6.70	3,464	89
Mean	2.24[d]	2.41[e]	5.42	13,011	155

[a]Reprinted from Eisenberg et al. (1984) with permission.
[b]Mean number of doses per full day minus one.
[c]Number of doses per year divided by daily dose frequency.
[d]Weighted by percentage of drug use at each hospital.
[e]Weighted by percentage of patient days at each hospital.

Illustrates financial consequences of ineffective treatment.

TABLE 11.13. Consequences of Ineffective Treatment[a]

Component	Typical cost
Increased length of hospital stay	$242 per day
Increased length of intensive care stay	$807 per day
Prolonged antibiotic therapy	$ 30 to $150 per day
Increased intensity of service	?
Increased risk of nosocomial complication	?
Increased risk of litigation	?

[a]Reprinted from Gladen (1986) with permission.

Illustrates financial consequences of medical complications.

TABLE 11.14. Typical Cost of Complications Used in Model[a]

Complication	Incidence	Estimated cost	Cost per course
Nephrotoxicity	14% of 4,023	$1,000	$140
Vestibular toxicity	3% of 535	$300	$9
Cochlear toxicity	8% of 1,895	$200	$16
Total			$165

[a]This model uses gentamicin as an example. Reprinted from Gladen (1986) with permission.

Illustrates financial consequences of drug resistance.

TABLE 11.15. Effect of Resistance on the Cost of Initial Empiric Therapy[a]

	Number of patients	Drug	Days	Cost (each)	Cost
Gentamicin as empiric initial therapy	1,000	Gentamicin	2	$ 47.28	$ 94,560
Susceptible to gentamicin (88.2%)	882	Gentamicin	8	47.28	333,610
Resistant to gentamicin (118) and susceptible to tobramycin (89.6%)	106	Tobramycin	10	58.66	62,200
Susceptible to amikacin only (99.6%)	12	Amikacin	10	66.58	7,990
Extra hospital days (236)				242.00	57,112
Total					$555,472
Tobramycin as empiric initial therapy	1,000	Gentamicin	2	$ 58.66	117,320
Susceptible to tobramycin (896) and susceptible to gentamicin (82.2%)	790	Gentamicin	8	47.28	298,810
Remainder susceptible to tobramycin	106	Tobramycin	8	58.66	49,744
Resistant to tobramycin (104) and susceptible to gentamicin (88.2%)	92	Gentamicin	10	47.28	43,498
Susceptible to amikacin only (99.6%)	12	Amikacin	10	66.58	7,990
Extra hospital days (208)				242.00	50,336
Total					$567,698
Amikacin as empiric initial therapy	1,000	Amikacin	2	$ 66.58	133,160
Susceptible to gentamicin (88.2%)	882	Gentamicin	8	47.28	333,610
Resistant to gentamicin and susceptible to tobramycin (89.6%)	106	Tobramycin	8	58.66	49,744
Susceptible to amikacin only (99.6%)	12	Amikacin	8	66.58	6,392
Extra hospital days (none)					0
Total					$522,904

[a]Effect of efficacy on empiric therapy costs. Comparison is made between regimens in which the initial empiric therapy is amikacin, gentamicin, or tobramycin. It is assumed that after two days antibiotic sensitivity patterns are available, which mirror those at the Baltimore Veterans Administration Medical Center in 1984, at which time therapy is changed to the one with the lowest daily cost. The lowest overall cost of therapy is obtained by starting with the highest priced (acquisition cost) antibiotic. Reprinted from Gladen (1986) with permission.

Illustrates drug costs obtained at different pharmacies.

TABLE 11.16. Monthly Cost of Antiglaucoma Medications (in Dollars)[a]

Pharmacy[b]	Pilocarpine 2% (15 ml)	Dipivefrin 0.1% (10 ml)	Timolol 0.5% (10 ml)	Methazolamide 50 mg (60 tablets)	Total cost	Discount to senior citizen	Free delivery
1	5.95	16.49	24.95	19.89	67.28	Yes	No
2	10.80	23.50	32.95	24.50	91.75	Yes	No
3	8.25	22.10	32.50	21.40	84.25	Yes	Yes
4	6.72	18.20	26.10	21.94	72.96	No	No
5	10.25	26.32	25.60	20.25	82.42	Yes	No
6	7.50	18.75	29.50	18.95	74.70	Yes	Yes
7	5.45	15.72	20.88	16.20	58.25	Yes	No
8	7.69	16.49	21.47	17.40	63.05	Yes	No
9	5.09	15.99	19.99	18.00	59.07	Yes	No
10	7.95	14.97	19.44	18.60	60.96	Yes	No
11	9.39	15.59	16.19	18.00	59.17	Yes	No
12	3.80	13.75	19.50	16.60	53.65	No	Yes

[a]Reprinted from Kooner and Zimmerman (1987) with permission.
[b]Pharmacies 1–6 belong to group 1; pharmacies 7–12 belong to group 2; pharmacy 12 belongs to the American Association of Retired Persons.

Illustrates cost versus benefit for selected procedures.

TABLE 11.17. Costs and Benefits of Selected Medical Services[a]

Medical service	Cost per patient ($)	Benefit per outcome ($)	Patients treatable (N)[b]	Gross benefit ($)[c]	Net benefit ($)[d]
Hip replacement	1,200	52,607	300	15,782,000	15,482,000
Duodenal ulcer treatment	2,500	1,000	144	144,000	−156,000
Screening for neural tube defects	5,200	19,900	69	1,373,000	1,073,000

[a]Benefits are defined in text.
[b]Number of patients refers to the number who can be treated with available resources.
[c]Gross benefit equals number of patients times benefit per patient.
[d]Net benefit, gross benefit minus $300,000 invested in the program.

Illustrates comparisons of different therapies for one problem.

TABLE 11.18. Estimates of Efficacy of Different Regimens in Clearing of Acne[a]

Therapy	Base case probability estimate	Sensitivity analysis range
Two topical agents given initially	.40	.20–.60
Alternative topical agents after initial topical agent therapy failed	.20	.10–.40
Tetracycline at first visit (combined therapy)	.75	.55–.90
Tetracycline after topical therapy failed	.49	.24–.62
High-dose tetracycline after initial dose tetracycline therapy failed	.50	.1–.9
Erythromycin after tetracycline therapy failed	.50	.1–.9
High-dose erythromycin after initial tetracycline therapy failed	.50	.1–.9
Minocycline after all previous systemic agent therapy failed	.50	.1–.9

[a]Reprinted from Stern et al. (1984) with permission.

Illustrates probability of adverse reactions occurring in different situations.

TABLE 11.19. Estimates of Probability of Adverse Reactions from Systemic Therapy[a]

Variables	Base case probability estimate[b]	Sensitivity analysis range
Risk of adverse reaction with exposure to initial course of systemic therapy	.05	.01–.30
Proportional change in risk of adverse reaction to other systemic agents; no adverse reactions to initial systemic agent used[c]	—	.50
Proportional change in risk of adverse reaction to other systemic agents, in reactions to the initial systemic agent used[c]	—	2.0
Fraction of patients with adverse reaction to systemic agent; requires physician	.10	.10–.50
Fraction of patients experiencing sufficient topical reaction to preclude continued therapy with topical agents alone	.10	.10–.50

[a]Reprinted from Stern et al. (1984) with permission.
[b]This number is in addition to survey of dermatologists.
[c]This is not used in sensitivity analysis.

Illustrates cost of different therapies.

TABLE 11.20. Estimates of Drug Cost per Week of Therapy with Different Regimens[a]

Variables	Base case cost estimate ($)	Sensitivity analysis range ($)
Tetracycline	1.33	0.84–3.08
Erythromycin	1.68	1.12–3.50
Minocycline	5.95	4.76–7.14
Benzoyl peroxide (low-cost topical agent)	0.50	0.25–1.00
Expensive topical agent (tretinoin, topical antibiotic)	1.00	0.50–2.00

[a]All drug costs are expressed as per week cost of initial (first exposure) dosage, and the increased dosage regimen cost equals twice the initial dose. Reprinted from Stern et al. (1984) with permission.

Illustrates a comparison of morbidity and costs for two routes of administration.

TABLE 11.21. Morbidity, Adverse Reactions, and Cost of Systemic and Topical Agent Strategies: Base Case Results[a]

Outcome	Strategy		
	Systemic	Topical	Systemic minus topical
Morbidity from acne, week to clearing	8.67	14.86	−6.19[b]
Adverse reaction episodes per 1,000 patients	60	34	26
Cost to clearing, $/patient	85.13	105.00	−19.87[b]

[a]Reprinted from Stern et al. (1984) with permission.
[b]A negative sign means that the systemic strategy's cost or morbidity was less than that of the topical strategy.

Illustrates three cases (high, base case, low) for changing outcomes of specific variables.

TABLE 11.22. One-Variable Sensitivity Analysis[a]

Variable	Change in outcome, %[b]		
	Morbidity from acne (week)	Episodes of adverse reactions	Money spent to achieve clearing
Probability of improvement with initial topical therapy			
High (.6)	−33%	+38%	−66%
Base case (.4)	0	0	0
Low (.2)	+33	−35	+66
Probability of improvement on altered topical regimen after failure of initial therapy			
High (.4)	—[b]	—[b]	−27
Base case (.2)	0	0	0
Low (.1)	—[b]	—[b]	+13
Weeks between visits			
High (12)	+100	—[b]	+47
Base case (6)	0	0	0
Low (4)	−33	—[b]	−17
Cost per week of topical agent			
High ($2)	—[b]	—[b]	−47
Base case ($1)	0	0	0
Low ($0.50)	—[b]	—[b]	−23
Cost per week of tetracycline			
High ($2.20)	—[b]	—[b]	−18
Base case ($1)	0	0	0
Low ($0.60)	—[b]	—[b]	—[c]
Probability of adverse reactions with initial exposure to a systemic agent			
High (.30)	—[b]	+585	—[c]
Base case (.05)	0	0	0
Low (.01)	—[b]	−86	—[c]

[a]Reprinted from Stern et al. (1984) with permission.
[b]In each of the sensitivity analyses shown, percentage change from base case result is shown for each of three outcomes, when value for a particular variable is assumed to be higher or lower than a base case.
[c]Less than 10% change in difference.

Illustrates comparative costs for different IV drugs.

TABLE 11.23. Comparison of Patient Charges for IV Antibiotic Prophylaxis[a]

Drug	Dose	Charge/patient ($)	Charge/year[b] ($)
Cefamandole	2 g preop & 2 g q6h × 5 d[c]	727.65	727,650
Cefamandole	2 g preop & 1 g q6h × 5 d	612.15	612,150
Cefazolin	2 g preop & 1 g q8h × 5 d	430.04	430,040
Cefamandole	2 g preop & 2 g q6h × 2 d	311.85	311,850
Cefamandole	2 g preop & 1 g q6h × 2 d	262.35	262,350
Cefazolin	2 g preop & 1 g q8h × 2 d	190.01	190,010
Cefuroxime	1.5 g preop & 1.5 g q12h (6 g)[d]	132.40	132,400

[a]Antibiotics used in cardiovascular surgery. Reprinted from Peterson and Lake (1986) with permission.
[b]Based on 1,000 patients/year.
[c]Previously used antibiotic regimen; g, gram; q, every; h, hour; d, day.
[d]Antibiotic regimen chosen by cardiovascular surgeons.

Illustrates a hospital-oriented financial analysis of drug use.

TABLE 11.24. Hospital Financial Analysis of Project[a]

Evaluation	Cefamandole[b]	Cefazolin[c]	Cefuroxime[d]
Total cost/patient ($)	182.88	89.56	76.02
Number of patients	1242	1242	1242
Total cost all patients ($)	227,137.96	111,233.52	94,416.84
Cost savings by not using cefamandole ($)		115,904.44	132,721.12
Margin/patient ($)	129.15	100.45	57.40
Number of patients paying margins	372	372	372
Total margins ($)	48,043.80	37,367.40	21,352.80
Loss in margins by not using cefamandole ($)		10,676.40	26,691.00
Net savings by not using cefamandole ($)		105,228.04	106,030.12

[a]Reprinted from Peterson and Lake (1986) with permission.
[b]Cefamandole 2 g preop and 2 g IV 6 h × 2 d (18 g).
[c]Cefazolin 2 g preop and 1 g IV q8h × 2 d (8 g).
[d]Cefuroxime 1.5 g preop and 1.5 g q12 h (6 g).

Illustrates cost-effectiveness of diagnostic tests.

TABLE 11.25. Costs of Diagnostic Tests (Table Headings Only)

No. of tests of stool guaiac	No. of cancers found	No. of cancers missed (false negatives)	Total cost of diagnosis ($)	Average cost per cancer ($)

TABLE 11.26. Marginal Results and Costs for Subsequent Stool Guaiac Tests (Table Headings Only)[a]

No. of tests of stool guaiac	Increase in no. of cancers found	Increases in total costs ($)	Marginal cost per cancer found ($)

[a]Table 11.26 provides a preferable means for assessing the value of conducting multiple tests than Table 11.25.

FIG. 11.1. Calendar results of three patients in a study for the month of June. ○, no drug taken that day; −, one less tablet taken than the correct dose; ●, correct dose taken (2 tablets per day); +, one tablet more than correct taken; *, two or more extra tablets taken that day.

• This type of display could be applied to many measures of efficacy or safety parameters.
• Could illustrate months 1, 2, 3 for one patient.
• Could present summary data in this format to look for patterns (e.g., poorer compliance on weekends).
• Could label each calendar with month, days, and year.

Illustrates use of a calendar format to present data (individual patients, single site or study).

Patient: 101 - Month: June

S	M	T	W	T	F	S
					-	•
•	•	•	•	•	•	•
-	•	+	•	•	-	•
•	•	-	•	•	•	-
•	•	•	•	-	★	•

Patient: 102 - Month: June

S	M	T	W	T	F	S
					-	•
•	•	•	•	•	•	•
•	-	○	○	○	○	○
-	•	-	•	•	•	•
•	•	•	•	•	•	+

Patient: 103 - Month: June

S	M	T	W	T	F	S
					•	○
○	•	•	+	•	+	•
★	-	•	•	-	•	•
•	•	+	+	•	•	-
-	○	-	+	-	•	★

12

Metaanalyses

Metaanalyses are statistically based evaluations of multiple independently conducted clinical studies. Studies are chosen to be evaluated because they address the same question or issue. An attempt is usually made to include all possible studies in the evaluation that meet specified criteria. In a perfect metaanalysis data are pooled, but this is rarely possible. Results are usually expressed in terms of odds ratios of either the drug or placebo being superior.

The general steps carried out in conducting a metaanalysis to address a specific question are:

1. Establish criteria of which studies will be included in the metaanalysis.
2. Determine the total pool of studies from various sources (e.g., computerized searches of data bases, personal letters sent to investigators) to evaluate for inclusion in the metaanalysis.
3. Score or assess each of the articles or reports according to specified factors (e.g., study design, blind) and possibly for their overall quality, utilizing a standard assessment tool. This step may be performed by two or more people who are blind to the purpose of the study and the identity of the authors of each study.
4. Identify which studies qualify for inclusion in the metaanalysis.
5. Conduct an independent assessment of those factors relating to the specific question(s) posed (e.g., is drug better than placebo?). This step may be performed by two or more people who are blind to the purpose of the study.
6. Combine the data from all studies evaluated.
7. Analyze the results.
8. Interpret the results.

The presentation of a metaanalysis includes data on some or all of these steps. Some tables or graphs present two or more of these steps. Nonetheless, most displays that are specific for metaanalyses focus on describing the studies included or presenting odds ratios of the summary results.

Tables 12.1 to 12.11 provide formats for presenting information about studies included in a metaanalysis. Tables 12.12 to 12.19 provide formats for presenting results obtained in metaanalyses. Figure 12.1 is a prototype for presenting information about studies. Other figures give examples for presenting results from individual metaanalyses.

Illustrates a simple list of studies included in a metaanalysis.

TABLE 12.1. Studies Included in a Metaanalysis

Study	Study drugs	Number of patients	Additional information
AT-105	Antihistamine #1	38	Conducted in San Antonio, Texas during mountain
	Antihistamine #2	37	cedar season
AT-106	Antihistamine #2	102	Conducted in Chapel Hill, North Carolina during
	Placebo	98	ragweed season
AT-117	Antihistamine #1	75	Conducted in Boise, Idaho during summer
	Antihistamine #2	64	
	Placebo	59	

• Studies could be identified by notation (e.g., ANTI-01), by investigator's name, by journal, or by drug.

• If pertinent, additional information such as study design (e.g., parallel, crossover), or type of study (e.g., pharmacokinetic), or quality score may be added.

Illustrates a summary of studies in a metaanalysis according to study design.

TABLE 12.2. Studies Included in the Metaanalysis Categorized by Type of Study Design

Study design	N[a]	Mean value of major parameter	SD	95% CI	Quality score of article
1. Crossover					
2. Parallel with placebo					
3. Parallel with active drug control					
4. Parallel with active drug control and placebo					

[a]Refers to number of randomized, double-blind (or other category) studies.

Illustrates another listing of studies included in a metaanalysis.

TABLE 12.3. Characteristics of Studies Included in the Metaanalysis

Study number or name of investigator	Drug dose(s)	Sample size	Compliance	Blind	Major efficacy parameters measured

Illustrates a more detailed list of studies included in a metaanalysis.

TABLE 12.4. Results of Five Selected Studies Reporting Rates of Sensitivity[a]

Study reference and year	Framework[b]	Timeframe	Admission criteria	Method of ascertainment	Diagnosis of study pts.	Total no. of pts.	Total no. sensitive (%)
Chafee and Settipane, 1974	Allergy clinic (PP)	Not specified	All patients with asthma or rhinitis	Record review	Asthma alone Asthma and rhinitis Rhinitis alone	1,133 642 2,006	47 (4.3) 29 (4.5) 13 (0.7)
Settipane et al., 1974	Allergy clinic (U & PP) Health testing center	Nov. 15, 1972–Jan. 15, 1973	Consecutive allergy patients Consecutive nonallergic patients	Direct interview Direct interview Direct interview	Asthma or asthma and rhinitis Rhinitis alone "Normal patients"	731 641 808	28 (3.8) 9 (1.4) 7 (0.9)
Rachelelfsky et al., 1976	Allergy clinic (U & PP)	Not specified	Consecutive patients	Oral challenge	Atopic asthmatics	50	14 (28)
Settipane et al., 1980	Allergy clinic (U & PP)	Not specified	All patients with asthma or rhinitis	Record review	Asthma or rhinitis (all with nasal polyps)	211	30 (14)
Settipane et al., 1980	Health testing center (U) Mobile pediatric unit (U)	Dec. 1972–June 1974 Oct. 1974–March 1976	Consecutive nonallergic patients Consecutive nonallergic patients	Direct interview Direct interview	"Normal adults" "Normal children"	1,974 618	6 (0.3) 2 (0.3)

[a]Reprinted from Kwoh and Feinstein (1986) with permission.
[b]PP, private practice setting; U, university setting.

Illustrates characteristics of studies included in a metaanalysis.

TABLE 12.5. Characteristics of Randomized Controlled Trials of Diuretics in Pregnancy[a]

Study	Design	Criteria for entry	Treatment regimen	No. followed up			Number withdrawn	Primary endpoints	Definition of pre-eclampsia[b]
				Total	Diuretic treated patients	Control patients			
Zuspan et al.	Double-blind	Rapid or excessive weight gain, Presence of edema	Hydrochlorothiazide 100 mg/day × 4 days or 100 mg/day × 2 days plus 50 mg/day dihydrotri-chlorothiazide 10 mg/day × 2 days plus 5 mg/day × 5 days	336	193	143	154	Weight gain	Not used as endpoint
Wesley and Douglas	Double-blind	Second or third trimester with ≥ 2.3 kg weight gain in 2 weeks or increasing edema of extremities	Chlorothiazide 100 mg/day until delivery	267	131	136	Nil	Pre-eclampsia, Proteinuric pre-eclampsia, Stillbirth, Neonatal death	CMW
Flowers et al.	Double-blind	< 30th week, Mean = 19th week	Chlorothiazide 250 mg/day, 500 mg/day, or 750 mg/day until delivery	519 (445)[c]	385 (335)[c]	134 (110)[c]	No details on perinatal deaths for 50 treated patients and 24 controls	Pre-eclampsia, Stillbirth, Neonatal death	Systolic blood pressure ≥ 140 mm Hg or diastolic blood pressure ≥ 90 mm Hg in previously normotensive patient, or appreciable change in hypertensive patient
Menzies	Open control: pheno-barbital	> 24th week with systolic blood pressure ≥ 140 mm Hg, diastolic blood pressure ≥ 85 mm Hg, or ankle edema, or weight gain ≥ 1.8 Kg in any 2 weeks after 24th week	Chlorothiazide 100 mg/day plus potassium chloride 2 g/day for a week and continued if indications persist or return	105	57	48	Nil	Pre-eclampsia requiring admission, Proteinuric pre-eclampsia, Stillbirth, Neonatal death	Systolic blood pressure > 145 mm Hg or diastolic blood pressure > 85 mm Hg or weight gain > 0.9 kg in week of treatment; or noninfective albuminuria; or substantial increase in edema

continued

TABLE 12.5. Continued

Study	Design	Criteria for entry	Treatment regimen	No. followed up			Number withdrawn	Primary endpoints	Definition of pre-eclampsia[b]
				Total	Diuretic treated patients	Control patients			
Fallis et al.	Double-blind	All primigravid. Expected date of delivery > 13 weeks. Diastolic blood pressure < 90 mm Hg. Free of edema and proteinuria	Hydrochlorothiazide 50 mg/day until delivery	78 (74)[c]	38 (34)[c]	40 (40)[c]	Two lost to follow-up. No details on perinatal deaths for four treated patients	Pre-eclampsia Stillbirth Neonatal death	CMW
Cuadros and Tatum	Double-blind; "rotational" allocation	≥ 30 weeks	Bendroflumethiazide 5 mg/day until delivery	1,771	1,011	760	Nil	Pre-eclampsia Proteinuria Eclampsia Stillbirth Neonatal death	Not available
Landerman et al.	Double-blind	28th to 32nd week	Chlorthalidone 50 mg/day until delivery	2,706	1,370	1,336	193	Pre-eclampsia Proteinuric pre-eclampsia Stillbirth plus neonatal death	CMW
Finnerty and Bepko	Open; "alternate" allocation	< 17 years. No history of renal disease or findings of edema, increased blood pressure, or albuminuria	Thiazide diuretics until delivery	3,083	1,340	1,743	201 treated patients transferred to control group for "noncompliance"	Pre-eclampsia Stillbirth Neonatal death	Edema of periorbital area and hands; > 10% rise in mean arterial pressure or noninfective albuminuria

Study	Design	Entry criteria	Treatment					Outcomes measured	Definition
Kraus et al.	Double-blind	< 24th week without idiopathic thrombocytopenic purpura, severe diabetes, or sickle cell anemia	Hydrochlorothiazide 50 mg/day until delivery	1,030	506	524	62 treated patients, 47 controls	Blood pressure, Pre-eclampsia, Stillbirth, Neonatal death	CMW
Tervila and Vartiainen	Single-blind	Primigravid > 16th week	Chlorthalidone 50 mg/day until delivery	211	108	103	15 treated patients, 19 controls (including two abortions)	Edema, Proteinuric pre-eclampsia, Blood pressure, Weight gain	Proteinuria ≥ 0.4 g/d, Blood pressure > 140/90 mm Hg
Campbell and MacGillivray	Open; two controls: 5 MJ diet, Normal care	Primigravid with weight gain > 0.6 kg/week 20th to 30th week	Cyclopenthiazide 0.5 mg/day plus potassium 1.2 g/day, or spironolactone, or clopamide-K	255	153	102	Nil	Pre-eclampsia, Proteinuric pre-eclampsia, Birth weight	Nelson

[a]Reprinted from Collins et al. (1985) with permission.

[b]Definitions of pre-eclampsia: CMW, Committee on Maternal Welfare: increase in systolic blood pressure ≥ 30 mm Hg or systolic blood pressure ≥ 140 mm Hg, or increase in diastolic blood pressure ≥ 15 mm Hg or diastolic blood pressure ≥ 90 mm Hg, with or without proteinuria or edema after 24th week. Nelson: Diastolic blood pressure ≥ 90 mm Hg after 26th week, with proteinuria (severe) or without (mild).

[c]Numbers of patients with follow-up for perinatal deaths.

Illustrates characteristics of studies included in a metaanalysis.

TABLE 12.6. Treatment Regimen and Trial Design in Hypertension Studies[a]

Study	Randomized	Double-blind	Single-blind	Placebo	Active treatment[b]
Veterans Administration	+	+		+	1 Hydrochlorothiazide + reserpine + hydralazine
Gothenburg					1 β blocker 2 Thiazide diuretic 3 Hydralazine 4 Spironolactone or bethanidine or high dose furosemide
Hypertension detection and follow-up program	+				1 Chlorthalidone or triamterene or spironolactone 2 Reserpine or methyldopa 3 Hydralazine 4 Guanethidine ± 2 or 3 5 Others
Oslo	+				1 Hydrochlorothiazide 2 Methyldopa or propranolol 3 Others
Australian	+		+	+	1 Chlorothiazide 2 Methyldopa or propranolol or pindolol 3 Hydralazine or clonidine
Multiple risk factor interventions trial	+				1 Hydrochlorothiazide or chlorthalidone 2 Reserpine or hydralazine or guanethidine or others
European	+	+		+	1 Hydrochlorothiazide or triamterene 2 Methyldopa
International prospective primary prevention study	+	+		+	1 Slow-release oxprenolol 2 Other non-β blockers
MRC	+		+	+	1 Bendrofluazide or propranolol 2 Methyldopa

[a]Reprinted from Wilcox et al. (1986b) with permission.
[b]All studies except for the Veterans Administration used step care treatment.

• The clarity of this table would be enhanced by adding a blank line between each of the studies.

Illustrates characteristics of patients included in a metaanalysis.

TABLE 12.7. Type of Patient, Blood Pressure, and Number of Patients
Included in Major Trials of Reduction of Blood Pressure[a]

Study	Patients	Blood pressure (mm Hg)	No. of patients
Veterans Administration	Men in hospital	Diastolic > 90	523
Gothenburg	Men aged 47–54	Systolic > 175 or diastolic > 115	635
Hypertension detection and follow-up program	Men and women aged 30–69	Diastolic > 90	10,940
Oslo	Men aged 40–49	150–179/> 100	785
Australian	Men and women aged 30–69	Diastolic 95–109	3,427
Multiple risk factor intervention trial	"High risk" men aged 35–59	Diastolic 90–115	12,866
European	Men and women over 60	Diastolic 90–119	940
International prospective primary prevention study	Men and women aged 40–69	Diastolic 100–125	6,357
MRC	Men and women aged 35–60	Diastolic 90–109	17,354
Total			53,827

[a]Reprinted from Wilcox et al. (1986b) with permission.

Illustrates study characteristics categorized by drug.

TABLE 12.8. Annual Duodenal Ulcer Recurrence Rates Reported in Double-Blind Studies[a]

Drug	Dose (mg)	No. of evaluatable patients	Recurrence rate (%)	Reference
Cimetidine	200 bid	83	39	45
	300 bid	150	23	45
	400 bid	24	25	53
		26	15	55
		29	16	56
		164	27	58
	400 hs	67	24	45
		46	43	47
		197	37	48
		23	39	51
		49	27	54
		179	22	58
		23	10	59
		20	15	60
		52	17	61
		26	35	62
Ranitidine	150 hs	138	35	49
		45	16	47
		207	23	48
		174	28	49
		22	18	52
		20	35	57
Famotidine	20 hs	86	23	50
		307	36	64
	40 hs	97	25	50

continued

TABLE 12.8. *Continued*

Drug	Dose (mg)	No. of evaluatable patients	Recurrence rate (%)	Reference
Nizatidine	150 hs	257	22	63
Placebo		70	50	45
		139	60	46
		165	68	49
		87	57	50
		325	76	64
		256	44	63
		23	83	51
		21	86	52
		27	93	53
		51	51	54
		14	100	55
		23	78	56
		17	88	57
		333	61	58
		24	70	59
		18	61	60
		39	69	61
		30	83	62

[a]In trials of longer than 1 year the recurrence rate at the end of the first year has been used in this table. Reprinted from Freston (1987) with permission.

• This presentation is not ideal because the reader cannot easily match-up placebo results with the active drug results from the same study.

• By lumping all of the results together for each group one can see between-study variability.

• "Reference" column relates to bibliography where additional study results can be found. This column is the only way to link within-study results.

• Weighted values could be given. This would be obtained by averaging the number of patients multiplied by recurrence rates across studies. A range could also be given.

Illustrates an emphasis on diagnostic characteristics of patients included in a metaanalysis.

TABLE 12.9. Diagnostic Characteristics Reported in Eight Studies of Patients with Urticaria and Angioedema[a]

Duration of ailment	Type of ailment	Precipitated by physical stimuli	Related to cholinergic factors	Dermatographic manifestations	Other
>6 wk	Ordinary	—	—	—	—
>6 wk	Chronic	—	0	0	0
>2 mo	Chronic	—	—	—	0
>2 mo	Ordinary	0	0	0	—
>3 mo	Urticaria	0	+	—	0
>3 mo	Recurrent	0	—	—	0
>4 mo	Recurrent	—	—	—	—
?	Urticaria	+	+	+	+

[a]Reprinted from Kwoh and Feinstein (1986) with permission.

Illustrates a summary of how data were acquired in various studies included in a metaanalysis.

TABLE 12.10. Method of Data Acquisition Cited in 47 Studies of Sensitivity Rates[a]

Method	No. of studies
Oral challenge	17
Direct questioning and then oral challenge in "solicited patients"	2
Direct questioning	7
Chart review, direct questioning, and physical examination	1
Chart review and direct questioning	1
Chart review	6
By history in some patients and challenge in others	7
Referring physician's report	1
Unclear	5

[a]Reprinted from Kwoh and Feinstein (1986) with permission.

• This is a good summary of the background nature of data collection. If the type of collection is related to data quality, this information is crucial to interpretation of the metaanalysis.

Illustrates data of studies to be included in the metaanalysis.

TABLE 12.11. Primary Results of Analyses[a]

Source of data	Year of report	No. of cases	Diagnostic criteria for myocardial infarction	Experimental study	Concurrent controls
Comparison of anticoagulation with no anticoagulation:					
Wright et al.	1948	800	0	+	+
Greisman & Marcus	1948	175	±	0	0
Tulloch & Gilchrist	1950	154	±	+	+
Bresnick et al.	1950	250	0	+	+
Holten	1951	430	0	+	+
Smith et al.	1951	920	0	0	0
Feldman et al.	1952	189	±	+	+
Rashkoff et al.	1952	287	+	+	+
Furman et al.	1953	311	±	0	0
Loudon et al.	1953	200	±	0	0
Schnur	1953	1350	±	0	+
Burton	1954	745	0	0	0
Manchester & Rabkin	1954	300	±	+	+
Manson & Fullerton	1956	314	0	0	+
Eastman et al.	1957	362	0	0	+
Honey & Truelove	1957	543	±	0	+
Richards	1958	267	±	0	0
Rosenberg & Malach	1958	264	+	0	+
Toohey	1958	326	0	0	0
McCluskie & Seaton	1959	226	+	0	+
Carleton et al.	1960	81	±	+	+
Hilden et al.	1961	800	+	+	±
Blake et al.	1962	128	±	0	+
Griffith et al.	1962	191	±	0	+
Gumpert	1962	104	0	0	±
Meltzer et al.	1964	761	+	0	+
Wasserman et al.	1966	147	+	+	+
Comparison of one anticoagulant with another:					
Fitzgerald	1962	484	+	0	+
Schumachet et al.	1962	193	±	+	+
Brown & MacMillan	1964	206	+	+	+
Cooperative study	1964	798	0	+	+
Strömgren	1964	99	0	0	+

continued

TABLE 12.11. *Continued*

Source of data	Hospital coordination	Random allocation	Stratified prognostic correlation	Diagnostic criteria for thrombo-embolism	Double-blind technique	Was anticoagulant therapy significantly better than none?
Comparison of anticoagulation with no anticoagulation:						
Wright et al.	0	0	0	0	0	Yes
Greisman & Marcus	+	0	0	0	0	Yes
Tulloch & Gilchrist	+	0	0	0	0	Yes
Bresnick et al.	+	0	0	0	0	No
Holten	0	0	0	0	0	Yes
Smith et al.	+	0	0	0	0	Yes
Feldman et al.	+	0	+	0	0	No
Rashkoff et al.	+	0	0	0	0	Yes
Furman et al.	+	0	+	0	0	No
Loudon et al.	+	0	+	0	0	Yes
Schnur	0	0	+	—[b]	0	No
Burton	+	0	+	0	0	Yes
Manchester & Rabkin	+	0	+	0	0	Yes[c]
Manson & Fullerton	0	0	0	0	0	Yes
Eastman et al.	+	0	+	—[b]	0	No[d]
Honey & Truelove	+	0	+	±	0	No
Richards	+	0	+	0	0	No
Rosenberg & Malach	+	0	0	—[b]	0	No
Toohey	0	+	0	0	0	Yes
McCluskie & Seaton	+	0	0	0	0	Yes
Carleton et al.	+	+	0	0	+	No
Hilden et al.	+	0	+	0	0	No[e]
Blake et al.	+	0	+	—[b]	0	No
Griffith et al.	+	0	+	—[b]	0	Yes
Gumpert	+	0	+	—[b]	0	No
Meltzer et al.	0	0	+	0	0	Yes
Wasserman et al.	+	+	+	0	0	No
Comparison of one anticoagulant with another:						
Fitzgerald	+	0	+	0	0	—[b]
Schumachet et al.	+	0	0	0	0	—[b]
Brown & MacMillan	+	+	0	—[b]	0	—[b]
Cooperative study	±	+	+	—[b]	0	—[b]
Strömgren	+	0	0	0	0	—[b]

[a]Reprinted from Gifford and Feinstein (1969) with permission.

[b]Not pertinent (see text).

[c]Benefit only for "bad-risk" group.

[d]Anticoagulants only slightly superior.

[e]No difference in mortality although lower rate of thromboembolism noted at autopsy.

Illustrates the results of a metaanalysis evaluating relative risk in three groups of patients.

TABLE 12.12. Results of Randomized Controlled Trials of Diuretics on Perinatal Deaths, Stillbirths, and Neonatal Deaths[a]

Study	No. of patients followed up		Perinatal deaths				Stillbirths				Neonatal deaths			
	Treated	Control	No. in treated patients	No. in controls	Treated patients O − E[b]	Variance	No. in treated patients	No. in controls	Treated patients O − E[b]	Variance	No. in treated patients	No. in controls	Treated patients O − E[b]	Variance
Weseley and Douglas	131	136	1	4	−1.5	1.2	1	2	−0.5	0.7	0	2	−1.0	0.5
Flowers et al.	335	110	6	3	−0.8	1.6	3	2	−0.8	0.9	3	1	0	0.7
Menzies	57	48	3	2	+0.3	1.2	1	1	−0.1	0.5	2	1	+0.4	0.7
Fallis et al.	34	40	1	3	−0.8	1.0	0	1	−0.5	0.3	1	2	−0.4	0.7
Cuadros and Tatum	1,011	760	14	13	−1.4	6.5	6	5	−0.3	2.7	8	8	−1.1	3.9
Landesman et al.	1,370	1,336	24	19	+2.2	+10.6	Not available				Not available			
Kraus et al.	506	524	14	16	−0.7	7.3	6	9	−1.4	3.7	8	7	+0.6	3.7
Tervila and Vartianen	108	103	0	0	0	0	0	0	0	0	0	0	0	0
Campbell and MacGillivray	153	102	0	0	0	0	0	0	0	0	0	0	0	0
Overall:														
Perinatal deaths	3,705	3,159	63 (1.7%)	60 (1.9%)	−2.7	29.4								
Stillbirths and neonatal deaths	2,335	1,823					17 (0.7%)	20 (1.1%)	−3.4	8.8	22 (0.9%)	21 (1.2%)	−1.5	10.3

	"Pooled" relative risk	95% confidence interval	Test for heterogeneity
Perinatal deaths	0.91	0.64, 1.31 (NS)	$X_8^2 = 3.5$ (NS)
Stillbirths	0.68	0.35, 1.31 (NS)	$X_7^2 = 1.0$ (NS)
Neonatal deaths	0.86	0.47, 1.59 (NS)	$X_7^2 = 2.5$ (NS)

[a]Reprinted from Collins et al. (1985) with permission.
[b]The number of patients allocated to treatment who were observed to develop a particular unfavorable event minus the number that would have been expected to do so if treatment had had no effect. O − E, observed − expected.

Illustrates a presentation of adverse reaction data in a metaanalysis.

TABLE 12.13. Reported Adverse Reactions in Randomized Controlled Studies of Diuretics in Pregnancy[a]

Adverse reaction	Study	Treated patients		Controls	
		N	N with adverse reaction	N	N with adverse reaction
Neonatal					
Thrombocytopenic	Menzies	97	1	48	0
purpura	Kraus et al.	506	0	524	0
Jaundice	Flowers et al. (random selection from complete study)	70	13	40	31
Maternal					
Pancreatitis,	No cases reported in randomized controlled trials				
hypokalemia,	Flowers et al.	No cases in 10% sample and all patients complaining of weakness			
hyponatremia, or both					
	Menzies	No significant difference in serum sodium or potassium concentrations			
	Cuadros and Tatum				
	Landesman et al.				
	Campbell and MacGillivray				
	Kraus et al. (Potassium concentration <3.5 mmol (mEq/l)	506	80	524	37
	Tervila and Vartiainen (Potassium concentration <2.7 mmol/l)	109	4	103	0

[a]Reprinted from Collins et al. (1985) with permission.

Illustrates adverse reactions observed in a metaanalysis.

TABLE 12.14. Adverse Reactions Observed in Studies Included in the Metaanalysis

Specific adverse reaction reported	Number of studies where adverse reaction was reported	Crude rate	
		Controls Number of events ——————————— Total number of patients	Treated patients Number of events ——————————— Total number of patients
1			
2			
3			
. . .			
N			

Illustrates how each study in a metaanalysis contributed to overall effect.

TABLE 12.15. Relative Contribution of Each Study to Overall Effect of the Metaanalysis

Study number	Size of the effect	Weighting factor	Size X weighting factor

Illustrates a comparison of published and unpublished studies.

TABLE 12.16. Results of Published RCTs Vs. Results of Completed Unpublished RCTs[a]

Trend/statistical significance	Number	Published RCTs percentage of total with trend specified	Number	Completed unpublished RCTs percentage of total with trend specified
Favors new therapy (p<0.05)	423	55.1	26	14.6
Trend favors new therapy	123	16.0	40	22.5
No difference between therapies	170	22.2	79	44.4
Trend favors control/standard therapy	25	3.3	23	12.9
Favors control/standard therapy (p<0.05)	26	3.4	10	5.6
Total number RCTs with trend specified	767	100.0	178	100.0
Number RCTs with trend of results not specified	274		26	
Total number RCTs	1041		204	

[a]RCT, randomized controlled trials. Reprinted from Chalmers et al. (1987) with permission.

Illustrates a comparison of ratings of two reviewers or two groups.

TABLE 12.17. Comparison of How Two Reviewers or Groups Classified Patients' Endpoints[a]

Ratings by group II	Ratings by group I				
	Cardiovascular disease	Coronary artery disease	Other disease	Unknown	Total
Cardiovascular disease	37	6	2	1	46
Coronary artery disease	3	76	9	2	90
Other disease	1	0	16	3	20
Unknown	0	1	3	2	6
Total	41	83	30	8	162

[a]One group could be the patient's classification of death on the death certificate.

Illustrates listing of studies that support and do not support a result.

TABLE 12.18. Contradictory Randomized Clinical Trials on 19 Cardiology Topics[a]

Topic	Years spanned by trials	Supportive results		Equivocal results		Nonsupportive results	
		Number	References	Number	References	Number	References
Anticoagulants and acute myocardial infarction	1960–1973	1	[6]	2	[7,8]	3	[9–11]
Anticoagulants after recovery from myocardial infarction	1960–1980	3	[12–14]	2	[15,16]	4	[17–20]
Beta blockers and acute myocardial infarction	1965–1983	4	[21–24]	1	[25]	7	[26–32]
Medical treatment of mild hypertension	1967–198–	2	[33–34]	0	—	4	[35–38]
Dipyridamole and venous thrombosis	1969–1980	1	[39]	0	—	2	[40,41]
Aspirin and stroke	1977–1983	2	[42–43]	1	[44]	1	[45]
Long-acting nitrates and angina pectoris	1969–1976	1	[46]	0	—	3	[47–49]
Lidocaine in acute myocardial infarction	1970–1976	5	[50–54]	0	—	4	[55–58]
Beta blockers after recovery from myocardial infarction	1970–1982	4	[59–62]	0	—	3	[63–65]
Low-dose heparin in venous thrombosis	1971–1980	3	[66–68]	0	—	1	[69]
Thrombolytic drugs and acute myocardial infarction	1971–1985	2	[70,71]	1	[72]	6	[73–78]
Lipid-lowering agents and ischemic heart disease	1971–1984	5	[79–83]	0	—	2	[84,85]
Medical vs. surgical treatment of stable coronary artery disease	1975–1980	3	[86–88]	1	[89]	1	[90]
Aspirin and myocardial infarction	1976–1980	2	[91,92]	0	—	1	[93]
Disopyramide and acute myocardial infarction	1976–1980	2	[94,95]	0	—	2	[96,97]
Sulfinpyrazone and myocardial infarction	1978–1982	1	[98]	0	—	2	[99,100]
Nitroprusside and acute myocardial infarction	1981–1982	1	[4]	0	—	2	[5,101]
Aspirin and venous thromboembolism	1972–1980	1	[102]	1	[103]	1	[104]
Steroids and shock	1963–1984	1	[105]	1	[106]	3	[107–109]

[a]Reprinted from Horwitz (1987) with permission.

Illustrates study characteristics and results in a metaanalysis.

TABLE 12.19. Previous Studies of Lp(a) and Coronary Heart Disease[a]

Source	Year	Cases	Controls	Method	Odds ratio	95% Confidence limits	Comments
Dahlen et al.	1972	68 men with angina by Rose questionnaire	218 negative by questionnaire from same population	LE	2.26	1.15–4.42	Stronger association found if clinical diagnosis of "typical or suspected" angina was used, but not clear if this was blind to laboratory results
Berg et al.	1974	46 Finns with CHD aged 23–57 yr	61 healthy Finns	DI	3.14	1.31–7.58	Cases and controls studied at different times
Dahlen et al.	1975	58 Swedish survivors of MI aged 36–74 yr	103 healthy Swedish men aged 50–92 yr	DI and LE	2.25	1.00–5.08	Odds ratio shown is for subjects with results of both tests positive
Albers et al.	1977	90 MI survivors	90 spouses	RIA	1.62	0.83–3.13	Odds ratio = 1.98 for cases with MI before age 50 yr (relative to spouses); results are significant if 95th percentile cut point is used
Frick et al.	1978	108 Finns aged 10–62 yr with atherosclerosis by coronary angiography	45 Finns with normal coronaries by angiography	DI and LE	3.28	1.41–7.72	Stronger association found for persons with "severe" atherosclerosis
Berg	1979	188 CHD patients	1109 Norwegian controls	DI (QIE in a subset)	3.60	2.57–5.06	In subset of patients with coronary angiography, higher Lp(a) levels were associated with more atherosclerosis
Kostner	1983	82 MI survivors aged 40–60 yr	115 controls matched for age, sex, and social status	QIE	a)1.56 b)2.29	0.84–2.90 0.93–5.68	Using cut point of 25 mg/dL (0.25 g/L) (64th percentile)[b] Using cut point of 50 mg/dL (90th percentile)[b]
Present data	1986	228 Japanese male MI survivors aged < 70 yr	311 population-based controls	QIE	1.82	1.26–2.63	Oldest age group excluded to make data more comparable with other studies; 75th percentile cut point used

[a]LE, lipoprotein electrophoresis; CHD, coronary heart disease; DI, double immunodiffusion; MI, myocardial infarction; RIA, radioimmunoassay; and QIE, quantitative immunoelectrophoresis. Reprinted from Rhoads et al. (1986) with permission.
[b]Percentiles estimated from controls.

Illustrates bar chart to present information about known quality of studies comprising the metaanalysis.

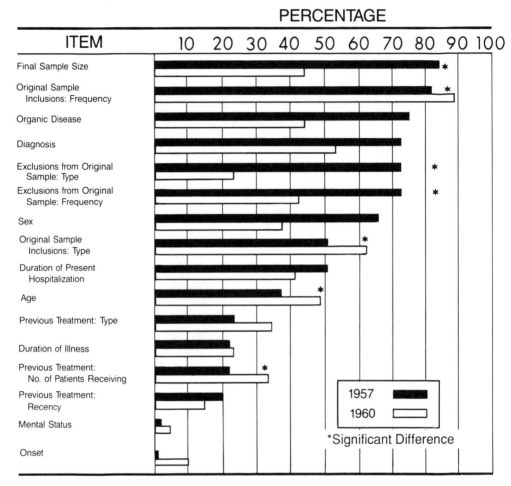

FIG. 12.1. Selection and description of patients: percent of articles reporting specific information.

    • Use of different shaded or colored bars allows for easy visual comparison of articles comprising the 1957 and 1960 analyses.

    • Use of asterisks indicates significant differences between the 1957 and 1960 data.

    • Similar bars could be used to illustrate items relating to design aspects (e.g., double-blind, control group), adverse reactions, efficacy parameters, or any other items of interest.

Illustrates use of bars (size based on 95% confidence interval for treatment effect) to present efficacy results from the studies included in the metaanalysis.

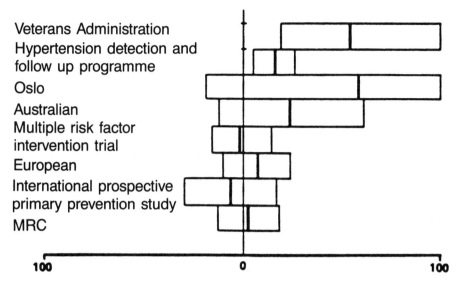

% Increase with active treatment   % Decrease with active treatment

EFFECT

FIG. 12.2. Hypertension trials: 95% confidence intervals for differences in mortality. Bold vertical bars indicate mean reduction (or increase). Reprinted from Wilcox et al. (1986b) with permission.

Illustrates use of bar charts to display the number of studies reporting precategorized response rates.

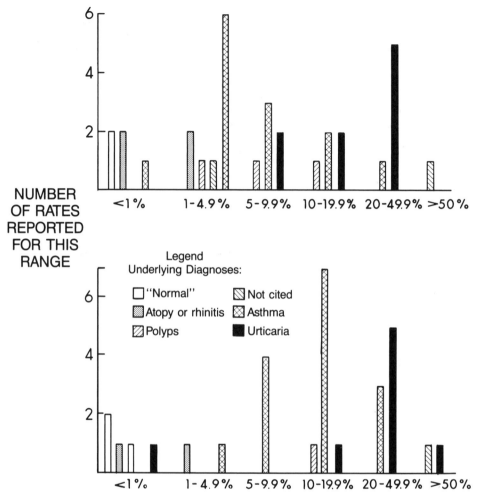

FIG. 12.3. Range of 63 rates reported in 47 studies of aspirin-sensitive reactions, arranged according to underlying diagnosis and method of ascertainment. **Top**, ranges of values reported for rates of sensitivity reaction (historical ascertainment). **Bottom**, ranges of values reported for rates of sensitivity reaction (ascertainment by oral challenge). Reprinted from Kwoh and Feinstein (1986) with permission.

• It is good to display data by underlying diagnosis to see if there was a difference.

• The graph would be improved if the different types of shading were more distinct so that the reader could more easily and immediately identify diagnosis.

• Presentation would be improved if the number of patients with each diagnosis were indicated, possibly as part of the legend.

• Note that category groupings on the horizontal axis are not of equal size. This is not necessarily a drawback, but does need to be noted.

• Note that category groupings are the same in both graphs. This is important and it would be misleading if the groupings were not the same.

Illustrates using straight lines to connect treatment group and control group response rates.

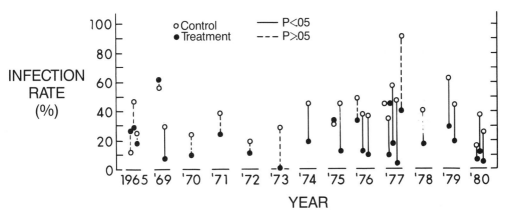

FIG. 12.4. Infection rates for both the treatment and control regimens for the individual trials by year reported, with statistical significance noted. Reprinted from Baum et al. (1981) with permission.

• Different symbols represent treatment and control; it is easy to identify them and to see which is higher.

• Lines connect treatment and control values: the solid line for statistically significant difference and the dotted line for difference that is not significant. It is easy to evaluate both magnitude (by length of line) and significance (by type of line) of difference.

• Unfortunately we are not told if the statistical comparisons are one or two sided.

• Note the vertical axis on both sides of the graph.

• Note that one year (1965) on the x-axis is noncontinuous.

METAANALYSES

Illustrates placing confidence intervals around mean differences in treatment differences over time.

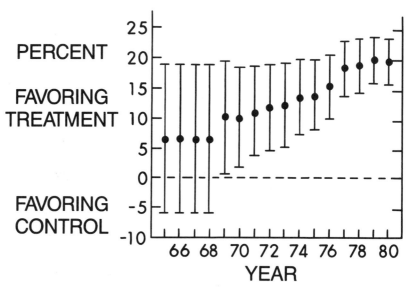

FIG. 12.5. The 95% confidence intervals on the true difference in infection rates, calculated cumulatively over time. Reprinted from Baum et al. (1981) with permission.

Illustrates printing sample sizes on graphs which provide efficacy results for individual groups of studies included in the metaanalysis.

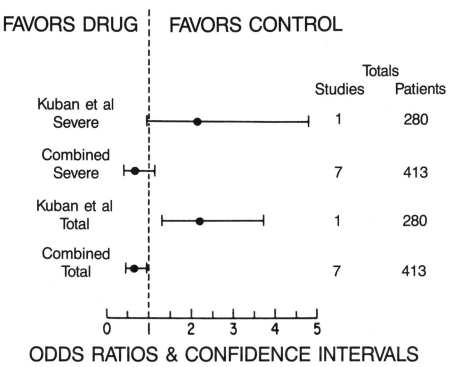

FIG. 12.6. Comparison of metaanalysis of seven small RCTs of phenobarbital in the treatment of neonatal intracranial hemorrhage with one large cooperative study (three institutions). Endpoints are total infants with hemorrhage and totals with severe hemorrhage (Grades III–IV) only. Reprinted from Chalmers et al. (1987) with permission.

Illustrates a comparison of two individual large drug study results with the combined results of multiple drugs of one specific type in 12 small studies.

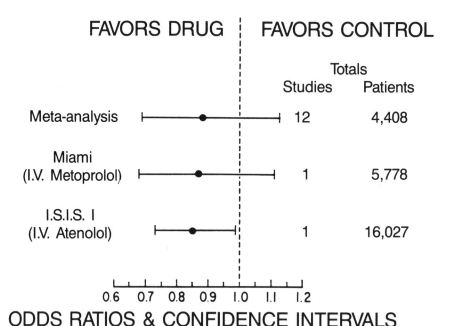

FIG. 12.7. Comparison of metaanalysis of 12 RCTs of IV mixed drugs (double-blind) with IV metoprolol (double-blind) and IV atenolol.

• Use of the vertical reference line is useful to indicate the "dividing point" between studies which favor drug and studies which favor control.
• A log scale may be used instead of an arithmetic one.
• Studies may be ordered based on the length of the confidence interval.
• Studies may present separate endpoints.

Illustrates various metaanalyses performed on a set of studies—each analysis is on a different grouping of those studies.

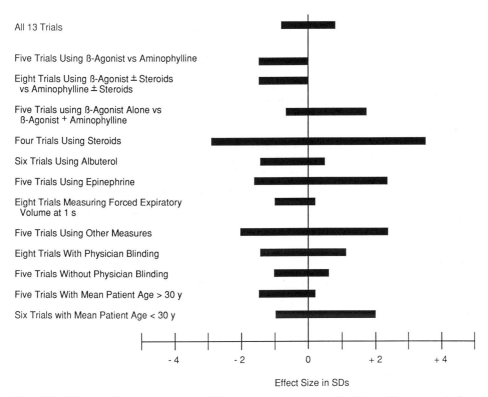

FIG. 12.8. 95% confidence intervals of the pooled subgroups. Positive effect sizes indicate that aminophylline regimen was more effective than control regimen. Negative effect sizes indicate that control regimen was more effective. Reprinted from Littenberg (1988) with permission.

• Individual studies within any category could be listed by author or by another identifier.

Illustrates results of individual studies.

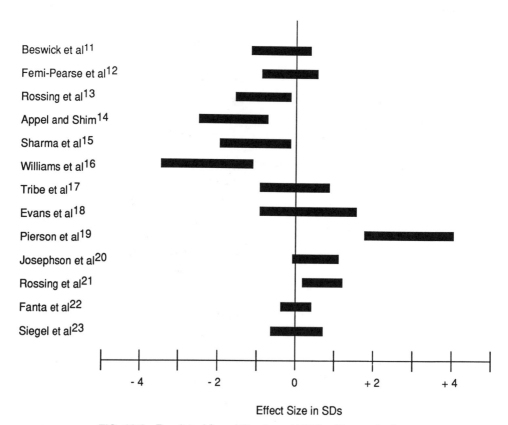

FIG. 12.9. Reprinted from Littenberg (1988) with permission.

• Studies shown could constitute one (or more) of the subsets shown in Fig. 12.8.

Illustrates the efficacy of various drugs of one type in past (i.e., early) versus present (i.e., late) studies.

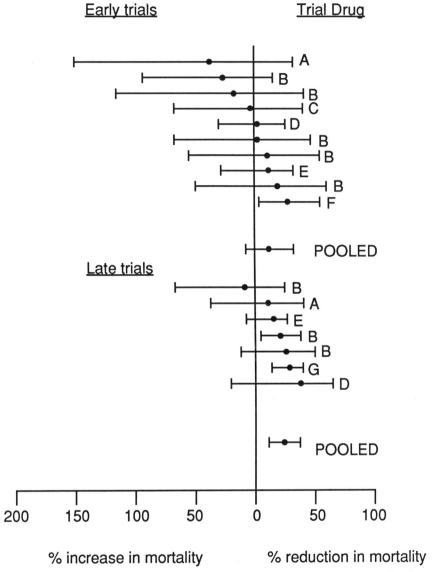

FIG. 12.10. Comparison of results obtained in early vs. late trials on specific drugs for disease X. Drugs (A to G) would be identified in the graph or legend.

Illustrates use of different symbols for showing odds ratios and related data.

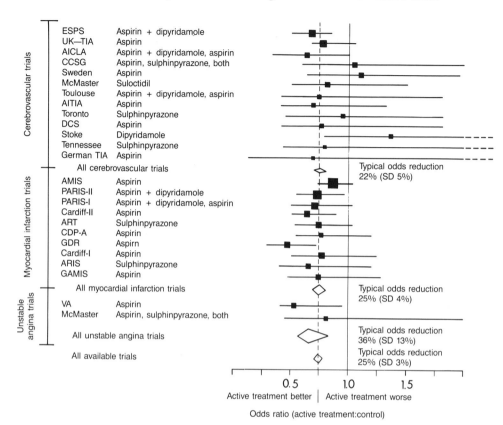

FIG. 12.11. Odds ratios (active treatment : control) for first stroke, myocardial infarction, or vascular death during scheduled treatment period in completed antiplatelet trials. ▬ ■ ▬ = Trial results and 99% confidence intervals (area of rectangle is proportional to amount of information contributed). Diamond shape equals overview results and 95% confidence intervals. Dashed vertical line represents odds ratio of 0.75 suggested by overview of all trial results. Solid vertical line represents odds ratio of unity (no treatment effect). Reprinted from Antiplatelet Trialists' Collaboration (1988) with permission.

Illustrates use of a symbol different than a straight line or bar to show confidence intervals.

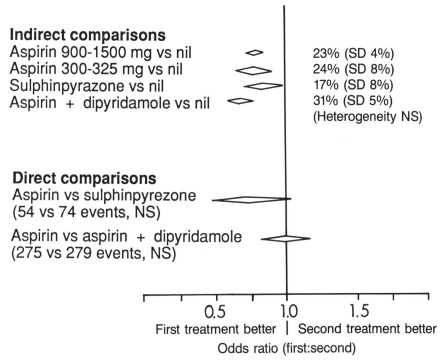

FIG. 12.12. Direct and indirect comparisons between reductions in new vascular event rates with different antiplatelet agents. Diamond shape equals 95% confidence intervals for typical odds ratios. Reprinted from Antiplatelet Trialists' Collaboration (1988) with permission.

Illustrates presenting an overall measure of the quality of study versus year of study.

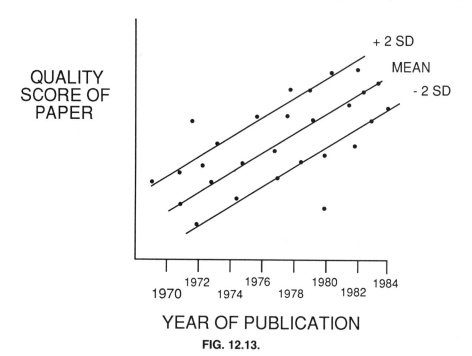

FIG. 12.13.

- The year that the study was conducted may be more relevant as an abscissa.
- The abscissa could be number of patients.
- The method of evaluating quality should be identified.
- Quality may be graphed vs. any parameter that influences it.

Illustrates a scatterplot based on the cross-classification of odds ratio obtained with a measure of the quality of the study.

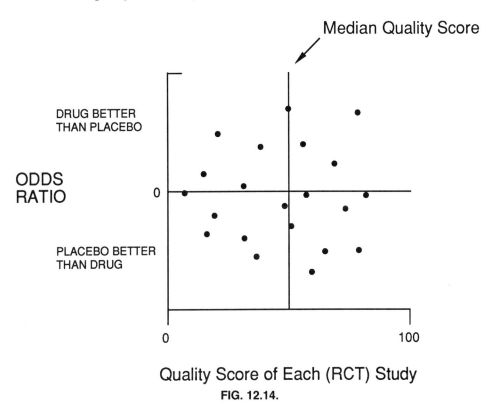

FIG. 12.14.

Illustrates another means of illustrating the quality score of papers of three separate groups, plus providing characteristics of each group.

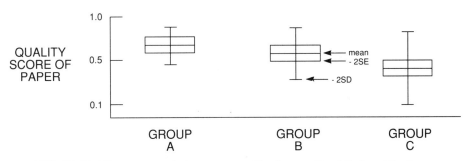

FIG. 12.15. Three groups being compared by the quality of their publications.

• Groups that may be evaluated include studies from different (1) eras, (2) type of funding, (3) type of practice, (4) specific journal, or (5) any other factors.

13

Complex or Confusing Presentations

This chapter is not intended to be a rogues gallery of major blunders, distortions, or errors in presenting clinical data. Nor is it meant to reflect problems in the content or nature of data presented. Rather, it is primarily intended as a selection of presentations that are either confusing or overly complex. Representative examples were chosen to illustrate pitfalls which should be avoided.

When data are not totally and accurately comprehended and interpreted, the problem may lie in the data presented, the presentation itself, or the individual reading the presentation. This chapter does not deal with problems of data or of the reader; it focuses primarily on the presentation format.

Many clear presentations of data lead to incorrect interpretations. This type of problem is not included in this chapter because it primarily relates to the type or amount of data shown (e.g., too few; too many) or inappropriate elements of the presentation. These elements include types of scales used on an axis (e.g., logarithmic or arithmetic), condensation or elongation of scales along an axis, parameters chosen to be graphed, and groups of patients whose data are graphed and compared. The influence that these and other elements have on the interpretation of clinical data is discussed in *Guide to Clinical Interpretation of Data* (Spilker, 1986).

Readers may not agree with some (or many) of the examples included in this chapter. That confirms the important point that varied opinions exist on defining appropriate presentations of clinical data. Some of these examples are taken from highly prestigious journals and their editors did not consider these figures to be overly complex or confusing.

The poor designs which were presented by their authors as appropriate graphs and figures are very slightly modified and not identified as to their original source. The figures were taken from *The New England Journal of Medicine, The Lancet, British Journal of Medicine,* and other well-respected journals.

WHY CERTAIN FORMATS ARE CONFUSING

1. Symbols are not identified, not easily read, or indistinguishable from each other.
2. Too much data are placed in a single table, graph, or figure.
3. Complex or sophisticated statistical analyses are used and the results make little or no sense to clinicians.
4. Too many graphs overlap each other.
5. Data that are usually or almost always illustrated in one manner are shown in a new way. For example, a dose-response curve with dose as the ordinate would be quite unusual.

6. Too many lines or extraneous material make the figure difficult to digest.
7. The label of the ordinate or abscissa is not lucid and the meaning of the data plotted will thus be obscured.
8. The visual impact of the format suggest one interpretation while the data suggest another.
9. The scales do not obey basic rules (e.g., logarithmic and arithmetic scales should not be mixed on the same axis).

Table 13.1 shows the same data using three formats. The top format is the most difficult to read, primarily because the vertical lines interfere with horizontal scanning. The middle presentation is an improvement, but breaking up the lines does not permit scanning as readily as in the lowest presentation.

Table 13.2 presents the data used to graph Fig. 13.1. This figure is highly misleading because it may be read as implying that each point represents a separate baby. Moreover, the apparent upward relationship over time is shown by looking at the individual patient data in Table 13.2 to be spurious.

GRAPHING DATA IN THREE DIMENSIONS

When three-dimensional objects of different sizes are used, the reader must ascertain whether differences in the actual data are accurately reflected. The presenter may have considered only one dimension (e.g., height) of the objects in determining relative sizes, or two dimensions (e.g., height and length) only. If the reader views the objects according to the same number of dimensions used by the presenter, then no distortion in interpretation results. But, readers usually interpret objects based on three-dimensional volumes and presenters often only consider one or two dimensions. This leads to a distortion referred to by Tufte (1983) as a lie factor. The lie factor was defined as the size of an object in a graph divided by the size in the data. For example, assume that a value increased from 5,000 to 10,000 and two objects are to be drawn in three dimensions to illustrate this growth. If both the height and length of the first three-dimensional objects are doubled, the area of the larger object will be four times as great as the smaller one and the volume will be eight times as great. The correct mathematical procedure to determine the dimensions of the second object is to divide the larger number by the smaller one, take the cube root of this number, and multiply both the height and length by the cube root.

Because a mathematically appropriate presentation of three dimensional objects is much less dramatic than presentations based on incorrect principles, correct presentations are rarely made. Incorrect presentations may be found in major newspapers and magazines on a daily basis.

A three-dimensional object may be used appropriately in a comparative graph when it is used as a one dimensional object (e.g., a bar graph using cigarettes of different lengths may be used to show changes in the number of cigarettes consumed). This is acceptable because the other two dimensions of a cigarette are thought of as being constant, and only the length varies.

TABLE 13.1. Studies Included in a Metaanalysis

	Group One	Group Two	Group Three	Sex
Parameter A	4364 2173	79 43	132 148	Male Female
Parameter B	7612 7930	96 112	77 92	Male Female
Parameter C	2230 1886	96 87	111 116	Male Female

		Group		
Parameter		1	2	3
A	Male	4,364	79	132
	Female	2,173	43	148
B	Male	7,612	96	77
	Female	7,930	112	92
C	Male	2,230	96	111
	Female	1,886	87	116

		Group		
Parameter	Sex	1	2	3
A	Male	4,364	79	132
	Female	2,173	43	148
B	Male	7,612	96	77
	Female	7,930	112	92
C	Male	2,230	96	111
	Female	1,886	87	116

TABLE 13.2. Proconvertin Levels in Newborn Babies Receiving Vitamin K[a]

	Day after birth											
Baby	1	2	3	4	5	6	7	8	9	10	11	12
1	12	14	10	15								
2		28		29	30		32	29	30			
3		16	20		14							
4							28	33	39	30	32	36
5	24	20		20	17	21	20		24			
6	13	11										
7			26			30						
8								38		36	38	
9					28	26						
10	14											
Mean	15.8	17.8	18.7	21.3	22.2	25.7	26.7	33.3	31.0	33.0	35.0	36.0

[a]Reprinted from De Jonge (1983) with permission.

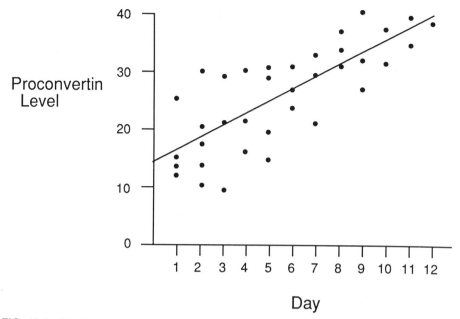

FIG. 13.1. Proconvertin levels in newborn babies receiving vitamin K; $r = 0.80$ (p<0.001).

• Note that the table of these data (Table 13.2) and the plot tend to contradict each other. The problem is the "day to day" variation in which patients provide data on what day.

• It is also important to be aware of proper interpretation of correlation coefficients. These coefficients measure the linearity of a relationship and not the significance of that relationship. Reprinted from De Jonge (1983) with permission.

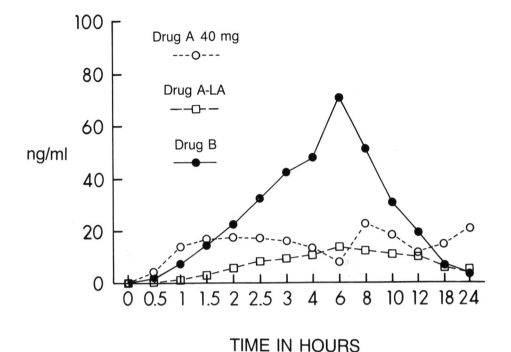

TIME IN HOURS

FIG. 13.2. Note the three changes in scale along the abscissa. The first six equally spaced sections are 0.5 hr, the next equals 1 hr, the next four equal 2 hr, and the final two equal 6 hr.

• The author of this graph created an arbitrary scale that makes interpretation of results more difficult.

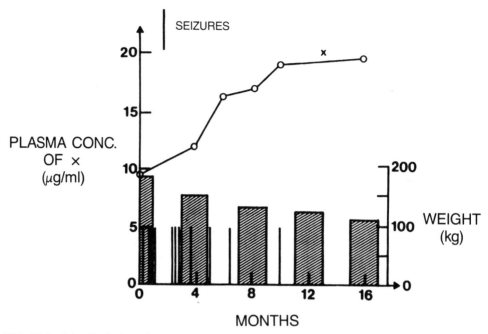

FIG. 13.3. A badly designed graph, based on examples from the scientific press. This graph was specifically constructed to illustrate the flaws. Reprinted from Reynolds and Simmonds (1984) with permission.

Problems:

- Inward facing scale calibrations add confusion to a confused picture.
- The key for seizures is separated from the part of the graph dealing with seizures.
- Arrows at the end of axes are irrelevant, as are the two zeros at the origin.
- Differently measured sets of data should not be superimposed on one graph, unless the resulting graph is clear.

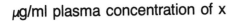

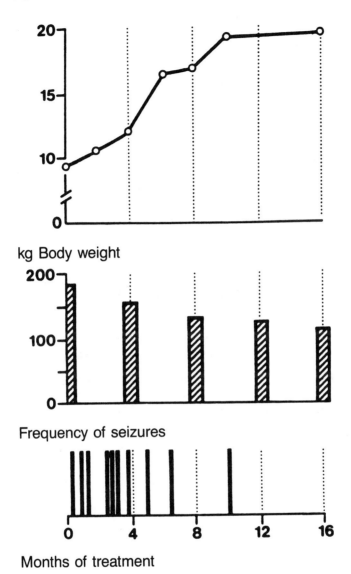

FIG. 13.4. The three sets of data shown in Fig. 13.3 each have been provided with their own scales linked through time. Reprinted from Reynolds and Simmonds (1984) with permission.

• The identity of the months of treatment are not stated in this improved version.

• The use of vertical dotted lines to identify months in all 3 related graphs helps the reader interpret these data.

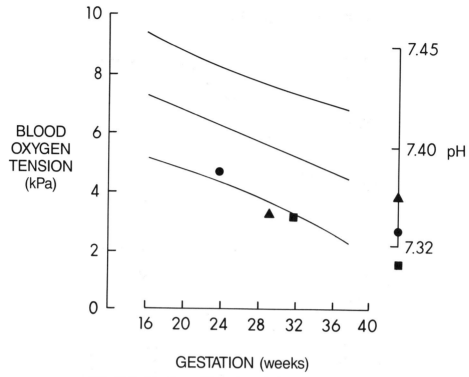

FIG. 13.5. The three different symbols are not identified.

• It is unclear whether the three symbols to the right are pH measures, and if so, why the bottom one is below the scale.

• The relationship of the symbols to the lines is unclear (i.e., why did the presenter place both symbols on the same graph?).

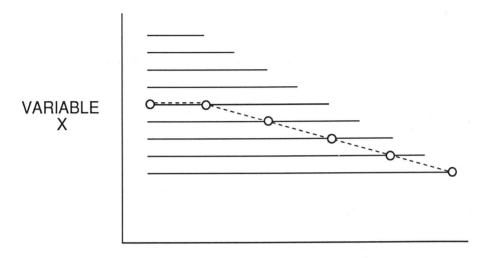

AGE

FIG. 13.6. Influence of selective mortality on age trends in cross-sectional data. The **X** denotes a risk factor associated with mortality. The **circles** represent mean cross-sectional values and show an apparent decline in X with age, which results from a progressive loss of subjects with high X levels in older age groups. The **horizontal lines** show that the level of X is not influenced by age.

• The legend (quoted verbatim from the paper) makes the point "that the level of X is not influenced by age." Nonetheless, the presentation makes it look as though it is.

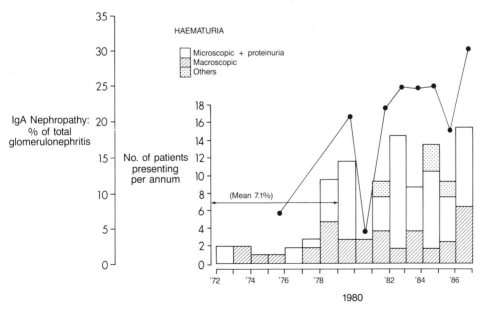

FIG. 13.7.

• Too complex to understand readily.

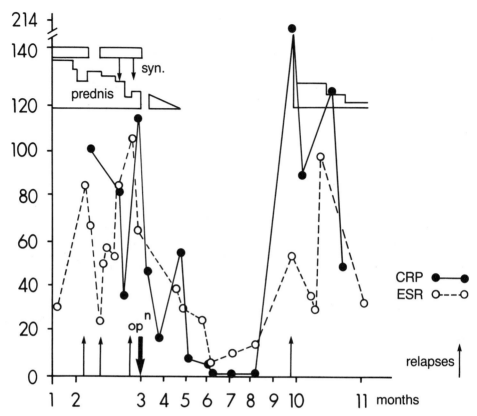

FIG. 13.8. Draft layout of data as originally conceived for a 35 mm slide. It is unscientific to compare two differently measured variables on the same axis. Therefore, ESR and CRP must be separated. A square format is a disadvantage since it will waste one-third of the slide area. Data reprinted from Reynolds and Simmonds (1984) with permission.

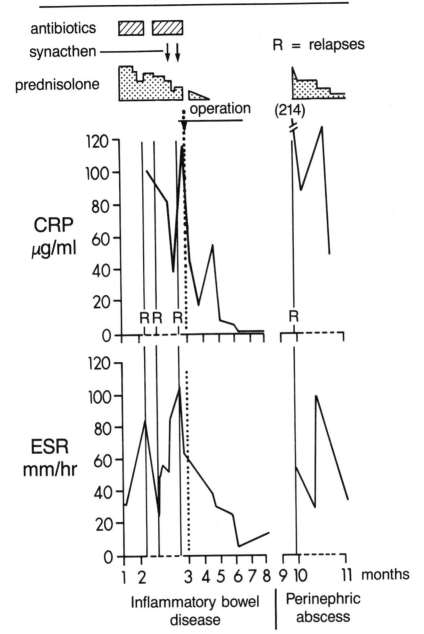

FIG. 13.9. Data in Fig. 13.8 redesigned. The full 2 : 3 slide format has been occupied. The two differently measured y-axis variables are now clear. Common events in time coincide vertically. The two disease phases are distinct. Treatment is not obscured by other data. Reprinted from Reynolds and Simmonds (1984) with permission.

• Additional efforts should be made to simplify this presentation further and enhance clarity.

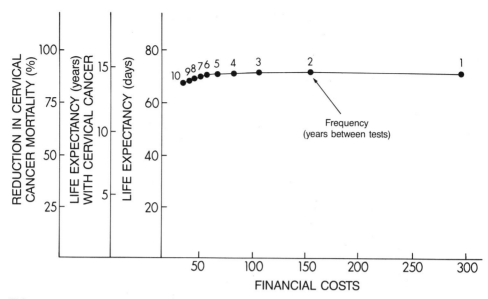

FIG. 13.10. This simple figure attempts to achieve too much and fails. A table or revised graph is preferable.

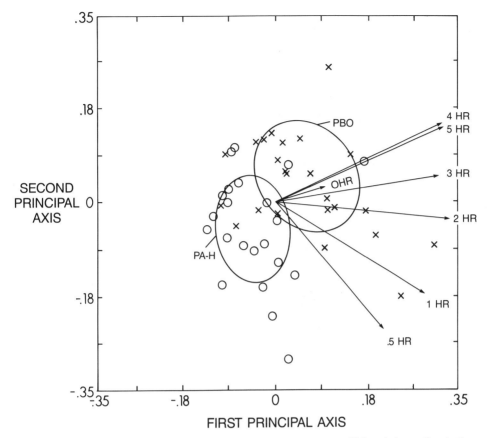

FIG. 13.11. This figure (from a clinical journal) does not convey sufficient information to those who are not intimately familiar with this obscure presentation.

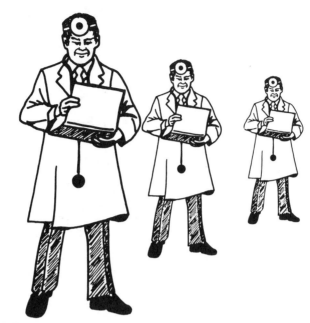

FIG. 13.12. Three-dimensional objects (see text for discussion).

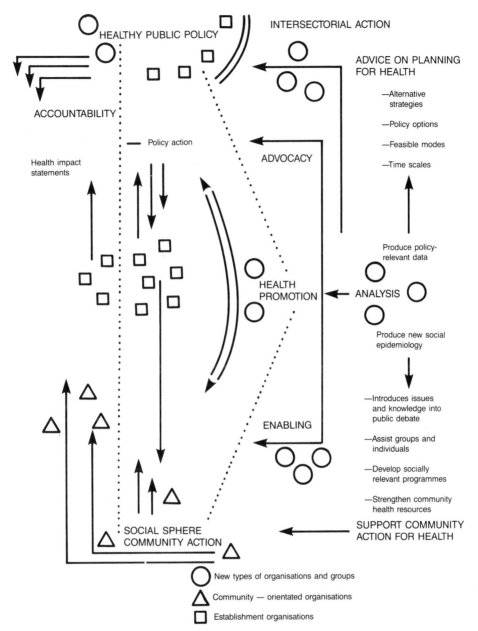

FIG. 13.13. This outrageous diagram prepared by the World Health Organization was spoofed by the *British Medical Journal.* Reprinted from anonymous, British Medical Journal (1986) with permission.

Bibliography

Anderson, I.D., Woodford, M., de Dombal, F.T., and Irving, M. (1988): Retrospective study of 1000 deaths from injury in England and Wales. *Br. Med. J.*, 296:1305–1308.

Anonymous (1986): WHO's kidding? *Br. Med. J.*, 293:1643.

Antiplatelet Trialists' Collaboration (1988): Secondary prevention of vascular disease by prolonged antiplatelet treatment. *Br. Med. J.*, 296:320–331.

Avanzini, F., Alli, C., Bettelli, G., Colombo, F., Conforti, L., Pirone, F., Spagnoli, A., Taioli, E., Tognoni, G., Villella, M. et al. (1987): Feasibility of a large prospective study in general practice: An Italian experience. *Br. Med. J.*, 294:157–160.

Bailar, J.C. III, and Mosteller, F. (Eds.) (1986): *Medical Uses of Statistics*. New England Journal of Medicine Books, Waltham, MA.

Baum, M.L., Anish, D.S., Chalmers, T.C., Sacks, H.S., Smith, H. Jr., and Fagerstrom, R.M. (1981): A survey of clinical trials of antibiotic prophylaxis in colon surgery: Evidence against further use of no-treatment controls. *N. Engl. J. Med.*, 305:795–799.

Becker, P.M., McVey, L.J., Saltz, C.C., Feussner, J.R., and Cohen, H.J. (1987): Hospital-acquired complications in a randomized controlled clinical trial of a geriatric consultation team. *JAMA*, 257:2313–2317.

Bellak, L., and Chassan, J.B. (1964): An approach to the evaluation of drug effect during psychotherapy: A double-blind study of a single case. *J. Nerv. Ment. Dis.*, 139:29–30.

Bigby, M., Jick, S., Jick, H., and Arndt, K. (1986): Drug-induced cutaneous reactions: A report from the Boston Collaborative Drug Surveillance Program on 15,438 consecutive inpatients, 1975 to 1982. *JAMA*, 256:3358–3363.

Blank, D.W., Hoeg, J.M., Kroll, M.H., and Ruddel, M.E. (1986): The method of determination must be considered in interpreting blood cholesterol levels. *JAMA*, 256:2867–2870.

Bombardier, C., Ware, J., Russell, I.J., Larson, M., Chalmers, A., and Read, J.L. (1986): Auranofin therapy and quality of life in patients with rheumatoid arthritis: Results of a multicenter trial. *Am. J. Med.*, 81:565–578.

Bowen, G.S., Griffin, M., Hayne, C., Slade, J., Schulze, T.L., and Parkin, W. (1984): Clinical manifestations and descriptive epidemiology of Lyme disease in New Jersey, 1978 to 1982. *JAMA*, 251:2236–2240.

Breslow, L., and Cumberland, W.G. (1988): Progress and objectives in cancer control. *JAMA*, 259:1690–1694.

Brodie, M.J., and Feely, J. (1988): Adverse drug interactions. *Br. Med. J.*, 296:845–849.

Brody, J.A. (1987): The best of times/the worst of times: Aging and dependency in the 21st century. In: *Ethical Dimensions of Geriatric Care: Value Conflicts for the 21st Century*. Spicker, S.F., Ingman, S.R., and Lawson, I.R. (Eds.), pp. 3–21. Reidel, Holland.

Brundage, J.F., Scott, R.M., Lednar, W.M., Smith, D.W., and Miller, R.N. (1988): Building-associated risk of febrile acute respiratory diseases in Army trainees. *JAMA*, 259:2108–2112.

Budnick, L.D. (1984): Bathtub-related electrocutions in the United States, 1979 to 1982. *JAMA*, 252:918–920.

Campbell, S.K. (1974): *Flaws and Fallacies in Statistical Thinking*. Prentice-Hall, Englewood Cliffs, NJ.

Castelli, W.P., Garrison, R.J., Wilson, P.W.J., Abbott, R.D., Kalousdian, S., and Kannel, W.B. (1986): Incidence of coronary heart disease and lipoprotein cholesterol levels: The Framingham study. *JAMA*, 256:2835–2838.

Centers for Disease Control Vietnam Experience Study (1988): Health status of Vietnam veterans: I. Psychosocial Characteristics. *JAMA*, 259:2701–2707.

Chalmers, T.C., Levin, H., Sacks, H.S., Reitman, D., Berrier, J., and Nagalingam, R. (1987): Meta-analysis of clinical trials as scientific discipline. I: Control of bias and comparison with large cooperative trials. *Stat. Med.*, 6:315–328.

Cleland, J.G., Dargie, H.J., McAlpine, H., Ball, S.G., Morton, J.J., Robertson, J.I., and Ford, I. (1985): Severe hypotension after first dose of enalapril in heart failure. *Br. Med. J.*, 291:1309–1312.

Cole, C.G., Walker, A., Coyne, A., Johnson, L., Hart, K.A., Hodgson, S., Sheridan, R., and Bobrow, M. (1988): Prenatal testing for Duchenne and Becker muscular dystrophy. *Lancet*, 1:262–266.

Collins, R., Yusuf, S., and Peto, R. (1985): Overview of randomized trials of diuretics in pregnancy. *Br. Med. J.*, 290:17–23.

Council on Scientific Affairs (1983): Medical evaluations of healthy persons. *JAMA*, 249:1626–1633.

Croog, S.H., Levine, S., Testa, M.A., Brown, B., Bulpitt, C.J., Jenkins, C.D., Klerman, G.L., and Williams, G.H. (1986): The effects of antihypertensive therapy on the quality of life. *N. Engl. J. Med.*, 314:1657–1664.

Dam, M., Gram, L., Philbert, A., Hansen, B.S., Lyon, B.B., Christensen, J.M., and Angelo, H.R. (1983): Progabide: A controlled trial in partial epilepsy. *Epilepsia*, 24:127–134.

Dattilo, J., and Nelson, G.D. (1986): Single-subject evaluation in health education. *Health Educ. Q.*, 13:249–259.

Davis, B.R., Furberg, C.D., and Williams, C.B. (1987): Survival analysis of adverse effects data in the beta-blocker heart attack trial. *Clin. Pharmacol. Ther.*, 41:611–615.

De Jonge, H. (1983): Deficiencies in clinical reports for registration of drugs. *Stat. Med.*, 2:155–166.

Delamothe, T. (1988a): First United Kingdom healthy cities conference, Liverpool. *Br. Med. J.*, 296:1117–1120.

Delamothe, T. (1988b): Nursing grievances. II: Pay. *Br. Med. J.*, 296:120–123.

DeLong, D.M., Delong, E.R., Wood, P.D., Lippel, K., and Rifkind, B.M. (1986): A comparison of methods for the estimation of plasma low- and very low-density lipoprotein cholesterol: The lipid research clinics prevalence study. *JAMA*, 256:2372–2377.

DeVries, W.C. (1988): The permanent artificial heart: Four case reports. *JAMA*, 259:849–859.

Dobbins, J.J., Johnson, G.S., Kunin, C.M., and DeVries, W.C. (1988): Postmortem microbiological findings of two total artificial heart recipients. *JAMA*, 259:865–869.

Doll, R., and Peto, R. (1977): Mortality among doctors in different occupations. *Br. Med. J.*, 1:1433–1436.

Dripps, R.D., Eckenhoff, J.E., and Vandam, L.D. (1982): *Introduction to Anesthesia: The Principles of Safe Practice*. Saunders, Philadelphia.

East, C., Grundy, S.M., and Bilheimer, D.W. (1986): Normal cholesterol levels with lovastatin (Mevinolin) therapy in a child with homozygous familial hypercholesterolemia following liver transplantation. *JAMA*, 256:2843–2848.

Eiseman, B. (1981): The second dimension [Editorial]. *Arch. Surg.*, 116:11–13.

Eisenberg, J.M., Koffer, H., and Finkler, S.A. (1984): Economic analysis of a new drug: Potential savings in hospital operating costs from the use of once-daily regimen of a parenteral cephalosporin. *Rev. Infect. Dis.*, 6(Suppl 4):S909–S923.

Eschenhof, V.E. (1973): Untersuchungen über das schicksal des antikonvulsivums clonazepam im organismus der ratte, des hundes und des menschen. *Arzneimittelforschung*, 23:390–400.

Ewbank, D. (1986): Population and public health. In: *Maxcy-Rosenau Public Health and Preventive Medicine*. Last, J.M. (Ed.), pp. 75–99. 12th ed. Appleton-Century-Crofts, Norwalk, CT.

Falliers, C.J., Redding, M.A., and Katsampes, C.P. (1978): Inhibition of cutaneous and mucosal allergy with phenyltoloxamine. *Ann. Allergy*, 41:140–144.

Freston, J.W. (1987): H2-receptor antagonists and duodenal ulcer recurrence: Analysis of efficacy and commentary on safety, costs, and patient selection. *Am. J. Gastroenterol.*, 82:1242–1249.

Gardner, M. (1982): *Aha! Gotcha: Paradoxes to Puzzle and Delight*. W.H. Freeman, New York.

Garnett, A.R., Ornato, J.P., Gonzalez, E.R., and Johnson, E.B. (1987): End-tidal carbon dioxide monitoring during cardiopulmonary resuscitation. *JAMA*, 257:512–515.

Gifford, R.H., and Feinstein, A.R. (1969): A critique of methodology in studies of anticoagulant therapy for acute myocardial infarction. *N. Engl. J. Med.*, 280:351–357.

Gladen, H.E. (1986): Cost-effective aminoglycoside therapy in surgical patients. *Am. J. Med.*, 80(Suppl. 6B):228–233.

Gottschalk, L.A., Gleser, G.C., Wylie, H.W. Jr., and Kaplan, S.M. (1965): Effects of imipramine on anxiety and hostility levels. *Psychopharmacologia*, 7:303–310.

Grobbee, D.E., Hackeng, W.H., Birkenhäger, J.C., and Hofman, A. (1988): Raised plasma intact parathyroid hormone concentrations in young people with mildly raised blood pressure. *Br. Med. J.*, 296:814–816.

Grundy, S.M. (1986): Cholesterol and coronary heart disease: A new era. *JAMA*, 256:2849–2858.

Harris, T., Cook, E.F., Garrison, R., Higgins, M., Kannel, W., and Goldman, L. (1988): Body mass index and mortality among nonsmoking older persons: The Framingham heart study. *JAMA*, 259:1520–1524.

Henneman, E., Somjen, G., and Carpenter, D.O. (1965): Excitability and inhibitibility of motoneurons of different sizes. *J. Neurophysiol.*, 28:599–620.

Hershko, C., Abrahamov, A., Moreb, J., Hersh, M., Shiffman, R., Shahin, A., Richter, E.D., Knoijn, A.M., Weissenberg, E., Graver, F., et al. (1984): Lead poisoning in a West Bank Arab village. *Arch. Intern. Med.*, 144:1969–1973.

Hirsh, J., and Levine, M.N. (1987): The optimal intensity of oral anticoagulant therapy. *JAMA*, 258:2723–2726.

Hooke, R. (1983): *How to Tell the Liars from the Statisticians*. Marcel Dekker, New York.

Hooshmand, H. (1975): Serum lactate dehydrogenase isoenzymes in neuromuscular diseases. *Dis. Nerv. Syst.*, 36:607–611.

Horwitz, R.I. (1987): Complexity and contradiction in clinical trial research. *Am. J. Med.*, 82:498–510.

Huff, D. (1954): *How to Lie with Statistics*, 1st ed. W.W. Norton, New York.

Jacobs, I., Stabile, I., Bridges, J., Kemsley, P., Reynolds, C., Grudzinskas, J., and Oram, D. (1988): Multimodal approach to screening for ovarian cancer. *Lancet*, 1:268–271.

Johnsson, G., Åblad, B., and Hansson, E. (1984): Predictions of adverse drug reactions in clinical practice from animal experiments and phase I-III studies. In: *Detection and Prevention of Adverse Drug Reactions. (Skandia International Symposia)*. Bostrom, H., and Ljungstedt, N. (Eds.), pp. 190–199. Almqvist and Wiksell International, Stockholm.

Kahn, P.C., Gochfeld, M., Nygren, M., Hansson, M., Rappe, C., Velez, H., Ghent-Guenther, T., and Wilson, W.P. (1988): Dioxins and dibenzofurans in blood and adipose tissue of Agent Orange-exposed Vietnam veterans and matched controls. *JAMA*, 259:1661–1667.

Kaplan De-Nour, A. (1982): Psychosocial adjustment to illness scale (PAIS): A study of chronic hemodialysis patients. *J. Psychosom. Res.*, 26:11–22.

Kaplan, R.M. (1982): *Human Preference Measurement for Health Decision and the Evaluation of Long-Term Care*. D.C. Heath and Co., Lexington, MA.

Kaplan, R.M., Bush, J.W., and Berry, C.C. (1976): Health status: Types of validity and the index of well-being. *Health Serv. Res.*, 11:478–507.

Kellner, R., Wilson, R.M., Muldawer, M.D., and Pathak, D. (1975): Anxiety in schizophrenia: The responses to chlordiazepoxide in an intensive design study. *Arch. Gen. Psychiatry*, 32:1246–1254.

Knell, A., Pratt, O., Curzon, G., and Williams, R. (1972): Arranging ideas in hepatic encephalopathy. In: *Eighth Symposium on Advanced Medicine*. Neale, G. (Ed.), pp. 156–170. Pitman Medical, London.

Kooner, K.S., and Zimmerman, T.J. (1987): The cost of antiglaucoma medications. *Ann. Ophthalmol.*, 19:327–328.

Kosinski, L.A. (1970): *The Population of Europe: A Geographical Perspective*. Longmans, London.

Koul, R., Razdan, S., and Motta, A. (1988): Prevalence and pattern of epilepsy (Lath/Mirgi/Laran) in rural Kashmir, India. *Epilepsia*, 29:116–122.

Krieg, A.F., Beck, J.R., and Bongiovanni, M.B. (1988): The dot plot: A starting point for evaluating test performance. *JAMA*, 260:3309–3312.

Krugman, S., and Ward, R. (1973): *Infectious Diseases of Children and Adults*, 5th ed. Mosby, St. Louis.

Kumar, N., Behari, M., Ahuja, G.K., and Jailkhani, B.L. (1988): Phenytoin levels in catamenial epilepsy. *Epilepsia*, 29:155–158.

Kunin, C.M., Dobbins, J.J., Melo, J.C., Levinson, M.M., Love, K., Joyce, L.D., and DeVries, W. (1988): Infectious complications in four long-term recipients of the Jarvik-7 artificial heart. *JAMA*, 259:860–864.

Kwoh, C.K., and Feinstein, A.R. (1986): Rates of sensitivity reactions to aspirin: Problems in interpreting the data. *Clin. Pharmacol. Ther.*, 40:494–505.

Langhoff, E., and Madsen, S. (1983): Rapid metabolism of cyclosporin and prednisone in kidney transplant patients on tuberculostatic treatment. *Lancet*, II:1303.

Lantz, D., and Sterman, M.B. (1988): Neuropsychological assessment of subjects with uncontrolled epilepsy: Effects of EEG feedback training. *Epilepsia*, 29:163–171.

Lawrence, L., and Christie, D. (1979): Quality of life after stroke: A three-year follow-up. *Age Ageing*, 8:167–172.

Leads from the Morbidity and Mortality Weekly Reports (1988a): Arborviral infections of the central nervous system—United States, 1987. *JAMA*, 260:1688–1694.

Leads from the Morbidity and Mortality Weekly Reports (1988b): Changes in premature mortality—United States, 1979–1986. *JAMA*, 259:1148.

Leads from the Morbidity and Mortality Weekly Reports (1986): Premature mortality due to malignant neoplasms—United States, 1983. *JAMA*, 256:821–828.

Littenberg, B. (1988): Aminophylline treatment in severe, acute asthma: A meta-analysis. *JAMA*, 259:1678–1684.

Lockwood, A. (1969): *Diagrams: A Visual Survey of Graphs, Maps, Charts and Diagrams for the Graphic Designer*. Studio Vista, London.

Loiseau, P., Bossi, L., Guyot, M., Orofiamma, B., and Morselli, P.L. (1983): Double-blind crossover trial of progabide versus placebo in severe epilepsies. *Epilepsia*, 24:703–715.

Mabey, D.C., Tedder, R.S., Hughes, A.S., Corrah, P.T., Goodison, S.J., O'Connor, T., Shenton, F.C., Lucas, S.B., Whittle, H.C., and Greenwood, B.M. (1988): Human retroviral infections in the Gambia: Prevalence and clinical features. *Br. Med. J.*, 296:83–86.

Macphee, G.J.A., McInnes, G.T., Thompson, G.G., and Brodie, M.J. (1986): Verapamil potentiates carbamazepine neurotoxicity: A clinically important inhibitory interaction. *Lancet,* I:700–703.

Mandelblatt, J.S., and Fahs, M.C. (1988): The cost-effectiveness of cervical cancer screening for low-income elderly women. *JAMA,* 259:2409–2413.

Markopoulos, C., Berger, U., Wilson, P., Gazet, J.-C., and Coombes, R.C. (1988): Oestrogen receptor content of normal breast cells and breast carcinomas throughout the menstrual cycle. *Br. Med. J.,* 296:1349–1351.

Mays, J.B., Williams, M.A., Barker, L.E., Pfeifer, M.A., Kammerling, J.M., Jung, S.Y., and De-Vries, W.C. (1988): Clinical management of total artificial heart drive systems. *JAMA,* 259:881–885.

McNeil, B.J., Weichselbaum, R., and Pauker, S.G. (1981): Speech and survival: Tradeoffs between quality and quantity of life in laryngeal cancer. *N. Engl. J. Med.,* 305:982–987.

McPherson, F.M., and Le Gassicke, J. (1965): A single-patient, self-controlled and self-recorded trial of Wy 3498. *Br. J. Psychiatry,* 111:149–154.

Meinert, C.L., and Tonascia, S. (1986): *Clinical Trials: Design, Conduct, and Analysis.* Oxford University Press, New York.

Meissner, I., Wiebers, D.O., Whisnant, J.P., and O'Fallon, W.M. (1987): The natural history of asymptomatic carotid artery occlusive lesions. *JAMA,* 258:2704–2707.

Miller, R.W., and McKay, F.W. (1984): Decline in US childhood cancer mortality: 1950 through 1980. *JAMA,* 251:1567–1570.

Mindel, A., Faherty, A., Carney, O., Patou, G., Freris, M., and Williams, P. (1988): Dosage and safety of long-term suppressive acyclovir therapy for recurrent genital herpes. *Lancet,* 1:926–928.

Mocarelli, P., Marocchi, A., Brambilla, P., Gerthoux, P., Young, D.S., and Mantel, N. (1986): Clinical laboratory manifestations of exposure to dioxin in children: A six-year study of the effects of an environmental disaster near Seveso, Italy. *JAMA,* 256:2687–2695.

Nakanishi, M., Yokota, Y., and Fukuzaki, H. (1988): Cardiovascular effects of dibutyryl cyclic AMP in patients with congestive heart failure: Comparison with dobutamine and captopril. *Jpn. Circ. J.,* 52:503–510.

Neville, R.G. (1985): Clinical algorithms. *Br. Med. J.,* 291:1819.

O'Neill, J.S., Elton, R.A., and Miller, W.R. (1988): Aromatase activity in adipose tissue from breast quadrants: A link with tumour site. *Br. Med. J.,* 296:741–743.

Oldham, R.K. (Ed.) (1987): *Principles of Cancer Biotherapy.* Raven Press, New York.

Openshaw, S., Craft, A.W., Charlton, M., and Birch, J.M. (1988): Investigation of leukaemia clusters by use of a geographical analysis machine. *Lancet,* 1:272–273.

Pääkkö, P., Anttila, S., Kokkonen, P., and Kalliomaki, P.L. (1988): Cadmium in lung tissue as marker for smoking [Letter to Editor]. *Lancet,* 1:477.

Peeters, M., Koren, G., Jakubovicz, D., and Zipursky, A. (1988): Physician compliance and relapse rates of acute lymphoblastic leukemia in children. *Clin. Pharmacol. Ther.,* 43:228–232.

Peters, W.P., Shogan, J., Shpall, E.J., Jones, R.B., and Kim, C.S. (1988): Recombinant human granulocyte-macrophage colony-stimulating factor produces fever [Letter to Editor]. *Lancet,* 1:950.

Peterson, C.D., and Lake, K.D. (1986): Reducing prophylactic antibiotic costs in cardiovascular surgery: The role of the clinical pharmacist. *Drug Intell. Clin. Pharm.,* 20:134–137.

Reynolds, L., and Simmonds, D. (1984): *Presentation of Data in Science. Publications, Slides, Posters, Overhead Projections, Tape-Slides, Television: Principles and Practices for Authors and Teachers.* Martinus Nijhoff, The Netherlands.

Rhoads, G.G., Dahlen, G., Berg, K., Morton, N.E., Dannenberg, A.L. (1986): Lp(a) lipoprotein as a risk factor for myocardial infarction. *JAMA,* 256:2540–2544.

Rippe, J.M., Ward, A., Porcari, J.P., and Freedson, P.S. (1988): Walking for health and fitness. *JAMA,* 259:2720–2724.

Ritschel, W.A. (1984): *Graphic Approach to Clinical Pharmacokinetics,* 2nd ed. Drug Intelligence Publications, Bethesda, MD.

Rodda, B.E. (1974): Sequential analysis in phase I and phase II clinical trials. In: *Importance of Experimental Design and Biostatistics.* McMahon, F.G. (Ed.), pp. 19–27. Futura, Mt. Kisco, NY.

Rossi, A.C., Bosco, L., Faich, G.A., Tanner, A., and Temple, R. (1988): The importance of adverse reaction reporting by physicians. Suprofen and the flank pain syndrome. *JAMA,* 259:1203–1204.

Rubenstein, L.Z., Josephson, K.R., Wieland, G.D., English, P.A., Sayre, J.A., and Kane, R.L. (1984): Effectiveness of a geriatric evaluation unit. A randomized clinical trial. *N. Engl. J. Med.,* 311:1664–1670.

Sackett, D.L., Haynes, R.B., and Tugwell, P. (1985): *Clinical Epidemiology: A Basic Science for Clinical Medicine.* Little, Brown and Company, Boston.

Sacks, J.J., Stroup, D.F., Will, M.L., Harris, E.L., and Israel, E. (1988): A nurse-associated epidemic of cardiac arrests in an intensive care unit. *JAMA,* 259:689–695.

Sage, W.M., Hurst, C.R., Silverman, J.F., and Bortz, W.M. II (1987): Intensive care for the elderly: Outcome of elective and nonelective admissions. *J. Am. Geriatr. Soc.,* 35:312–318.

Schade, D.S., Mitchell, W.J., and Griego, G. (1987): Addition of sulfonylurea to insulin treatment in poorly controlled type II diabetes: A double-blind, randomized clinical trial. *JAMA,* 257:2441–2445.

Schipper, H., and Levitt, M. (1985): Measuring quality of life: Risks and benefits. *Cancer Treat. Rep.,* 69:1115–1125.

Selevan, S.G., Lindbohm, M.-L., Hornung, R.W., and Hemminki, K. (1985): A study of occupational exposure to antineoplastic drugs and fetal loss in nurses. *N. Engl. J. Med.,* 313:1173–1178.

Siest, G., Schiele, F., Henny, J., and Young, D.S. (Eds.) (1985): *Interpretation of Clinical Laboratory Tests: Reference Values and Their Biological Variation.* Biomedical Publications, Foster City, CA.

Simmonds, D. (Ed.) (1980): *Charts & Graphs: Guidelines for the Visual Presentation of Statistical Data in the Life Sciences.* MTP Press, Lancaster.

Smith, G.R. Jr., and O'Rourke, D.F. (1988): Return to work after a first myocardial infarction: A test of multiple hypotheses. *JAMA,* 259:1673–1677.

Sogliero-Gilbert, G., Mosher, K., and Zubkoff, L. (1986): A procedure for the simplification and assessment of lab parameters in clinical trials. *Drug Info. J.,* 20:279–296.

Spear, M.E. (1969): *Practical Charting Techniques.* McGraw-Hill, New York.

Spilker, B. (1988): Choosing formats for presenting clinical data. *Drug News Persp.,* 1:282–283.

Spilker, B. (1984): *Guide to Clinical Studies and Developing Protocols.* Raven Press, New York.

Spilker, B. (1986): *Guide to Clinical Interpretation of Data.* Raven Press, New York.

Spilker, B. (1987): *Guide to Planning and Managing Multiple Clinical Studies.* Raven Press, New York.

Spilker, B. (1989): *Multinational Drug Companies: Issues in Drug Discovery and Development.* Raven Press, New York.

Spilker, B., and Segreti, A. (1984): Validation of the phenomenon of regression of seizure frequency in epilepsy. *Epilepsia,* 25:443–449.

Spilker, B. (Ed.) (1990): *Quality of Life Assessments in Clinical Trials.* Raven Press, New York.

Stern, R.S., Pass, T.M., and Komaroff, A.L. (1984): Topical v systemic agent treatment for papulo-pustular acne: A cost-effectiveness analysis. *Arch. Dermatol.,* 120:1571–1578.

Stevenson, J.M., Maibach, H.I., and Guy, R.H. (1987): Laser doppler and photoplethysmographic assessment of cutaneous microvasculature. In: *Models in Dermatology 1987. Volume 3.* Maibach, H.I., and Lowe, N.J. (Eds.), pp. 121–140. Karger, New York.

Stiller, C.A. (1988): Treatment of osteosarcoma [Letter to Editor]. *Lancet,* 1:931.

Strong, J.M., Dutcher, J.S., Lee, W.-K., and Atkinson, A.J. Jr. (1975): Pharmacokinetics in man of the *N*-acetylated metabolite of procainamide. *J. Pharmacokinet. Biopharm.,* 3:223–235.

Stuck, A.E., Frey, B.M., and Frey, F.J. (1988): Kinetics of prednisolone and endogenous cortisol suppression in the elderly. *Clin. Pharmacol. Ther.,* 43:354–362.

Sugarbaker, P.H., Barofsky, I., Rosenberg, S.A., and Gianola, F.J. (1982): Quality of life assessment of patients in extremity sarcoma clinical trials. *Surgery,* 91:17–23.

Thompson, W.L., Brunelle, R.L., Enas, G.G., and Simpson, P.J. (1987): Routine laboratory tests in clinical trials: Interpretation of results. *J. Clin. Res. Drug Dev.,* 1:95–119.

Tufte, E.R. (1983): *The Visual Display of Quantitative Information.* Graphics Press, Cheshire, CT.

Uno, H. (1987): Stumptailed macaques as a model of male-pattern baldness. In: *Models in Dermatology 1987. Volume 3.* Maibach, H.I., and Lowe, N.J. (Eds.), pp. 159–169. Karger, New York.

Vere, D.W. (1976): Risks of everyday life. *Proc. R. Soc. Med.,* 69:105–107.

Washington, A.E., Cates, W. Jr., and Zaidi, A.A. (1984): Hospitalizations for pelvic inflammatory disease: Epidemiology and trends in the United States, 1975 to 1981. *JAMA,* 251:2529–2533.

Watkins, J., Abbott, E.C., Hensby, C.N., Webster, J., and Dollery, C.T. (1980): Attenuation of hypotensive effect of propranolol and thiazide diuretics by indomethacin. *Br. Med. J.,* 281:702–705.

Wilcox, R.G., Hampton, J.R., Banks, D.C., Birkhead, J.S., Brooksby, I.A., Burns-Cox, C.J., Hayes, M.J., Joy, M.D., Malcolm, A.D., Mather, H.G., et al. (1986a): Trial of early nifedipine in acute myocardial infarction: The Trent study. *Br. Med. J.,* 293:1204–1208.

Wilcox, R.G., Mitchell, J.R., and Hampton, J.R. (1986b): Treatment of high blood pressure: Should clinical practice be based on results of clinical trials? *Br. Med. J.,* 293:433–437.

Wolery, M., and Harris, S.R. (1982): Interpreting results of single-subject research designs. *Phys. Ther.,* 62:445–452.

Woo, E., Chan, Y.M., Yu, Y.L., Chan, Y.W., and Huang, C.Y. (1988): If a well-stabilized epileptic patient has a subtherapeutic antiepileptic drug level, should the dose be increased? A randomized prospective study. *Epilepsia,* 29:129–139.

Woo, S.L.C., Lidsky, A.S., Güttler, F., Thirumalachary, C., and Robson, K.J.H. (1984): Prenatal diagnosis of classical phenylketonuria by gene mapping. *JAMA,* 251:1998–2002.

Subject Index

Subject Index

A

Abscissa
  of dot plot, 38
  independent variable on, 7, 8
  of single-axis graph, 9
Administration route, tabular presentation, 416
Adverse reactions data, 265–306
  categorizing mortality, 267–268
  definition, 265
  dictionaries, 269
  by dosing regimen, 292, 302
  by drug administration route, 291
  frequency distribution, 265–267, 273–283
    by body system, 273–283
    in clinical practice, 290
    by exposure duration, 276–277
    by relationship to drug, 280–281
    relative frequency, 290
    by severity of report, 278–279, 285
    by study phase, 274–279
    by treatment action, 282–284
    by withdrawal from study, 285–286
  group data, 271–283, 286, 288–292, 294–299, 301–302, 304–305
  incidence, 274–277, 286, 288–289, 291, 294, 296–298, 300–301
  individual patient data, 269–270, 284–285, 287, 293
  interpretation difficulties, 114
  in metaanalyses studies, 498
  number of, 265–267
  onset/duration patterns, 293, 295, 304–305
  as patient accountability factor, 143
  prevalence, 272
  probability, 480
  as quality-of-life indicator, 455
  relative risk, 294
  summarization, 271–272
  superimposition of study design indicators, 300
  terminology, 269

by treatment time, 303
Age cohort comparison, 388
Age distribution, of a population, 337
Algorithm, 52, 60
Analytes profile, 258
Anatomical diagrams, 52, 54–55
  of efficacy data, 390
Annotations
  on bar graph, 225
  on demographic tables, 131–132
  of dosage efficacy data, 112
  footnotes for, 131
  on histogram, 226
  of study design, 120
Appendix
  of demographic data, 133
  of pharmacokinetic data, 433
Autoradiograph, thin layer chromatography, 443
Axes, *See* Graphs, axes

B

Bar(s), step arrangement, 73
Bar chart/graph; *See also* Histogram
  of adverse reactions data, 296–297
  annotations, 225
  circular, 44
  definition, 15
  error bar, 224
  of individual patient data, 224
  individual site summary statistics, 224
  of metaanalyses data, 502–504
  of quality-of-life data, 456–457
  sample size, 457
  vertical axis break, 457
Baseline data/values
  alternating pattern, 368
  demographic, 129, 131–133
  multiple, 369
  normal range, 255
  percent change, 242